348

The Best
Medicine

Also by Robert Arnot, M.D.

Sportselection

The Best Medicine

How to Choose the Top Doctors,

the Top Hospitals,

and the Top Treatments

Robert Arnot, M.D.

Addison-Wesley Publishing Company

Reading, Massachusetts ▪ Menlo Park, California ▪ New York
Don Mills, Ontario ▪ Wokingham, England ▪ Amsterdam ▪ Bonn
Sydney ▪ Singapore ▪ Tokyo ▪ Madrid ▪ San Juan ▪ Paris
Seoul ▪ Milan ▪ Mexico City ▪ Taipei

This book is meant to educate and should not be used as an alternative to appropriate medical care. The author has exerted every effort to ensure that the information presented is accurate up to the time of publication. However, in light of ongoing research and the constant flow of information it is possible that new findings may raise questions about some of the data presented here.

None of the specific opinions stated in any of the chapters of this book should be attributed to any one expert or source unless otherwise stated.

Many of the designations used by manufacturers and sellers to distinguish their products are claimed as trademarks. Where those designations appear in this book and Addison-Wesley was aware of a trademark claim, the designations have been printed in initial capital letters.

Hospital lists from HEALTH CARE USA by Jean Carper. Prentice Hall Press, New York, 1987. Reprinted by permission.

Hospital lists from THE BEST IN MEDICINE by Herbert J. Dietrich, M.D. and Virginia H. Biddle copyright © 1986 by Herbert J. Dietrich, M.D. and Virginia H. Biddle. Reprinted by permission of Harmony Books, a Division of Crown Publishers, Inc.

Hospital lists from US NEWS & WORLD REPORT © August 1991. Reprinted by permission.

Hospital lists created by Lexecon Health Service reprinted by permission.

Jacket design © 1992 by Steve Snider
Jacket photograph © 1992 by Simon Metz
Text design by Editorial Design / Joy Dickinson
Production services by Michael Bass & Associates
Set in 11 point Minion by Recorder Typesetting, San Francisco

Library of Congress Cataloging-in-Publication Data
Arnot, Robert Burns.
    The best medicine : how to choose the top doctors, the top hospitals, and the
    top treatments / Robert Arnot.
        p.   cm.
    Includes index.
    ISBN 0-201-57792-5
1. Medicine, Popular.   2. Consumer education.   I. Title.
[DNLM: 1. Hospitals—United States—popular works.   2. Physicians—United States—popular works.   3. Quality of Health Care—United States—popular works.   W 84 AA1 A68b]
362.1'0973—dc20
NDLM/DLC
for Library of Congress   92-17849
                                                                       CIP

1 2 3 4 5 6 7 8 9-MA-96 95 94 93 92
First printing, July 1992

Addison-Wesley books are available at special discounts for bulk purchases by corporations, institutions, and other organizations. For more information, please contact:
Special Markets Department, Addison-Wesley Publishing Company, Reading, MA 01867
(617) 944-3700 x2431

Dedication

This book is dedicated to my parents for their lifelong pursuit of excellence in medicine.

My mother takes great pride in her family's tradition of medical excellence. Both her mother and aunt were strong, bold, and courageous leaders in American nursing. My mother was the Red Cross Field Director for a 5,000 bed hospital during World War II. She has worked for over 50 years as a psychiatric social worker, putting a compassionate, human face on the treatment of the mentally ill. She pioneered day care and elder care in our area long before they became fashionable. In addition to raising six children, she has volunteered her time endlessly, from the care of displaced children to delivering "meals on wheels." She has passed this tradition on to us. Long before President John F. Kennedy made famous the line "Ask not what you can do . . . ," mother told all of us as children: "To whom much is given, much is expected." Now in her late 70s she continues to help psychiatric patients overcome the numerous discriminatory obstacles they face.

My father has been a psychiatrist for nearly 50 years. As different schools of psychiatry have come and gone, he has steadfastly remained true to his belief that mental illness should be treated just like any other illness, as a fundamental change in a biological process. He has always treated those suffering psychiatric diseases with the same respect and sympathy as a patient with a heart attack or brain tumor. While others have procrastinated with months to years of digging into a patient's remote past, he has treated mental illness as aggressively and quickly as a life-threatening medical illness. Letting mental illness fester could be as detrimental in the long run as allowing a pneumonia to go untreated. My father has steered his course through all the fads of modern psychiatry and fought endless bruising battles to do the right thing for the patient. That has often meant heated exchanges with those who promoted the politically correct therapy of the moment. He is one of the few physicians his age who has not tired of the never-ending struggle against bureaucracy and outside interference in the practice of medicine. He is always pushing for the best possible way to treat a patient, looking for what tomorrow's state-of-the-art treatment will be, but with a discriminating eye that can tell fad and fantasy from fact.

Contents

Chronic Diseases

Acknowledgment

The Best Medicine was an extraordinarily difficult book to research. I thank Jill Werman for being my partner, in the truest sense of the word, in this research effort.

Jill is a journalist who spent the last year and a half coaxing, pulling, and prying data and expert knowledge from academics, government agencies, private research foundations, physicians, professional associations, and others. Even when her research efforts hit dead ends or blind alleys, she exhausted every possible avenue to secure the right answer for this book. There was no lead too thin, no job too difficult. During the Gulf War, she tracked me down in Kuwait and Saudi Arabia to review her most recent research.

Jill's efforts were ceaseless and tireless. Her dedication has been extraordinary. I offer her my sincerest congratulations for a terrific job.

Excellence
in Medicine

From my earliest days as a medical student, I have had the greatest admiration for the patients who became real winners, who were cured or achieved a significantly improved quality of life through their own efforts. They were not rich or even well connected. They did have several traits in common that inspired everyone around them. They were curious, and were driven by an insatiable desire to find excellence in their medical care. They were also optimists. Even in the face of dreadful illness and, sometimes, insuperable odds, they were actively engaged in a battle to overcome the obstacles in their way. They drove their doctors and nurses to work even harder on their behalf. I believe that every patient can improve his or her future, and I want you to fight for yours.

The more you know about medical care, the better prepared you will be to make that fight. I've written this book to share with you the basic rules of thumb that the experts themselves use to find excellence for their families and their patients. I've based these guidelines on discussions with some of the country's most highly respected medical specialists, who also have reviewed these chapters for accuracy.

This book also gives you hard facts you can use to distinguish one hospital from another and one doctor from another. That data has been painstakingly assembled from the country's top research firms, think tanks, and medical schools. The statistics were drawn from the American College of Surgeons, the American College of Cardiology, medical schools, research companies such as Value Health Sciences, MediQual, and Lexecon, and articles published in medical journals. In addition, the specialists interviewed for this book contributed their expert judgments based on their years of treating patients and, many of them, chairing departments at major university-affiliated teaching hospitals.

Some statistics, such as hospital death rates, are well established, while those for doctors, such as the number of operations a surgeon should perform annually, represent what I have found to be the consensus of the medical establishment. By and large, researchers have devoted more time to analyzing surgical procedures and are farther along in developing objective measures of excellence than they are in assessing the treatment of chronic disease. That's why there are more statistics in the chapters on operations and procedures than in those on managing chronic disease. The important added value is that you will have hard data and expert knowledge you can use to evaluate your own health care team's performance. It's what distinguishes this book from those previously published for patients.

To date, much of the consumer health movement has focused on the patient as an auditor. You are expected to pepper doctors, nurses, technicians, and others with hundreds of questions. During former Senator Paul Tsongas's 1992 campaign to be the Democratic nominee for president, I asked him what advice he had to offer cancer victims. (He himself had contracted cancer eight years previously.) He said, simply, choose the best doctors and the best hospital and let them do their job. That's the philosophy of this book.

You needn't be an idle bystander, but you will accomplish much more by starting at the best hospital with the best doctors than by second-guessing your care after you've landed in a second-rate institution. It's an approach open to anyone. You don't need a special education, and you won't need to learn but a handful of technical terms. The difference in your care can be dramatic. I am constantly referring patients for treatment. When I look at the care they were receiving and compare it to the care they get at a center of excellence, I am just astounded at the difference in quality.

I have designed this book so you can judge if your care is state-of-the-art. The more you know, the more respect you'll gain from those that treat you and the better chance you'll have at survival. With this book, you'll know you're in trouble before it's too late. Use it as a defensive weapon! Patients have a great fear of "bucking the system." But remember that "the system" kills every day. I can recall numerous cases in which a patient refused to back away from an operation that was not clearly indicated. Why? Because it would upset the doctor. But I believe most health care professionals will admire you and support your efforts. Besides, it's much more likely that the new breed of health care managers, not your doctor, is calling the shots. Your doctor should be on your side, not theirs. Remember, America was made great by individual initiative. Why let the government, your employer, your insurer, or your claims clerk decide what health care you get or don't get. You should be more of an expert in what you need than they are, and you should be willing to fight for it!

The Dangers of
Cut-Rate Medicine

American medicine, once celebrated as the best in the world, is in a precipitous and catastrophic decline. For the past eight years, as a medical correspondent for CBS News, I have witnessed the meteoric rise of high tech medicine paralleled by life-threatening changes in the actual delivery of medical care. The triumph of high tech has overshadowed the darker side of American medicine. For several years I hoped that the investigative stories we reported of death and disability caused by flaws in the delivery of care were dangerous exceptions. But the more stories I reported, the more a pattern began to emerge.

The Flaws in Our Current Health Care System

As I interviewed hundreds of leading doctors across the country, I was troubled to learn that from Harvard to Stanford medical schools, from the best hospitals in New York to the Mayo Clinic and beyond, the experts shared my belief that our national system of health care is deeply wounded and bordering on chaos. And that's if you can get into the system. Access to care for the poor, the uninsured, and even the well insured can be far more limited than most of the industrial world. Why isn't more being done? Industry, Washington, and the media focus largely on the exorbitant, skyrocketing cost of medicine. A hurried, even panicked national "solution" will cause the quality of care in America to plummet even further. I've written this book as part of the solution and to protect you from fundamental flaws in American medicine. These flaws are hidden from public view and put you and your family at serious risk of disability or death as the focus sharpens on cost cutting alone. They are as follows: failure to determine when surgery works and who should do it; failure to manage chronic disease; failure to prevent illness; failure to pursue quality; cut-rate medicine. Let's look at these flaws one at a time.

Failure to Determine When Surgery Works and Who Should Do It

Twenty-five percent of all surgery in the United States is unnecessary. That's what Dr. Arnold Relman, editor emeritus of the prestigious *New England Journal of Medicine*, states. Unfortunately, no one has identified the one in four operations that shouldn't be done. Not only are those unnecessary operations a waste of money, they're also dangerous. One hospital can have a death rate from an operation that is 20 times higher than another in the same town, and yet most patients don't know one hospital from another. You could be scheduled for an operation you don't need in a hospital where one of every five patients dies during that kind of surgery! A friend of ours needed an open heart operation. Doctors replaced her heart valve instead of repairing it. The hospital did few of these operations to begin with. She suffered a catastrophic stroke and lived, paralyzed, in a nursing home until she died. Unnecessary operations and procedures cost as much as $135 billion a year.

Failure to Manage Chronic Illness

The vast majority of patients are not treated in a hospital bed; they are treated as outpatients in clinics, doctors' offices, and formal outpatient departments of hospitals. But many medical schools and residency training programs teach outpatient medicine poorly, if at all. Training programs are geared to teach doctors how to treat patients once they are sick enough to require hospitalization. The government, insurers, and provider organizations are accused of putting little value on outpatient medicine. There's little incentive for doctors to take the time and effort to plan and follow through with a long-term treatment program for disease.

I remember my own stints in outpatient departments. Patients would come to us with enormous charts. They'd see a different doctor each visit. I was one of those different doctors. There was no time allotted to review an entire chart thoroughly. There was no continuity in their care. No one knew which drugs patients were on, why they were on them, if one drug interacted with another, if there was any real plan. Each successive doctor just put another patch on a quilt of medical care. One problem might be solved, but it could worsen the treatment of another illness. Outpatient departments in many large hospitals are crowded. There's often little interest shown in the welfare of these patients—the walking ill—as compared to high-tech intensive care units or surgical suites. The results are catastrophic.

Sometimes, patients with asthma wait until they can barely breathe on their own before seeing a doctor. I remember one poor man admitted to the emergency department at Lincoln Hospital in the Bronx, New York, with acute and chronic asthma. He experienced respiratory arrest and had to be resuscitated and put on a ventilator. A modest change in his medications several days prior could have prevented the entire episode. A well-thought-out program of education, regular use of home self-tests, and a customized drug treatment program might have prevented *any* hospitalization, *ever.* Technology has driven the advances in medicine over the last 20 years. But little attention has been paid to improving the quality of the actual care that is delivered. Outpatient medicine is the victim of that trend.

What experts across the country in leading academic centers told me repeatedly was that American medical education has failed to provide a wide base of general doctors who can provide state-of-the-art care to the majority of Americans who suffer from serious chronic diseases. There's little time and incentive for doctors to learn outpatient medicine on their own. From conducting interviews with leading specialists, I learned that that was the issue that surfaced again and again. There hasn't been a master plan for medical education in generations. The training of doctors has evolved in its own peculiar way. One medical leader after another, including former surgeon general C. Everett Koop, said that medical training doesn't focus on producing doctors who can take care of the most common medical problems. It does turn out competent doctors who are capable of memorizing lots of complex biochemistry and operating star wars technology but who cannot keep up with the complexities of the latest techniques for managing a wide variety of chronic diseases.

The irony is this: The sicker you are, the better the care you are apt to get. That's because doctors in medical school and postgraduate training treat, almost exclusively, hospitalized sick patients. They learn how to treat very sick patients quite well. They don't learn how to treat outpatients. They may spend lots of time treating these patients, but they are taught very little about the complex business of managing their various illnesses over a lifetime. As general internists and family practitioners, they often don't learn how to add and subtract drugs, when to order a new diagnostic workup, when they're in over their heads and need specialists.

Senior neurologists told me that few pediatricians will refer a seizure patient to a specialist. Most family practitioners will not order a diagnostic workup for a new case of high blood pressure. Many internists won't begin "remittive therapy" for newly diagnosed arthritis patients until many months to a year has gone by.

Since there is usually no apparent threat to the lives of these patients, there is no urgency to do much. Even some doctors in large teaching hospitals may be unfamiliar with state-of-the-art outpatient care. The typical department chair might do 30 hours of administration, 20 hours of research, and only a few hours of patient care. I went to rounds with a department chief at a leading medical school. In a room of 12 specialists, he could point out only three doctors he considered great clinical practitioners.

Failure to Prevent Illness

American medicine fails in achieving the two most important goals of any health care system: a low infant mortality rate and a high life expectancy for all citizens. Any way you cut it, America outspends the rest of the world for health care. Americans spend more money per person, both in total dollars and as a percentage of the gross domestic product, than any country on earth. We lag behind over a dozen countries in infant mortality, and achieve poor life expectancy for many of our citizens. A black man in Harlem has a life expectancy that is less than that of a man born in Bangladesh, one of the world's four poorest countries. Several years ago our infant mortality rate was roughly equivalent to a Third World Caribbean nation.

So why does our system fail in so many ways? Simple. There is no system. There are thousands of individual unconnected fiefdoms: insurers, medical colleges, community hospitals, clinics, health maintenance organizations, and governments (from local to federal). Some individual systems are truly awesome in their scope and excellence of medical care. But no single system ties them all together, and there is no guarantee of quality. It's nearly impossible for the consumer to differentiate between good and bad health care.

Failure to Pursue Quality

Technology has driven the major advances in medicine over the last generation. There has been no parallel drive to improve the quality of medicine, nor has the quality of medicine improved. Dr. Alan Brewster, an expert in medical excellence at the health data firm MediQual Systems, argues that our current quality assurance system is one of inspection control. Quality control inspectors police hospitals to make certain they don't fall below an average level. When a hospital does sink below average, tough disciplinary measures are taken. In other words, American hospitals are urged to strive not for excellence but for the average, for mediocrity.

Japan creates high-quality products by changing the process of production. There is a continuous improvement in the process from the inside. In American medicine, managers, bureaucrats, and inspectors stand outside the process to impose their changes on it. They don't understand how to deliver excellence in medicine. I believe those working to deliver care are the ones who understand the process best. They are the ones who need to look at how they can constantly improve medical care. The benchmarks they need to pursue are those of the *best* hospitals in America, not the average.

Here's an example: A large Midwest hospital looked at the process of delivering care. The hospital always passed accreditation inspection with flying colors and had excellent nursing and a first-rate medical staff. By most measures they were an excellent institution. They had all the latest technology, including magnetic resonance imaging (MRI) and other scanning devices. They discovered, however, a higher-than-expected death rate from pneumonia, a very low-tech illness. A close look at the care delivery to pneumonia patients found numerous flaws in the system. Little time was taken to get a quality sputum sample from the patient. The lab gave little effort to examining the sputum sample because its quality was so poor. Doctors blindly prescribed antibiotics without proper lab tests. Often, the wrong antibiotics were prescribed. Patients died as a result. This detailed measurement of the process of delivering care uncovered nearly a dozen errors.

This hospital changed its system. It added a respiratory therapist in order to help patients bring up good-quality sputum samples. A microbiologist promptly and accurately examined the sputum under a microscope to identify the bacteria most likely to cause the pneumonia. Each step in the process was measured. The sputum sample had to be produced within one hour. The lab technician had to issue a report on the probable bacteria within an hour. The doctor had to look at the results and choose an antibiotic as soon as the lab report was available. The result? A dramatic drop in death rates from pneumonia at this hospital.

Cut-Rate Medicine

Of all these flaws, there is one that threatens the very foundation of American medicine. It also represents a pernicious danger that has changed the character of medical practice. I'm referring to cut-rate medicine, which represents a slash-and-burn approach to cutting health care costs. It works by reducing the amount and quality of medical care that you get. It's usually insidious. You probably have no idea that so many decisions that affect your care are based on dollars and cents rather than on your welfare.

Throughout the nearly 2,400-year history of medicine, success has been measured by a single standard—the best possible result for the patient. But in the last decade that standard has been superceded by another, one that has ominous consequences for patients—the cost of medical care. If the trend that began in the

1980s continues through the 1990s—and all available evidence indicates it will—Americans will have worse medical care by the start of the twenty-first century than they do now.

It's a paradox. Although the United States spends more money on health care every year, the quality of that care is diminishing. In 1980 about $248 billion was spent on health care; in 1992 such spending had nearly tripled to over $804 billion. Yet, because of a patchwork system of medicine, there has been no tangible improvement in many measures of health care. As a result of these rising costs, the health care system—the people who pay for the care with the help of those who provide it—have instituted stringent cost-containment measures, poorly understood by patients, that jeopardize care. That's equally true for executives earning $300,000 a year and for the nation's 37 million uninsured.

While costs could be cut by improving efficiency or cutting the enormous fraud and waste in the system, by and large that has not happened. Instead, the effort to control costs has been directed at reducing access to health care in a variety of ways. Medical bureaucrats, accountants, and financial analysts have been put in charge of critical decisions about your care, replacing the doctors who once made those determinations. As a result you may find that treatments are withheld, specialists are unavailable, and high-tech diagnostic tests are denied. The cost-cutters have assembled a powerful coalition of forces that are united against you, the patient. Doctors who once sought only the best for their patients have been enlisted as so-called gatekeepers whose primary purpose is to hold down costs by refusing treatments. In fact, unless you are seriously ill, you may not see a physician at all. You'll be shunted to a physician assistant or a nurse practitioner. If you are allowed to see a doctor, it will be a primary care doctor rather than a specialist. You won't see a cardiologist for chest pain or an orthopedic surgeon for a knee problem, for example.

Corporations that were once generous in their employee health care plans have reduced benefits in an effort to improve profits. Health care benefits now cost many companies up to 25% of earnings and 50% of net profits. American automobile manufacturers, for instance, say they are spending more per car on health care benefits than on steel. Those costs add $700 to a car's sticker price. They argue that they can't compete with Japan, Europe, or even Canada if health care costs continue to increase at current rates. In some industries, company health care costs are rising 30% a year. In order to contain those costs, corporations are forcing employees to give up their family doctors, physicians who may have cared for their families for 30 years and longer. Has that cut the spiraling cost of health care. No!

To me this is the greatest single tragedy of cut-rate medicine. The right to a personal physician of your own choosing has always been a basic tenet of health care in this country, as American in its own way as Mom or apple pie. The family doctor was your advocate, knew you, was there in times of tragedy. He or she was willing to get up in the middle of the night for you. He or she also kept health care costs down. Your doctor could distinguish stress or emotional upset from alarming new symptoms requiring extensive and expensive workup.

The new doctors work 9 a.m. to 5 p.m. and are paid to hold down costs. Some even receive a bonus if they "keep costs low"—a euphemism for "rationing care." You have a right to wonder if the doctor is making the right decision, if she or he is doing what you want or doing what corporate America wants. In 1981, 95% of those insured had traditional insurance that gave them complete freedom to select their own doctors. Today, less than 24% have that freedom.

Ironically, some corporations have become concerned that cut-rate medicine may eventually hurt their bottom line, causing the quality of health care to deteriorate so that it spawns malpractice suits. Seminars are now being held on the "darker side" of cost containment. Corporations are seeking legal protection from the liability of employees in cut-rate health plans. Uwe Reinhardt, a leading health economist and James Madison, Professor of political economy at Princeton University, observes that those corporations who fail to control runaway health care costs are the same ones who poorly control costs in their basic business. They then point the finger at the health care industry as the villain. Uwe says there's nothing inherently wrong with spending lots of money on health care if that's what we as a nation choose to do—as long as we get our money's worth.

How Cut-Rate Medicine Fights Excellence in Health Care

Here are some of the ways that cut-rate medicine is negatively influencing your health care.

Access to Care Is Denied

If you aren't treated, your health care plan won't have to pay. Health insurers can save the maximum amount of money by refusing access to hospitals and specialists. It's that simple. The new, salaried physicians are called "gatekeepers" because they are expected to keep patients out of hospitals, even those who genuinely belong there. Even though the doctor may have legitimate fears that you could die, he or she may send you on home, gambling that you don't share such fears.

Take the case of a 41-year-old mother of two who arrived at a hospital emergency room, complaining of chest pains. When her doctor appeared, she was told to leave the hospital and to drive to his office seven miles away. There, an EKG was performed and blood tests run to determine if she was having a heart attack. Then she was sent home. During the next few hours she called the doctor to complain of increasingly severe chest pain, nausea, and vomiting and to report that she was also feeling cool and clammy. In short, she was exhibiting all the classic signs of a heart attack. Yet the doctor made no attempt to admit her to the hospital—or even to reexamine her. She died that day of a heart attack. The doctor had gambled that her condition was not serious, even though her symptoms would have been obvious to a medical student. Although she should have been evaluated fully in the emergency room and admitted to the hospital, the doctor was financially motivated to do otherwise. At the end of the year, he, like the other physicians who participated in his health plan, would receive a bonus for holding the number of patients requiring hospitalization to an absolute minimum.

Some doctors go to near-heroic limits, not to save patients' lives, but to deny care. A 17-year-old girl who had undergone surgery for cervical cancer developed postoperative complications after she returned home. In a matter of hours, her vaginal bleeding became profuse. Alarmed by the intensity of the bleeding, her mother called the family doctor and asked him to meet them in the emergency room. He refused. The mother said she was calling an ambulance anyway. While the ambulance was en route to their house, the doctor, angered by the mother's determination to get medical help, called three times to berate and to threaten her. Fortunately, the mother ignored him. By the time the daughter arrived in the emergency room, she had no blood pressure and was in shock. She was resuscitated, and she survived. Had the mother followed the doctor's orders, the daughter would have died.

In a similar fashion patients are often denied access to specialists by the gatekeeper, or even denied access to their own doctors by a secretary or nurse. A 32-year-old mother who suffered a spontaneous miscarriage at the beginning of her second trimester didn't lose her life, but she might have. When the woman sought help in the hospital emergency room, she was directed to her physician's office, where he performed a cervical dilatation and uterine curettage (D and C) to remove substantial remaining remnants of the placenta and fetus, under local anesthesia. That in itself was unusual. When a woman more than three months' pregnant has a D and C, the procedure typically is done in the hospital.

When the woman returned home, she was nauseated and in severe pain. For two weeks she complained to the doctor's secretary that she was bleeding, in pain, unable to sleep, and increasingly weak. Still the doctor's secretary refused to put her call through to her obstetrician. Finally, unable to endure the pain any longer, she returned to the emergency room, where she was admitted and scheduled for emergency surgery. During that operation the surgeon discovered that the obstetrician had failed to remove significant amounts of fetal tissue. She could have died from a life-threatening infection or continuing hemorrhage.

In this case the health maintenance organization tried to save money in several different ways—by doing the first D and C in the doctor's office, by the secretary's refusing to put her calls through, and by the doctor's failure to schedule follow-up appointments. But in the end this strategy was unsuccessful. In fact, it cost money because the procedure had to be repeated in a hospital operating room. Poor-quality care costs more money, not less. Dr. Alan Brewster of the MediQual corporation points out that poor care costs more money in the short term *and* in the long run. Bureaucratizing medicine adds to the total cost, lowers quality, and cuts the amount of care delivered.

Conflicts of Interest Are Generated

In all of the instances just discussed the doctors had financial interests that conflicted with their duty to provide the best possible care to their patients. Such conflict of interest is the result of growing pressure on doctors. When medical students are asked why they chose a medical career, they usually respond that they want "to help people." But when they enter practice, they discover that the incentive has changed.

In many health care plans doctors are paid a fixed annual amount for each patient. If the patient becomes seriously ill or needs hospitalization, for instance, the fee, called *capitation,* remains the same. Capitation plans are a strong inducement to provide no care. It is certainly a reason to avoid preventive tests such as mammograms, Pap smears, and stress tests. Why? Because at $150 per patient per year, a typical capitation fee, a physician can't order even a mammogram, Pap smear, or stress test without risking the year-end bonus.

Consider the case of the sexually active 34-year-old woman who consulted a family practitioner suggested by her health maintenance organization. Although she requested a Pap smear (following health care guidelines for an annual exam), her doctor refused, claiming it wasn't necessary. In reality, it was because he knew it would cost him money. During three other visits he also refused. Two years later another doctor did a Pap smear, which suggested cancer. Further tests and surgery led to the discovery that the cancer had spread beyond the uterus and was no longer curable.

Because most consumers aren't aware of this bonus system, lawyers and medical ethicists believe that capitation is both deceitful and immoral. Capitation has done more to destroy the doctor-patient relationship than anything that has happened since the first malpractice suit was filed. Do insurers care? They state flatly that doctors are expected to have sufficient goodwill to treat their patients properly.

But goodwill alone is not enough. Today doctors have little time to talk to patients about their problems and their care. Many physicians are poorly paid for the extraordinary amounts of time needed to take a detailed medical history and a thorough physical examination. In some health maintenance organizations, doctors are required to see so many patients that they must schedule restroom breaks. The situation is not much better for doctors who see privately insured patients. The existing health care system pays far more to doctors for performing procedures and operations than for counseling and educating patients. There is little financial incentive to spend time with patients, even with revised federal guidelines. The general practitioner spends seven minutes talking to the average patient. Whereas in England you will still hear surgeons talking about great cases and interesting patients in the locker room, in the United States that's rare. Most of the conversation revolves around cutting costs, the high price of malpractice insurance, and bureaucratic bungling. Doctors will tell you the fun has been taken out of practicing good medicine. And they're right!

Every Illness Has Its Credit Limit

Even with the best health insurance, you may be discharged days before it is completely "safe." Virtually every health plan now puts a "price" on your illness. This is reflected in what are called diagnosis-related guidelines (DRGs). In effect, the DRG is a price tag for the treatment of disease. The problem is that the price tag assumes that your case is routine and without excessive complications. While DRGs are based on averages, there is no average patient. Once the hospital reaches its DRG price limit, administrators are eager to discharge patients—quickly. At that point the patient starts costing the hospital money that won't be reimbursed. As a result, if you develop pneumonia or a urinary tract infection after surgery, for instance, and many patients do, you could be discharged without proper care.

A young doctor at a highly regarded New York City hospital ran up a $200,000 bill in a recent year because he let patients stay in the hospital overly long. Now he's badgered and pressured to release patients against his medical judgment. In Vermont, a 64-year-old man broke his hip and was hospitalized for 10 days. The morning of his scheduled discharge he was short of breath and complained of a sharp pain in his chest. He said he felt as if he were going to die. The hospital discharged him despite his complaints, since the money spent on his care already exceeded the insurance company's payment. At home he became increasingly ill and suffered a major blood clot in his lung, called a pulmonary embolus.

When you become sick, you start costing your insurance company money. And if it's an expensive illness, many companies will try to raise your rates or those of your business in the hopes that you will leave the plan. In some instances companies have ruthlessly doubled rates every quarter, reaching $8,000 a quarter. If you can no longer afford to be insured, your health care choices will be diminished significantly. For example, a successful entrepreneur of a small company offered a comprehensive insurance plan with excellent benefits for his 25 employees. Then he was diagnosed with a form of cancer called malignant lymphoma. During the first few months his treatment was the best that money could buy. But as he began his third regimen of chemotherapy, the insurance company balked. His business's insurance premium doubled, then tripled. Then his business was forced to drop him from the plan in order to maintain coverage for his other employees. His savings were not enough to pay for the experimental chemotherapy that offered the only hope of a cure. Finally, in order to get help he had to sell his house and business. Another family recently had their insurance premium raised to $16,000 a year because their daughter was at risk of developing an illness in the future. The insurance industry costs medicine $20 billion in marketing, management, and underwriting overhead. Much of that is spent on figuring out who not to insure and what bills not to pay.

Doctors Don't Call the Shots

Your most valuable asset as a patient is your doctor's clinical experience, which is the result of years of treating similar cases. There is no substitute for this experience. But as the medical bureaucrats substitute their cut-rate mentality for your doctor's judgment, you are being deprived of that resource. Take the case of a patient with diabetes who was admitted to the hospital with severe complications, including poor circulation that was already affecting her limbs. The doctor planned 10 days of treatments including physical therapy, antibiotic drugs, and bed rest to bring her diabetes under control. A representative of a managed care firm who had no medical training told the doctor that the patient needed to be discharged. When the doctor objected, the representative demanded, "Discharge the patient; we will not pay." The doctor acquiesced and the patient was sent home, only to be readmitted a week later. By then she had lost most of the use of her lower leg. Two days later it was amputated. By discharging the patient early the managed care plan had saved $4,000 in hospital expenses. A court later ruled that the patient would not have lost her leg if she had remained hospitalized.

Care Is Rationed, Patients Are Dumped

It is not only private insurers who are trying to hold down costs. City, county, and state governments, strapped for revenues, are also seeking ways to contain health care expenditures. In the late 1980s, the city of Los Angeles closed two-thirds of its acute care burn beds to lower the cost of treating burn patients, whose care can easily reach $350,000. It funded only 11 acute care burn beds for a city of 8.5 million. When the city needed extra beds, other facilities were asked to provide care. But since the city was willing to pay only $4,500 a case, few hospitals wanted to accept those cases.

That price tag can make the difference between life and death. Take the case of two small boys riding in the back of a pickup truck when a drunk driver slammed into the rear end. The truck exploded and the boys were severely burned. Medical insurance made the difference in their outcomes. The boy who sustained burns over 80% of his body had private insurance that paid for his care at a top burn center. To date his care has cost more than $800,000. But the boy lives. The other boy, who had 40% of his body burned, was insured by a state insurance program for the poor. He was sent to a facility that didn't specialize in burns, and he died. While the taxpayers saved a small fortune, a 2½-year-old boy who might have had a normal life expectancy lost his life.

Like many other metropolitan areas, Los Angeles has closed half its trauma centers completely, while the remainder have closed on a selective basis—because of overload, some say to avoid admitting uninsured patients. Badly injured accident or gunshot patients who lack health insurance represent a substantial drain on hospitals. A young man shot in the chest during an argument in downtown Los Angeles was bleeding copiously when the paramedics arrived. Working feverishly, they inserted two intravenous lines and applied MAST trousers as a tourniquet to his entire lower body. The paramedics thought they could keep him alive long enough to reach the nearest hospital, just minutes away, where he could undergo immediate surgery. But that hospital refused, saying it was closed to emergency patients. He died in the ambulance.

The closing of emergency rooms threatens the lives of all patients, uninsured and insured alike. Since a hospital can't know a patient's insurance status in advance, you are endangered whether you smash your Rolls-Royce Corniche or your pickup truck into a bridge pylon. From the standpoint of the health care system, everyone becomes indigent.

The most dramatic example of rationing is the experiment the state of Oregon is trying to run. Oregon's thesis is a good one. Why let 25–30 children die each year of preventible causes when you can deliver low-tech well-child care to every child? But at the beginning, the state chose to stop funding liver transplants for children in its Medicaid program. Restricting access to care may make sense when life expectancy and quality of life are unlikely to be improved by expensive care, such as prolonged intensive care for the terminally ill. (One-third of our national health budget is spent on care for those in the last few months of life.) But in the case of children needing liver transplants or burn care, it's hard to justify cost-cutting, even when the savings are huge.

Oregon has since begun paying for pediatric liver transplants. They do not want to pay for adult liver transplants in those with liver disease secondary to alcohol. Oregon has begun to make tough choices, but those choices are made aboveboard for all to see. Although rationing is widely practiced in America, it is largely invisible to the American public.

In Arizona, a second-grader developed leukemia. The state insurance program delayed approving treatment for months. They did finally approve treatment, but the boy died shortly after treatment was started. Cost-cutters are notoriously brave when it comes to cutting lifesaving treatment for children. In several of the news stories I have covered, cost-cutters hit children the hardest.

Fewer Enter Medicine, Ongoing Practices Close

Cut-rate medicine affects the quality of care of all Americans because fewer top college graduates are attracted to medicine as a career. Many of the best and the brightest are now lured into investment banking, law, or business. After decades of nearly exponential growth, medical school applications plummeted from 36,141 in 1979 to 26,915 in 1989, the lowest point in history. There were 2.8 applicants for every medical school opening in 1979 but only 1.7 applicants in 1989.

As the number of applications has fallen, medical schools have become willing to accept students with lower grade-point averages, a decline from 3.52 to 3.4 during that period. Medical school graduates are also choosing to enter the higher-paying specialities of radiology, surgery, opthalmology, and orthopedics. A declining number are entering internal medicine, the key diagnostic speciality. Half of the graduating class at Cornell Medical College in New York City once went into internal medicine; now only 12% choose that field.

Thousands of general practitioners, internists, and family doctors, exhausted by the daily struggle with the medical bureaucracy, are closing their practices. In Massachusetts 20% of the family doctors have quit, in large measure because the state pays too little too late. One departing physician I visited told me she received $4 from Medicaid for a patient visit, then waited two years to collect. One anesthesiologist was so disenchanted by medicine that he opened a laundromat; another now sells life insurance. By some estimates one-third of the family doctors in the United States will no longer be practicing in five years. In rural areas, where reimbursement is even lower, the exodus is more rapid. An estimated 20% of general practitioners may leave medicine by 1993. The loss of these caring doctors is a tragedy to our health care system as a whole but most of all to their patients.

Patients Are Increasingly Dissatisfied

Although Americans may not comprehend the new medical bureaucracy, with its jargon of "managed care," "preferred provider organizations," and "DRGs," they are expressing profound unhappiness with their care. By the end of 1991 there were increasing signs that Americans were ready for major changes in the health care system. In September of that year half the Americans surveyed said the nation's health care system needed fundamental changes, and another 40%, going even further, said that it needed to be completely rebuilt. Pennsylvania voters elected Harris Wofford, a Democrat who started out far behind in the polls, to the United States Senate against a clearly favored Republican candidate after he made national health insurance the major issue in the campaign. And in a poll conducted shortly after Wofford's election, only 19% of the people said the present health care system should be left alone, while over 41% said the federal government should adopt a new national health care plan to cover all Americans.

By and large Americans still believe the United States has the best medical care in the world. But in growing numbers they no longer have confidence that the best of medicine will be available to them. Few politicians in Washington understand the need to change the quality of care. They choose to focus on who will pay. They often suggest managed care and "pay or play" solutions, not excellence.

Solutions: Our Last Chance for Quality

Anyone who has lived through the last several years of bloodletting in American businesses knows that many American managers have little idea of how to cut costs effectively. Thousands of businesses that have ruthlessly fired their employees are not more efficient, more effective, or more competitive now than before layoffs began. Many managers used an axe rather than surgical precision to cut. Rather than pruning, they severed limbs. It's the same unfortunate story with health care. There are huge opportunities for cost cutting. The sad fact is that by and large cost-cutters don't know how to get under the hood and see what *needs* cutting.

America wastes sinful amounts of money on medicine. Each year, we lose a minimum of $70 billion to fraud, $135 billion to unnecessary operations, $20 billion to defensive medicine, $2 billion to malpractice, and $175 billion to a huge, inefficient, and bloated bureaucracy that is breaking the backs of doctors and nurses. There is an enormous overcapacity of everything from hospital beds and MRIs to open heart teams and transplant centers.

Could you imagine this enormous scale of inefficiency and waste in airline operations, mass merchandising, or even automobile manufacturing? No! Why? America is a land of very good consumers, even if we have to buy foreign products. Good consumers demand high quality at low prices. When it comes to cars, food, consumer electronics, and airfares, smart consumers get quality and low prices because they demand it. In medicine, that demand is curiously absent. Would you allow someone else to decide what car you drive, where you go on vacation, which size TV you watch, and what you eat? Why is there sticker shock

for a $40,000 car but not a $57,000 hospital bill? Because patients are not active consumers. Aggressive health care consumers can slash costs and improve quality.
    Here's how:

■ By being absolutely certain you need an operation, procedure, or medical test you cut out part of the $70 billion wasted on fraud and the $135 billion spent on unnecessary operations and procedures.

■ By carefully choosing where you will have an operation and who will operate, using the basic steps provided in this book, you drive doctors, hospitals, insurers, and your employers to focus on quality. Your insistence on treatment at a center of excellence will drive low quality, low volume, high cost hospitals out of services they perform poorly, which cuts overcapacity and promotes the survival of high quality, high volume, low cost providers. You cut health care costs further by getting it done right the first time. At least 25% of surgeries correct problems caused by a first surgery.

■ By paying for some of your own care and making decisions about the cost a Rand Corporation study showed you cut costs 30%.

■ By aggressively maintaining your own good health, you can cut your yearly health care costs as much as a third.

■ By choosing what kind of insurance you really need you also cut costs. At Quaker Oats, hospital use declined 46% when employees chose their own health plans.

We're at a critical juncture in medicine that will determine for the coming decades whether America gets first-rate or cut-rate care. At present, others—your employer, insurer, insurance claims adjuster, the government, or a paid company doctor—choose care for you. That person is a classic double agent. They can choose the care you get based on quality or price but you don't know which. Dr. Stanley Reiser stated in the *Journal of the American Medical Association* that creating consumer competence and responsibility in health care choices is the key to health care reform in the United States. "The concept of placing authority and responsibility in the hands of individuals has been an important factor in shaping American history—but not in American health care. Health care, the experts explain, needs judgments taken on behalf of consumers by experts." Unfortunately, these "experts" don't know you and don't have your interests uppermost in their minds. This book will help you make your own choices.

    The saving grace is that there is *great* medicine in America. The best is the best in the world. You need not have expensive insurance or a hundred thousand dollar salary to get great care. You do need to make the right choice. You're not going to luck into great health care. This book will provide the results, the experience, and other measures of quality that you can expect and demand of your doctors and hospitals. Look for continuous improvement in these results from one year to the next, which shows that the doctors, nurses, and technicians at that hospital care about quality. Some medical centers have long looked at the process of delivering high quality medicine. Massachusetts General Hospital has been examining the outcomes of operations since before World War I. The Mayo brothers began studying the process of improving care near the turn of the century, which is why they continue to be the best in so many fields. By looking first for quality, some businesses and managed health care firms are cutting costs and providing first-rate health care. Not all managed health care firms are bad. Some have courageously made the right choices. How? They're not afraid to get under that hood and look. They keep patients away from unnecessary surgery and save money by choosing quality providers, thus avoiding additional hospital costs and the cost of complications from surgery.

If you are at a hospital that delivers second-rate care, no amount of questioning, badgering, and checking is going to make your care first-rate. That's why this book is providing a simple roadmap to help you make *the* right choice. If you have a family physician, go over these steps with him or her. These steps are not as complex as evaluating a new VCR but they are much more important and deserving of your time and effort. If you buy the wrong VCR, you may miss copying the movie of the week. If you make the wrong health care decision, it could mean your life. With the help of this book, the medical centers mentioned here, and your family doctor, you can make smarter, better decisions than the cost-cutters. You can guarantee the best medicine for yourself and your family.

Clearly, consumerism alone isn't going to fix all of American medicine, but it is the arena most roundly ignored and most sorely needed. There can be a new vision for health care in America, but only if you're part of it. Unless you, the consumer, understand the dangerous flaws in our system of medical care and push for the right solutions, the government and industry will impose more and more pure cost cutting reforms . . . further endangering you and your family. You can be a big part of the solution; the next sections will tell you how.

How to Use
This Book

This book is divided into two main parts. One part is a consumer's guide to operations and procedures; the other is a guide to chronic diseases. Each part presents the steps you follow to find the best care for you and your family. I consider these steps road maps, because they give you a clear, simple, step-by-step approach to excellence. They are intended to provide the information and expert knowledge that will enable you to take charge of your health and to determine its direction.

There is a note of warning: Medicine is still far from standardized. While your care may not conform exactly to the suggestions in this book, it should be close. If there are wide variations, you should ask your physician for the reasons. Perhaps there are idiosyncrasies in your case that justify those differences. But if you have a first-rate doctor and are at a first-rate hospital, the discrepancies will probably be minor.

Introduction to the Chapters on Operations and Procedures

An operation by the wrong doctor at the wrong hospital for the wrong reason can increase your risk of dying by as much as 500%. If you don't clearly need the operation, that's a terrible chance to take. The chapters in this part can lower that risk substantially.

Chapter Organization

Here's an outline of how the discussion of each operation or procedure is organized:

GENERAL BACKGROUND
Likelihood of Unnecessary Surgery (or Procedure)
Potential Risk
What It Is

CONSUMER STEPS
Step 1. Make Sure You Need the Surgery (or Procedure)
Step 2. Consider an Alternative
Step 3. Get a Specialist's Opinion
Step 4. Choose a Hospital
Step 5. Choose a Doctor

Here's what each section describes.

Likelihood of Unnecessary Surgery (or Procedure)

This section estimates what percentage of the operations or procedures under consideration may be unnecessary. Since up to 25% of all operations are unnecessary, and all operations carry risks, ranging from minor complications to death, it's important to do what you can to avoid any surgery that is not absolutely necessary. Taking all my sources into account, I've compiled a ranking of the risk of unnecessary surgery, from low to extremely high. As you scan a chapter, you should get a sense of where your priorities should lie. If an operation or procedure carries a high likelihood of being unnecessary, you should direct most of your effort to determining if you really need it. Before agreeing to surgery in such a case, you should get a second opinion from a specialist and exhaust alternative treatments. Here are examples for each of the rankings:

RANKING	EXAMPLE
Extremely high	Cesarean section
Very high	Carotid endarterectomy
High	Coronary artery bypass surgery
Moderate	Gallbladder surgery
Low	Flexible sigmoidoscopy

Sources
In addition to articles published in medical journals, the numbers of inappropriate surgeries come from the following sources.

MediQual Systems Inc. is a developer of clinical software systems and databases for health care clients. It is a leading research organization in the field of improving the quality of care. You will see that the other statistics in this section are determined from guidelines drawn up for a surgeon's use when deciding whether or not to operate. MediQual statistics are based on what surgeons actually find when they go in to operate. The number shown represents the percentage of operations in which no problem was found. This is apt to be a lower number than other statistical numbers because it means there was no reason found to justify the operation. Some surgeons believe the percentage of inappropriate surgeries as prepared by other research organizations is high. The MediQual figure is provided here because I consider it the most conservative. MediQual has also provided data on average length of stay and hospital cost that are used as measures of excellence in the book.

Value Health Sciences, a company that identifies and seeks to deter medically inappropriate procedures for insurers, employers, managed health plans, and utilization review committees. It has found on average that about 10–15% of all recommended procedures are unnecessary. Value Health uses a proprietary database. Some doctors dispute certain criteria used to determine appropriateness. For the purposes of this book, Value Health gives an excellent indication of the percentage of unnecessary procedures.

What the Numbers Mean

When interpreting the several different statistics cited in each chapter, remember that some of these may be hotly debated by surgeons. What's important is to look for a general sense of what the numbers mean—the trend. For instance, estimates of the number of inappropriate hysterectomies vary from 25–50% to over 90%, depending on the source. The point is that most authorities cite a very high number of unnecessary surgeries, and you should be extremely wary of agreeing to a hysterectomy without extensive consultation.

Be aware that certain operations are performed at above-average rates in specific regions of the country. If you live in an area where that number is high, you need to seek proof that the particular operation can offer significant benefits. I will alert you to the country's danger zones. Here, for instance, is how different parts of the country rank on the frequency with which back surgery is performed:

REGION	RANKING
Northeast	Low
Midwest	High
West	Higher
South	Highest

There probably is an excessive number of operations performed in the Midwest, West, and South.

This brings up the question of whether there are areas of the country where too *few* operations are done. The answer isn't clear, but most experts agree that fewer operations across the board would reduce the number of deaths. In the case of prostate surgery, for instance, the answer is clear: The Rand Corporation, a research think tank, looked at what would happen if the entire country performed as few procedures as the region that currently did the least. They concluded that several thousand lives could be saved each year by the decreased number of prostate surgeries nationwide!

Potential Risk

This section rates the risk of complication or death from the procedure or operation, on the following rating scale:

RANKING	EXAMPLE
Very high	Emergency angioplasty
High	Angiogram
Moderate	Routine gallbladder surgery
Low	EKG stress test

If an operation or procedure carries a very high risk of death or disability, you should direct a great deal of effort into finding a doctor and a hospital that have the lowest complication rates and the highest success rates.

For an overall evaluation of an operation's or procedure's appropriateness and risk, you should look at these first two sections together (Likelihood of Unnecessary Surgery, and Potential Risk). If the procedure or surgery is uncomplicated and is rarely performed when it should not be, you have little need to worry. Sigmoidoscopy is an example. But if both measures are high, you'll want to give careful consideration before you consent. And if you do consent, you'll want to find the best possible hospital and doctor.

What It Is

This section gives a brief description of the operation or procedure and its objectives so you'll know what is involved. You need *not* have a sophisticated understanding of the technical aspects of your operation or procedure to use this book.

Step 1. Make Sure You Need the Surgery (or Procedure)

Clearly, you are not expected to decide by yourself whether you do or do not need an operation. You'll want to decide with your doctor and with the help of a second opinion from an expert specialist. This section alerts you to the possibility that the surgery or procedure may be unnecessary. Read through the lists in this section to see where your diagnosis places you within the following appropriateness categories.

I've drawn together these guidelines from leading medical journals, medical school professors, the research firm Value Health Sciences, the professional colleges and academies, and the consensus conferences of the National Institutes of Health. These conferences bring together top doctors to debate and to reach agreement on health care issues.

In some cases, you will need to know your diagnosis and the results of your doctor's examination, plus lab test results, x-rays, and scans. Ask your doctor to review your record with you or to send you a written summary.

Appropriateness Categories

Here's an explanation of the appropriateness categories.

APPROPRIATE PROCEDURE   Based on the best available evidence, this operation should provide definite benefits. If your condition is not listed here, you should seek a specialist's opinion before undergoing the operation or procedure. The word *appropriate* is used rather than *necessary* because the operation may be justified but not absolutely necessary for your continuing good health, for instance, cataract surgery.

UNCERTAIN IF PROCEDURE IS APPROPRIATE   Medicine is an inexact science. In this category research just hasn't determined whether or not the operation could benefit you.

PROBABLY AN APPROPRIATE PROCEDURE   On the basis of the medical literature and your own medical history, it appears the operation or procedure should help you but its benefits have not been proven through rigorous, scientific tests.

PROBABLY NOT AN APPROPRIATE PROCEDURE   Under the right circumstances this operation might help, but you should consult additional experts and medical literature before you proceed. If you have other risk factors, such as advanced age or generally poor health, you may decide to try a more conservative, noninvasive approach. Remember that an operation or procedure in this gray category may not help you and could actually hurt you.

NOT AN APPROPRIATE PROCEDURE   You should not have this operation. Consult your doctor and consider alternative treatments.

Step 2. Consider an Alternative

Before agreeing to surgery, you need to explore the alternatives. Nonsurgical treatments have an unfortunate reputation of being less effective. In truth, you may have a better result with substantially lower risk. The pain and disability of coronary artery disease, for example, may respond to drugs, eliminating the need for surgery. There are more than a dozen alternative therapies for hysterectomy, an operation too often performed unnecessarily. You and your doctors will want to individualize your treatment based on the severity of your illness, age, and general health. I will suggest low-risk treatments that may enable you to avoid operations that have only a limited chance of success. If you are reading about any of the heart procedures, be certain to read about your illness in the chronic disease portion of the book for more information on alternative treatments.

Step 3. Get a Specialist's Opinion

Many doctors refer patients to other doctors within a fairly close-knit network. Some call it an "old boy network." Chances are many of these doctors don't know exactly what kind of experience a surgeon has or what kind of results he or she gets. This network may hurt you. Let's say you live in a major urban area near a community hospital and are acquainted with many of the physicians who practice there. Chances are, that if you ask five of those doctors for a second opinion about your operation, each one will refer you to someone at that hospital or one of its affiliates. If your community hospital is Boston's Massachusetts General Hospital, an affiliate of Harvard Medical School, you're in good shape. But if your community hospital does only a handful of the proposed operations, you may well be ill-served.

This section is designed to help you break out of the usual referral network and to get a fresh perspective. It's not meant to denigrate community physicians and what they do. Many of them are extraordinary physicians, trained at first-rate medical centers, who have chosen a community hospital out of a desire to treat patients full time. When my own son gets sick in Vermont, we take him to the community hospital in Morrisville, without hesitation. When a producer friend of mine found himself sick at the same hospital with meningitis, I recommended he stay there and not transfer to the well-respected facility at the University of Vermont. These country doctors are trained at great places and are up-to-date. By breaking a pattern of referral, I simply mean that you and your doctor need to do some comparison shopping. Look around at the alternatives, evaluate credentials, experience, and results. If you end up back at your own hospital, that's great. You know you've made an excellent choice.

Notice that I recommend a *specialist's* opinion, not just any second opinion. A second opinion is just that—another opinion. (You should always have a second opinion even before minor or clearly indicated surgery.) By contrast, a specialist's opinion should provide an overview of all your options and the state-of-the-art therapies. This section will explain when you need an expert opinion. In general, a specialist's opinion is required if your procedure is not clearly indicated or lacks a high chance of success, the diagnosis is unclear, or certain medical treatments have not been tried. The specialist should have no financial interest in the operation. That means choosing a specialist who will not be performing your operation and is not a member of the same group practice or hospital as the physician who rendered the first opinion.

I will list the kind of specialists that are best for a second opinion. Sometimes there are several choices. For instance, if you are considering an operation on your carotid artery, either a neurosurgeon or a vascular surgeon who routinely performs the operation is a good choice. However, a neurologist who sees a large number of patients with near strokes, called *transient ischemic attacks,* would also be a good candidate. When you consult another doctor, you should discuss the medical alternatives, other procedures or operations, even a wait-and-see stance. The expert should carefully review your medical history and test results to be certain your diagnosis is correct. By choosing a medical specialist for a second opinion, you are seeing someone with an interest in making conservative therapy work. For example: I'll often send a back patient to a neurologist or a physical medicine specialist, before referring them to a back surgeon. The physical medicine specialist is a physician and an expert in rehabilitation medicine. This gives a back patient a good shot at conservative therapy. Many surgeons will do the same. Many patients will push their surgeons to operate without taking a close look at conservative medical treatment. Don't be one of them!

I've long believed that its worth the 100 or so dollars it costs to see a specialist at a top university-affiliated hospital. You're not committed to having your surgery there; nor does it mean you are abandoning your family doctor or community hospital. But when the stakes are high and you face major surgery or a risky procedure, it's worth taking the time to see the best. Keep in mind that these specialists are not necessarily better doctors than your own. What they do have is a huge wealth of experience dealing in one small area of medicine. No internist or family doctor could possibly hope to keep up with all that's changing in medicine today. If you live too far away from a specialist or just can't afford to see one, I've included the numbers of organizations that can help you over the phone.

Where to Find a Specialist

CENTERS OF EXCELLENCE   These medical centers have some of the best reputations in the country for the treatment of a specific illness. They're an excellent choice if your condition is complicated, you have a rare condition, or you are at high risk because of other existing illnesses or your age. If these centers are too far away to visit personally, you can call and ask to speak to one of the staff physicians about your condition. I emphasize the word *reputation* in referring to these centers of excellence. As more and more hard data becomes available, future authors will be able to say with a high degree of certainty what are the best hospitals, based on fact, not opinion. Preliminary evidence indicates that many of those "best" hospitals will be community hospitals. Lists of many nationally renowned hospitals appear in each chapter in *Step 4. Choose a Hospital.*

UNIVERSITY-AFFILIATED HOSPITALS   If you have absolutely no idea where to turn with a complicated medical problem or you need a specialist's opinion, university-affiliated teaching hospitals are an excellent place to seek help. They have a medical school affiliated with them and teaching programs for young doctors in a variety of specialties. All doctors train at teaching hospitals. If your complaints or problems have been brushed aside elsewhere, you will find the curiosity and interest here a pleasant change. When my wife and I first picked a pediatrician in New York for our infant son Bobby, we chose someone with a busy practice and an excellent reputation. We found him, however, too busy to spend any time answering our questions. Unfortunately, our son was having a problem with his formula that went undiagnosed despite our phone calls and visits. We then chose a pediatrician at New York Hospital–Cornell Medical Center. As an academic specialist, this doctor has the time, interest, and inclination to spend quality time with us and our son. When problems arise, he can get our son to the best specialist at that hospital or others.

How do you call a teaching hospital out of the blue? Some, like the Cleveland Clinic or Mount Sinai Hospital in New York, have self-referral numbers. All have clinics you can call for an appointment. With a little detective work, you can home in on a specific physician. You can call the chairman of the department of medicine or surgery. You probably won't reach him or her, but the chief's secretary or administrative assistant will probably help you with names of specialists. You may have good luck by calling the public relations department for a recommendation. Nurses will often be able to give you an excellent, inside, word-of-mouth recommendation. Ask for respected doctors trained there who may now be at a hospital closer to you. All this, of course, is made much easier if your family doctor will provide the introductions. There is a complete list of university-affiliated teaching hospitals in the Appendix.

Each chapter has a menu of organizations that serve people with the disease you suffer from. Many times they'll help you with referrals and further information. Perhaps the very best of those is the National Cancer Institute. Their 800/4-CANCER hot line will customize information over the phone that is specific to the kind and stage of cancer you have. They'll set up referrals and put you in touch with experimental programs if you have an incurable cancer for which conventional therapy no longer works. Some advocacy groups, like HERS for potential hysterectomy candidates, will bend over backwards to help you avoid an unnecessary operation. I've included these organizations for two reasons: (1) You may be reluctant to refer yourself until you know more. With more knowledge, you'll have more confidence. (2) You may be uninsured or underinsured. These organizations will be enormously helpful even if you don't have a dime.

If you can't afford to make long distance calls or are timid talking to health care professionals on the phone, I've also included addresses for you to write to. One good rule of thumb is this: The National Institutes of Health will respond to *any* legitimate question about an illness if you write to them. They will also send you a printout of the latest information about your illness by calling CRISP (Computer Retrieval of Information on Scientific Projects). If you want a hard copy, you can call 301/496-7543 and receive a computer printout of all the NIH-funded research (abstracts of the research as well as where they are taking place) for your particular disease, surgery, or procedure.

Other Resources for Locating Specialists

Here are some other organizations that may be helpful in seeking a specialist's opinion.

AMERICAN COLLEGE OF SURGEONS   This organization will provide names of fellows in your geographic area who can offer expert opinions. Its number is 312/664-4050.

EMPLOYER RESOURCES   Some employers and insurance companies maintain first-rate services that can offer expert advice about inappropriate operations. Others are concerned only with cutting costs and will be of little help. Call your benefits or personnel office to learn more about second-opinion services that may be available to you, such as Value Health Sciences.

DIRECTORY OF MEDICAL SPECIALISTS   This guide, available in most libraries, lists certification, fellowship training, and medical staff appointments of most doctors in the United States. You can study the qualifications of these physicians and call for an appointment. They are listed by city and state.

AMERICAN BOARD OF MEDICAL SPECIALTIES   This group will check physician credentials for you. The toll-free number is 800/776-2378.

Step 4. Choose a Hospital

If you and your doctor have decided that a procedure or surgery is needed, the next step is to choose a hospital. Your hospital can be even more important than your doctor. Studies have found that, by the end of the hospital stay, only 20% of an operation's outcome can be attributed to the surgeon. The hospital, including the quality of the nursing staff and infection control, is responsible for the remaining 80%. Once your doctor has written an order, the rest is out of his or her hands. A great doctor can't produce great results without a great team. That's why I recommend finding the team first, by choosing the hospital. If you know a great doctor by reputation, chances are that he or she operates out of a great hospital.

Hospitals can be dangerous places. As many as 15 of every 100 hospitalized patients can expect some mistake to complicate their recovery. The wrong hospital can turn danger into disaster. California patients who underwent bypass surgery at one hospital in southern California had a 17.6% risk of death in 1988 compared to only 1% at the Kaiser Foundation Hospital in San Francisco. Heart patients who went to the first hospital had no idea that their chance of dying had jumped from one in a hundred to nearly one in five! This section will help you evaluate which hospital you should choose.

There's nothing that makes most doctors angrier than seeing a list of "best hospitals" or "best doctors." I have to admit I'm one of them. Since these lists are based largely on opinion, many experts discount them entirely. The list of hospitals found in most chapters of this book is provided only as a convenient starting place in your search for excellence. Most are recommended on the basis of reputation, not experience and results. The lists are not an endorsement, nor are they comprehensive. There may be hospitals just as excellent that have been omitted. You should apply the guidelines for experience, results, and other measures of excellence to any hospital you choose, whether or not it is on this list.

Here's what to do. Select the hospitals you'd like to consider based on proximity, convenience, cost, personal preference, your health plan's eligibility, and your physician's recommendations. Although it need not be a long list, you should include in it a variety of types—the local community hospital and a nearby center of excellence or a university-affiliated hospital. For some procedures a hospital is not necessary. A clinic setting may be more convenient and less expensive. Be certain that if you use a clinic, it has the same safeguards as a hospital.

Kinds of Hospitals

Here are the kinds of hospitals from which you can choose.

CENTERS OF EXCELLENCE   At hospitals such as Massachusetts General Hospital in Boston, the Mayo Clinic in Rochester, Minnesota, or one of several dozen other hospitals in the United States with comparable reputations, your chances of surviving most operations are dramatically superior. You must be certain, however, that the hospital does a high volume of the operation and has an excellent record.

UNIVERSITY-AFFILIATED TEACHING HOSPITALS   These hospitals concentrate a high degree of excellence and expertise under one roof. Few of them are strong in all specialties so you will want to make certain that they have a strong department for the operation you are considering. These hospitals are also called *tertiary* hospitals because they accept referrals of difficult or unusual cases. If your operation is expected to be complicated, you belong at one of these hospitals or at a national center of excellence. University-affiliated hospitals also serve the surrounding community and accept routine cases. The complete list is found in the Appendix.

COMMUNITY HOSPITALS   There are great community hospitals that you should consider. These are nonprofit hospitals financed by tax dollars and usually operated by a public board. Although they may be quite large, they don't often offer the complete range of services and expertise of a university-affiliated hospital. However, they have advantages that may be important to you: They are convenient and may have a low rate of in-hospital infections. At many, you will be treated by your physician, not residents or interns. If you are undergoing a routine gall bladder operation, for instance, your community hospital may be a perfectly acceptable choice.

SMALL HOSPITALS   Hospitals with less than a hundred or so beds simply can't keep up with the rapid pace of medical research or the high cost of new technology. One cannot expect a small, rural hospital, for instance, to be able to perform enough heart bypass operations to maintain proficiency. In many states these hospitals are forming alliances with major medical centers. Those alliances allow small hospitals to deliver excellent primary care and to refer unusual and complicated cases to the major center.

Sources for Hospitals Lists

For each chapter of this book, I've compiled a list of hospitals taken from the following sources.

EXPERTS' LISTS   I asked my own group of experts to recommend centers of excellence. In most cases less than a dozen medical centers were cited in each category. To expand the number of hospitals, lists from the other sources are included.

NATIONAL INSTITUTES OF HEALTH   Many chapters list National Institutes of Health (NIH)-designated research centers. In the case of cancer, for instance, participating medical centers must undergo rigorous qualifications that make them the best in the country.

U.S. NEWS & WORLD REPORT   The National Opinion Research Center, a social science research group at the University of Chicago, sampled 1,501 physicians in 15 specialties, ranging from AIDS to urology, drawn from a list of 138,000 physicians in the American Medical Association's files. The 965 doctors who replied gave high marks to 45 of the nation's 6,700 hospitals.

HEALTH CARE USA   This excellent book lists hospitals in different areas of the country for a wide variety of medical treatments. The lists were developed in consultation with medical societies, hospital accreditation bodies, health associations, and government agencies.

LEXECON HEALTH SERVICE   LHS, a health-information company located in Chicago, evaluates the price, cost, and quality of care for health care providers. Their analysis is based on hospital databases. These lists (which you will find in the chapters on Coronary Artery Bypass and Angioplasty) are the future. They list experience, results, cost, and length of stay for the leading hospitals in America. This kind of list takes the guesswork out of shopping for hospitals. Be warned that some hospitals and experts hotly dispute the accuracy of these lists.

THE BEST IN MEDICINE   This book consists of lists of doctors and hospitals throughout the United States. The lists were developed from results of a questionnaire that asked top doctors: "Where would you go if you or a member of your family were in need of the best available health care?" Questionnaires were sent to 10 representative doctors in each of the 25 medical specialty categories covered in the book.

The compilation of hospitals was done for your convenience only, and each source is clearly identified by the following symbols or by a credit line in the text.

SOURCE	SYMBOL
U.S. News & World Report list	US
List based on the author's extensive personal research	EX
The Best in Medicine list	BIM
National Institutes of Health list	NIH
Health Care USA list	HC

The listed hospitals are not ranked in order of care quality—for example, the best is not necessarily first. They are arranged by state and then alphabetically within the state. Although hospitals from different sources have been combined into one list, the compilation in no way implies that one source has endorsed the hospital list of another source.

Again, remember that the hospitals listed in this book are offered only as a place to start your search. There may be hospitals just as fine for your operation, procedure, or illness that you won't find here. I have outlined the experience, results, and other measures of excellence that will help you evaluate hospitals in your own area or any hospital you may be considering.

Measures of Excellence

Once your own list is complete, the next step is to compare experience, results, and other measures of excellence. If you've chosen a national center of excellence for your operation, you've already improved your chance of a successful outcome. But for all the hospitals on your list you still need to do this basic homework.

Experience

In this section I will give you, where available from the sources mentioned earlier, the minimum number of operations that I believe are necessary to attain a basic level of competency and produce excellent results. You should be able to obtain the figures for any particular hospital from its administrator, your referring physician, or in some cases your health insurer. Study after study has documented the relationship between a high volume of surgery and successful outcomes. For example, the death rate declines steadily for coronary artery bypass surgery as the number of operations per year increases from 150 to a high of 2,000. Any hospital that won't share its results isn't interested in showing you how it is improving the process of care. It's a place you don't belong.

Results

The only real proof of excellence is success. In this book we look at three different measures. The first is *death rate* (also called *mortality rate*). For major surgery, a low death rate is the best measure of success. In bypass surgery, a death rate of less than 2% for healthy young patients demonstrates that a hospital has excellent results.

If the procedure has such a low death rate that you can't distinguish one hospital from another, we'll look at the *complication rate*. A low complication rate is a very good measure of a great surgeon and a great hospital. What about *success rates* as a measure of excellence? Curiously, success as a measure of excellence appears infrequently. In some cases, such as gall bladder surgery, having no complications *does* mean it was successful because, after all, the gall bladder is out! For others, like disc surgery, success can be easily measured.

You may want to look for results on your own. They are published by the U.S. Department of Health and Human Services, local and regional newspapers, and state cost-containment councils, among other sources. You may find a hospital via a hospital comparison chart for your state or city. However, such reports are enormously controversial. Why? When the government published its first statistics, the facility with the highest death rate was a hospice for dying patients! Other hospitals complained bitterly that they had high death rates because they had the courage to treat sicker, older, poorer patients. In the last several years, researchers and statisticians have tried to work out formulas. Because formulas are so hard to develop, many doctors prefer the old-fashioned way of evaluating a hospital, by reputation and experience.

This book doesn't use formulas either. For death rates or complication rates, I give you a single number you can use for your own comparison with other hospitals. For instance, I recommend that the death rate for endarterectomy not exceed 2%. In some cases this number is qualified. For instance, the death rate quoted for bypass surgery is less than 2% for healthy patients under 65. It's not unreasonable to ask your hospital to dig out a similar number for comparison. You need not become a statistician to use these numbers. If you discover a death rate far higher at a hospital you are considering, find out why. If it operates on many older, sicker, high-risk patients, it still may be an excellent hospital, especially if you are an older, sicker patient yourself and the hospital does a larger number of cases and fits the other standards of excellence. But if the hospital does a low number of surgeries and has unexplained death and complication rates, watch out!

SOURCES FOR MORTALITY AND COMPLICATION RATES   You can find the mortality rates and complication rates by consulting one of the following sources:

■ The hospital administrator

■ The Medicare hospital mortality information published by the Health Care Financing Administration (HCFA). The ones for your region are available free by calling 301/966-1133.

■ Cost-containment councils. Some states (Pennsylvania is one of them) release hospital data to the public.

■ Your health insurance company

■ The peer review organization that oversees hospitals in your state for the Medicare program. They have excellent comparative data. Some will not provide any data; others can be very helpful.

If a hospital has high death-rate statistics, most hospital administrators are eager to clear the record and answer your questions. However, if they won't provide satisfactory answers, you're in the wrong place! If a hospital's death rate is above average, ask the hospital administrator the following questions:

■ Why are the death and complication rates so high?

■ What was the hospital's response to the findings of the Health Care Finance Administration? (Each hospital is given the opportunity to explain its statistics, and the replies are included in the published reports. You also can ask the hospital for them.)

■ Has the hospital taken any actions to improve its performance?

■ Do certain doctors account for a disproportionate share of the bad numbers? Is your doctor one of them?

Hospitals have legitimate reasons for a high death rate in roughly 50% of cases. The other 50% probably deliver substandard care.

Other Measures of Excellence

Volumes have been written on how to choose a hospital. Much of it is based on criteria that don't guarantee the outcome of your surgery. That's why hard, objective criteria like experience and results are so important and emphasized so strongly in this book. If several hospitals on your list appear about equal based on the numbers, you may wish to look at other criteria. I have included these as other measures of excellence. Here are some examples.

STABLE, HIGH-QUALITY NURSING STAFF   Pretty much everyone agrees that a great nursing staff is critical. A high ratio of Registered Nurses to Licensed Practical Nurses is one such criterion. Another is the turnover rate of nurses—the lower, the better.

SPECIALIZED TRAINING PROGRAM   For cardiac surgery, for example, it's vital that the hospital have a training program in heart surgery. That guarantees you round-the-clock coverage for surgical emergencies.

EXCELLENT BACKUP DEPARTMENTS   For any operation, a great department of anesthesia is critical. Other key backup departments include: a neonatal intensive care unit, for a woman with a high-risk pregnancy; a "pump" team that does a large volume of open-heart cases and has been together a year or more, for bypass surgery; recovery room and intensive care unit teams that are high on experience.

EXPERTISE WITH DIFFICULT CASES   Be sure your hospital is expert at handling difficult cases.

AVERAGE LENGTH OF HOSPITAL STAY, AND HOSPITAL CHARGES   Many great hospitals actually cost *less*. They are more efficient, and you will, on average, suffer fewer complications. An abnormally long hospital stay may betray a high number of complications. High charges may reveal a low-volume hospital that lacks the efficiency or the economy of scale typical of better programs. The charges listed in this section are all hospital-based charges, not doctors' fees. The charges and lengths of stay were provided by the research firm MediQual. Note that these are 1991 figures. Since health care costs can increase 20–30% in one year, you will want to ask afresh what the average length of stay and average charges are at each hospital on your list.

In a January 22, 1992, lead story, the *Wall Street Journal* reported that a high-cost, low-quality producer should be doomed. Unfortunately, in medicine that is not always the case. Here's an example of two neighboring hospitals in Pennsylvania that the newspaper cited:

	HOSPITAL A	HOSPITAL B
Actual deaths	4	8
Expected deaths	7.75	2.95
Cost	$22,907	$33,906

Hospital A not only had fewer deaths than expected, it cost 50% less. Let's read this table carefully. Hospital B estimated that three patients would die, but eight actually did. That's not good. Hospital A expected almost eight patients to die, but only four did. Hospital A exceeded expectations. Now look at the cost. Hospital A's costs were nearly $11,000 less than Hospital B's. Cost is a surprisingly good indicator of excellence. The best programs don't necessarily cost more. With fewer complications and greater efficiency, better programs can be a lot cheaper. Be sure to ask about cost when you comparison shop.

HOSPITAL OWNERSHIP   Hospital ownership is another measure of excellence. A recent study in the *New England Journal of Medicine* rated hospitals by ownership. Here's how they were ranked, in descending order:

University teaching hospitals (best overall)

University-affiliated hospitals (rated high, but with some exceptions)

Not-for-profit hospitals

Osteopathic hospitals

For-profit hospitals

Public hospitals

Clearly, you can't choose a hospital based solely on ownership. But you can say that a hospital's status as a nonprofit university-affiliated teaching hospital is a well-established marker of excellence.

CONTINUING EFFORT TO IMPROVE   A last critical measure of excellence is whether the hospital is continually striving to improve the quality of care. You can tell this is so if a hospital's results improve each year. For instance, once results for bypass surgery became public in New York City, there was a dramatic improvement the following year in every hospital surveyed, with death rates falling as much as 300%! Look for improvement.

THE BOTTOM LINE   Can you get too detailed? Yes! You can easily lose sight of the forest for the trees and become the auditor I described earlier. A first-rate specialist's opinion and selecting a hospital and a doctor based on experience and results will guarantee you a very high level of care. These additional measures of excellence are important, but they are only icing on the cake if you've done your other homework.

Step 5. Choose a Doctor

You should choose a hospital before you choose the surgeon or specialist who will perform your procedure. As stated earlier, when you are discharged, 80% of the success of your operation is determined by the care you received in the hospital. However, choosing a first-rate hospital alone is not enough. Hospitals don't operate; surgeons do. While there are large variations among hospitals, there are even larger differences among surgeons, according to recent studies in Maryland and New England. Even some world-class medical centers have staff surgeons with very poor surgical records, so Step 5 is very important.

Measures of Excellence

CREDENTIALS   For operations, your surgeon should be board certified by the American College of Surgeons. For procedures, your physician should be certified by the appropriate board of the American Boards of Internal Medicine. I will provide you with the appropriate certifications in each chapter. To determine if a doctor is board certified, you can consult the following:

Directory of Medical Specialists

Your referring physician

The hospital administrator

The present medical referral system is based partly on hearsay and partly on reputation. We are moving into a new era in which referrals are made on the basis of objective performance. Performance is judged on two criteria, experience and results. The two usually go hand in hand. The more experience a surgeon has doing an operation, the better he or she is likely to be. To make certain that is true we need to measure results.

EXPERIENCE   Statistics can be a cruel science. Years of careful study and preparation are measured, in the end, by the sheer volume of operations that a surgeon performs. In many cases, the more operations the better. In cases where solid numbers are available from sources mentioned in the beginning of this chapter, I have listed the volume of procedures a surgeon should perform during training and during each year in practice. The exception is the surgeon who does a large volume of inappropriate operations. For instance, you're not looking for an obstetrician at a community hospital who delivers 50% of his or her low-risk patients by Cesarean section. Even if you ignore all my other advice, you should still heed this: Choose the doctor who has the best record based on experience, excellent results, and a low mortality rate. I'll list the figures that can be expected for your operation. For instance, an eye surgeon shouldn't have more than one postoperative infection in a year. Likely sources for this information are:

The surgeon

The state peer review organization

The hospital administrator

The referring physician

Many great surgeons keep their own records to review and to improve themselves. It's a measure of excellence. They are willing and proud to share their record with you. For the most commonly performed major surgeries, the required experience is quite clear. For lesser procedures or for operations performed less frequently, guidelines are not available as a matter of record. In those situations, we consulted the leading professional academies and colleges and the leading surgeons. In such cases, your surgeon may, legitimately, say that she or he has commensurate experience in other similar procedures. For instance, a neurosurgeon may not do a large number of endarterectomies but may have vast experience operating on blood vessels in and around the brain.

RESULTS   Look for at least the same excellent results in choosing a surgeon as you would in choosing a hospital: success rates, death rates, and complication rates. In many chapters, the rate given for choosing a surgeon is the same as the rate given for choosing a hospital. Assuming you have chosen a great hospital, just make sure the surgeon you have chosen is among the top performers. Even world-famous medical centers have the occasional surgeon who performs poorly.

If you have serious concerns about your surgeon's competence or behavior, here are the two best sources:

■ The Washington, D.C.-based Public Citizen Health Research Group publishes a list of nearly 7,000 doctors who have been disciplined by the state disciplinary boards. Make sure your doctor isn't on it.

■ Your state disciplinary board may be able to tell you if any action has been taken against the doctor.

Introduction to the Chapters on Chronic Diseases

If you have a chronic disease, chances are high that your care has been compromised by cost-cutters. The difficulty with chronic diseases is that it's very hard to prove that these cost-cutting measures have shortened *your* life. But research is under way that proves just how nefarious cost-cutting for those who have chronic diseases can be. In one study, patients with osteoporosis who had suffered hip fractures were discharged from hospital six days earlier than was customary, and with half of the physical therapy they needed. At the end of six months, many more of them were still in nursing homes than before cost-cutting was instituted. Just six more days in the hospital and many of these patients could have continued a normal life in their own homes.

The cost-cutters will try to wear you down. My own son had a debilitating hearing problem. After surgery, he needed a great deal of work with his speech, which was delayed about a year. As you might predict, our insurance company refused to pay for speech therapy. In fact, they cited a letter from the wrong doctor as evidence that he didn't need speech therapy! When I called the company they said, "It doesn't matter what the doctor's letter says—we still won't pay for it!" Through the usual series of letters and telephone calls, they did agree to pay for part of his speech therapy. But every six months they'd cut off the payment and say, "He's fine. He no longer needs speech therapy!" Now, that example pales by comparison with those of patients with cancer or AIDS who have been cut off by the insurers, but it does illustrate how cost-cutters approach every area in medicine with a hatchet and hope to wear you down.

In this part I've described briefly what most specialists agree is a reasonable standard of care for each of the major chronic diseases. If you notice big discrepancies between your care and this standard, ask your doctor why. The secret with chronic diseases is probably not some new high-tech procedure; it's having a specialist who will carefully *think* about your disease and plot a long-term, winning strategy.

Chapter Organization

Here's an outline of how the discussion of each chronic disease is organized:

GENERAL BACKGROUND
Risk for Inappropriate Care
What It Is

CONSUMER STEPS
Step 1. Make Sure You Get the Best Care
Step 2. Look for Shortcomings
Step 3. See a Specialist
Step 4. Become Your Own Expert

Here's what each section describes. (Note: Much of the Introduction to the Chapters on Operations and Procedures applies here as well.)

Risk for Inappropriate Care

This section estimates the likelihood that you will receive care that is not state-of-the-art.

What It Is

This section gives a brief description of the particular chronic disease.

Step 1. Make Sure You Get the Best Care

From thousands of phone calls and tens of thousands of letters over my years at CBS News, I have been continually astounded at the number of viewers whose care doesn't begin to approach state-of-the-art. In many cases they don't even know treatment exists for their condition! Viewers call who suffer horrendous side effects from medications for high blood pressure that were prescribed a generation ago. Over the last few months, hundreds of asthma patients have called who each year use dozens of a kind of inhaler that has been shown to have a high risk of death. They've never heard of inhaled corticosteroids, the new state-of-the-art treatment for moderate-to-severe asthma. Millions of Americans treat their stomach upsets themselves with antacids. Some have unrecognized heart disease. Others have undiagnosed ulcers or tumors that remain undiagnosed as long as they continue to treat themselves.

This section is intended to help you find obvious, glaring errors in your care. Don't be surprised if some of these errors are your own! For instance, you may have insulin-dependent diabetes and fail to take regular, daily blood sugar readings.

Risk Factors

You should be aware of the risk factors and early warning signs for various diseases. That's especially true if a disease runs in your family, increasing your own susceptibility to it. Many patients fail to get the best care because they don't get medical attention quickly enough, ignoring symptoms for months or even years. You should never delay seeking help.

When you do consult a doctor, you should help your doctor help you. Too many patients hide information from their physician. Your doctor should be aware of all the medications you are taking and all other health problems you have. Then the doctor should make an accurate diagnosis, using up-to-date tests that can provide accurate assessment of your condition. Many diseases are misdiagnosed because the doctor prescribes treatment after *assuming* a particular cause of your symptoms instead of ordering an objective assessment. As a result, you may be underdiagnosed and undertreated. This section outlines the therapy, treatment, and drugs that are considered state-of-the-art.

Step 2. Look for Shortcomings

From Step 1, I hope you will get a good feeling about your treatment, and that you understand much of it better. I'm sure you'll find differences between your care and that recommended by the experts. There is some obvious room for difference of opinion. What you are looking for are big gaping holes in your care.

Mistakes in Diagnosis or Treatment

This next section recaps Step 1 by stating some of the most common and potentially dangerous problems as specific mistakes. If you notice several such mistakes in your care, be sure to discuss them with your health care provider. But if the number of mistakes you find is high, then you need to sit down with a specialist.

In addition to the mistakes made in the management of specific diseases, there are errors that are common to all medical problems. You should be aware of them also. While there are a great many ingenious and sophisticated treatments, most patients suffer because they don't receive the basics. Simple problems can do more to decrease your quality of life than a lack of the latest high-tech treatments.

Many of these problems are within your own control and can be prevented. Certain behaviors, such as smoking, poor nutrition, and drinking to excess, can create health problems on their own or aggravate existing conditions. If you are at high risk for a certain disease because of your family history and other factors, you should be tested regularly. Diagnostic tests are increasingly sophisticated. If your close female relatives have had breast cancer and you have experienced premature menopause, for instance, you should adhere to the American Cancer Society's guidelines for mammograms. Too often people who have medical problems delay treatment, assuming that the problems will go away. Serious problems don't; they only get worse. You should never be ashamed to seek help or assume that treatment will be too expensive. Even if you are worried that your insurance won't cover your care, you should get help. Treatment may be less expensive than you anticipate, ongoing research projects may provide free care, or your doctor may be able to persuade your insurance plan to cover your care. You will never know if you don't schedule the initial appointment. The worst thing you can do is to treat yourself without consulting a doctor or to alter your treatment without prior discussion with your physician.

Some of the most frequent mistakes occur in drug therapy. If your doctor has prescribed medications, you should take those drugs faithfully and not discontinue them abruptly if you experience unpleasant side effects. You should discuss your medications with your doctor and make sure that none of these common errors are being made:

- Your medications interact adversely.

- Your medications are not state-of-the-art.

- You're receiving more than one medication at a time.

- Your medication doses are too frequent or they aren't being added one at a time.

You should also make sure your doctor doesn't underestimate the seriousness of your disease and fail to order the proper test that will provide the proper assessment of your care.

Step 3. See a Specialist

In this section I'll tell you the circumstances under which you should insist on referrals, the credentials you should look for in a specialist, and where to find state-of-the-art care. You'll also find lists of hospitals with excellent reputations, which can help you with your illness.

As a patient with a chronic illness, you need a careful, lifelong strategy for managing it. You need to know when to change drugs, when to consider surgery. You need to keep ahead of your disease.

With a complex, chronic illness, it can be impossible for a general practitioner to know enough to treat you for the long run. Even specialists have trouble keeping up-to-date on their narrowed focus. Take an epilepsy specialist I interviewed. He reads five monthly general neurology journals, three monthly epilepsy journals, plus two general weekly journals. Each week he reads 60 abstracts, 20–30 articles cover to cover. This takes him eight hours a week. He goes to two hours of lectures per week and three–four hours of conferences per week. *And all this is just barely enough to keep up!*

Even doctors in general practice who read their journals religiously don't have the time to scrutinize how every study was done or if they apply to his or her patients. Superspecialists treat many outpatient diseases extremely well. Rheumatologists, neurologists, cardiologists, gastroenterologists, diabetologists, epileptologists . . . they know all the exquisite fine points of managing your care in the most elegant fashion imaginable. They can map out a well-thought-out strategy of diagnosis and treatment.

But where does that leave your family doctor? Many academic doctors have a biased opinion. They can't imagine how any doctor knows a particular area unless that doctor eats, sleeps, and dreams about it. Their sentiment is: "I don't believe in GPs. No man can know five to six subjects." Are such specialists always "better" than a family doctor? No. But the superspecialist does have more experience in the narrow area of immediate concern.

Now, does this mean you should abandon your family doctor for a superspecialist in your disease? No! The family doctor sees you as a whole patient. He or she should be an expert on coordinating your care.

Step 4. Become Your Own Expert

Because of medicine's new cut-rate orientation, you have to be responsible in large measure for your own care. But you need not be alone. Even if you don't have the money to pursue Step 2. See a Specialist, there's lots more help out there, and much of it is free. There are organizations that will give you more than a sympathetic ear. Some of them are advocacy groups that will take you in hand and guide you through every step of what you need to do. Some will offer you financial advice. If you do nothing else after reading this book, start using the phone to line up help. You'll be surprised how much of your own expert you can become by just asking questions. Many of the numbers are toll free. Education is a powerful weapon. In medicine, it can save your life.

Choosing a Family Doctor

While it's important to select the right doctor to perform your operation or the right specialist to manage your chronic disease, you need to take equal care in choosing a family or primary care physician who will oversee your general health care and refer you to specialists when necessary. All the steps in this book are made quantitatively easier by having a physician as your partner. That's why I have written this special section.

The best doctor for you depends on your age, sex, risk factors, and medical history. If you're a 34-year-old woman starting a family, for instance, you'll want a doctor associated with a hospital that has great departments of obstetrics, gynecology, and pediatrics. If you are in your seventies, your doctor should be a gerontologist or an internist who specializes in gerontology. If you are generally healthy, you may want to choose from the key primary care specialties: internal medicine, family practice, pediatrics, and gynecology. If you have a single chronic disease that requires multiple doctor visits each year, you might choose a specialist for that disease as your primary physician. If you're a 67-year-old man with coronary artery disease, you'll want a doctor who has access to a hospital with an excellent department of cardiology. That doctor should be able to act as a broker: Should you have a heart attack, he or she should be able to quickly get you a bed in a first-rate cardiac intensive care unit. He or she should know who the most skilled and successful cardiac surgeons and cardiologists in your area are and be able to get you to them at any time of day or night.

It's critical to have that "quarterback" to make certain that multiple medications from different physicians don't interfere with each other or cause intolerable side effects. Generalists can catch problems that might otherwise fall through the cracks. It's also a good idea for any specialists involved in your care to coordinate with your internist or family physician and to have her or him write all your prescriptions.

If your health care plan is an HMO or other managed health care plan, your options will be more limited. But the same principles still apply. Choose your HMO for the doctors and hospitals you will be allowed to use. My sister-in-law needed gall bladder surgery during her last pregnancy. She belonged to a Harvard HMO that used one of the very best hospitals in the world for obstetrics and surgery, Brigham and Women's Hospital. She wouldn't have done any better with the best private insurance. Too many people choose an HMO without looking at their choice of hospitals and doctors should the very worst happen. They want convenience and low cost for trivial illnesses but neglect to think about who will take care of them if they become seriously ill.

What qualities should you expect in your doctor? Look for objective criteria of excellence and the personal qualities that make you comfortable. Let's start with objective criteria. Look for training at first-rate medical schools and teaching hospitals. Check to see if your doctor is board certified. Seventeen of the 23 different boards of internal medicine recertify doctors every 7–10 years, for new members. If your doctor has run into trouble, you can check that, too. Each year the Public Citizen Health Research Group in Washington, D.C., publishes a list of doctors who have been disciplined by the state disciplinary boards.

Some patients want and need a tough, authoritarian, old-school doctor who's going to tell them exactly what to do and make them stick to it. Others are looking for a health care partner who will make each decision with them. You need to decide in advance what kind of personality you want, then interview your doctors of choice. Prepare a set of questions from chapters in this book. For instance, if you have asthma, be sure that objective testing is used regularly in the doctor's practice and that patients with moderate and severe asthma are taking inhaled steroids as a first-line drug of choice. Find out how willing the doctor is to help you seek expertise at other hospitals and from other doctors. If he or she is not, you're in trouble. One thing I've learned in my current job is humility. No matter how much I think I know about a subject, I learn much, much more talking to a specialist about a specific problem. It's just not possible to keep up on everything, but it is possible to know where and how to look. Your doctor need not know everything, but he or she does need to know where to look for the best available information and treatment. If your doctor isn't offended by lots of probing questions in your "tryout" appointment, it's a pretty good guarantee she or he won't be offended down the road.

You want a doctor who instills in you a sense of optimism about your future, even if you have a chronic or a fatal disease. That optimism will catch on and help you, your family, nurses, and others on the health care team try harder. When a doctor withdraws hope, he or she withdraws support. Nurses and family sense that and often withdraw from the patient, leaving him or her alone.

For some illnesses there are no accepted cures. Your doctor should have his or her feet solidly on the ground and offer you the best of proven treatments. But he or she should know if and when to look at the experimental. In AIDS and cancer, for example, your doctor must be familiar with promising clinical trials that could benefit you. He or she should look to the future. This last year we did a segment on "CBS This Morning" on the use of interferon for macular degeneration. We never had more phone calls. The treatment hasn't passed all the hurdles, and long-term safety and effectiveness isn't yet proven. But with macular degeneration and other presently incurable illnesses, it's important for your doctor to learn when you have nothing to lose and when to refer for evaluation.

I am a physician and the son of a physician. Both my father and I, as well as many of our colleagues, find the oversight accompanying this new era of cost containment very painful. It's a distinct departure from the long history of the rugged, independent individuals who pioneered medicine in America. However, as a result of this scrutiny, new information has become available that all consumers should include in their health care decisions. I am certainly not encouraging you to think of every hospital as a death trap nor every physician as a criminal. But, given the data now available, you should use those facts to your advantage. Remember, in many cases, you're not second guessing the doctor, you're second guessing an insurer, a company benefits manager, a claims adjuster, or a government bureaucrat. Who would you rather have decide your fate?

The guidelines in this book apply to any procedure, surgery, or chronic illness. The following chapters of this book are written about specific operations, procedures, and chronic diseases. Much of the information is cutting-edge and so is not available for every operation or disease. I selected these specific illnesses and procedures for their prominence as problem areas in medicine and because data and knowledge existed from which to draw first-rate advice.

REFERENCES AND SUGGESTED READING

A great deal of this book is based on rules of thumb gathered from leading experts and data generated by research organizations. The references listed at the end of each chapter are meant to credit the most important sources and to guide you to further reading.

Berwick, D. M., and Wald, D. Hospital Leaders' Opinions of the HCFA Mortality Data. *Journal of the American Medical Association,* Vol. 263, No. 2 (Jan. 12, 1990), pp. 247–249.

Chassin, M. R., and others. Does Inappropriate Use Explain Geographic Variations in the Use of Health Care Services? A Study of Three Procedures. *Journal of the American Medical Association,* Vol. 258, No. 18 (Nov. 13, 1987), pp. 2533–2537.

Dubois, R. W., and others. Hospital Inpatient Mortality: Is It a Predictor of Quality? *New England Journal of Medicine,* Vol. 317 (Dec. 24, 1987), pp. 1674–1680.

Dubois, R. W., and Brook, R. H. Preventable Deaths: Who, How Often, and Why? *Annals of Internal Medicine,* Vol. 109 (1988), pp. 582–589.

Epstein, A. E., and others. Do the Poor Cost More? A Multihospital Study of Patients' Socioeconomic Status and Use of Hospital Resources. *New England Journal of Medicine,* Vol. 322 (April 19, 1990), pp. 1122–1128.

Fletcher, Robert H., and Fletcher, Suzanne W. Internal Medicine: Whole or in Pieces? [editorial] *Annals of Internal Medicine,* Vol. 115, No. 12 (Dec. 15, 1991), pp. 978–979.

Forrow, Lachlan, and others. Absolutely Relative: How Research Results Are Summarized Can Affect Treatment Decisions. *American Journal of Medicine,* Vol. 92, No. 2 (Feb. 1992), pp. 121–124.

Frater, Alison, and Costain, David. Any Better? Outcome Measures in Medical Audit [editorial]. *British Medical Journal,* Vol. 304, No. 6826 (Feb. 29, 1992), pp. 519–520.

Garber, A. M., and others. Case Mix, Costs and Outcomes: Differences Between Faculty and Community Services in a University Hospital. *New England Journal of Medicine,* Vol. 310 (May 10, 1984), pp. 1231–1237.

Ginzberg, E. High-Tech Medicine and Rising Health Care Costs. *Journal of the American Medical Association,* Vol. 263, No. 13 (April 4, 1990), pp. 1820–1822.

Grant, K. A. M. Leading for Health: Responses—Which Model for Delivering Care? *British Medical Journal,* Vol. 304, No. 6826 (Feb. 29, 1992), pp. 566–568.

Green, J., and others. The Importance of Severity of Illness in Assessing Hospital Mortality. *Journal of the American Medical Association,* Vol. 263, No. 3 (Jan. 12, 1990), pp. 241–246.

Hannan, E. L., and others. Investigation of the Relationship Between Volume and Mortality for Surgical Procedures Performed in New York State Hospitals. *Journal of the American Medical Association,* Vol. 262 (1989), pp. 503–510.

Hartz, A. J., and others. Hospital Characteristics and Mortality Rates. *New England Journal of Medicine* (1989), pp. 1720–1725.

Health Services Research Group. Small-Area Variations: What Are They and What Do They Mean? *Canadian Medical Association Journal,* Vol. 146, No. 4 (Feb. 15, 1992), pp. 467–470.

Jecker, Nancy S., and Schneiderman, Lawrence J. Futility and Rationing. *American Journal of Medicine,* Feb. 1992, pp. 189–196.

Kellie, E. S., and Kelly, J.T. Medicare Peer Review Organization Preprocedure Review Criteria: An Analysis of Criteria for Three Procedures. *Journal of the American Medical Association,* Vol. 265 (1991), pp. 1265–1270.

Kelly, J. T., and Kellie, S. E. Appropriateness of Medical Care: Findings, Strategies. *Archives of Pathology and Laboratory Medicine,* Vol. 114 (Nov. 1990), pp. 1119–1121.

Kosecoff, J., and others. Prospective Payment System and Impairment at Discharge: The Quicker-and-Sicker Story Revisited. *Journal of the American Medical Association,* Vol. 264, No. 15 (Oct. 17, 1990), pp. 1980–1983.

Laupacis, Andreas, and others. How Attractive Does a New Technology Have to Be to Warrant Adoption and Utilization? Tentative Guidelines for Using Clinical and Economic Evaluations. *Canadian Medical Association Journal,* Vol. 146, No. 4 (Feb. 15, 1992), pp. 473–481.

Luft, H. S., and others. Does Quality Influence Choice of Hospital? *Journal of the American Medical Association,* Vol. 263, No. 21 (June 6, 1990), pp. 2899–2906.

McCullough, L. B. An Ethical Model for Improving the Patient-Physician Relationship. *Inquiry,* Vol. 25 (Winter 1988), pp. 454–469.

Michaels, Evelyne. Doctors Can Improve on Way They Deliver Bad News, MD Maintains. *Canadian Medical Association Journal,* Vol. 146, No. 4 (Feb. 15, 1992), pp. 564–566.

NBC News/Wall Street Journal telephone poll (of 1,004 adults), Dec. 6–9, 1991.

Reiser, Stanley J. Consumer Competence and the Reform of American Health Care. *Journal of the American Medical Association,* Vol. 26, No. 11 (Mar. 18, 1992).

Sade, Robert M. The Different Drummer, the Double Agent, and Future Dilemmas in Bioethics. *Annals of Thoracic Surgery,* Vol. 53, No. 2 (Feb. 1992), pp. 183–190.

Sox, Harold C. Jr., and Griner, P. L. An Invitation to Join a Controversy [editorial]. *Annals of Internal Medicine,* Vol. 116, No. 5 (Mar. 1, 1992), pp. 422–423.

Stoeckle, John D., and Reiser, Stanley J. The Corporate Organization of Hospital Work: Balancing Professional and Administrative Responsibilities. *Annals of Internal Medicine,* Vol. 116, No. 5 (Mar. 1, 1992), pp. 407–413.

Operations and Procedures

Coronary Artery Bypass Surgery

Likelihood of Unnecessary Surgery   HIGH

Some experts say that as many as 25% of the 350,000 bypass surgeries performed each year are not clearly necessary. Dr. Thomas B. Graboys is Director of the Lown Cardiovascular Center and a professor at Harvard Medical School. His group carries out extensive work in second opinions for those who may need coronary artery bypass surgery. Dr. Graboys says, "We should all think it a little strange that in the last decade the number of bypass operations being performed has increased while the prevalence of the disease has decreased and medications are better than ever." He says that at least 50% of the second opinions he sees don't need surgery at all. This has led to some gallows humor I overheard between two Harvard professors. One said to the other: "I'm worried to death, I've been told I need bypass surgery. What should I do?" The other answered, "See Dr. Graboys. He'll tell you you don't need one!" You too should ask why you *don't* need the surgery.

The research firm MediQual has the more conservative figure. In 1991 they reported that 13.54% of bypass surgeries they studied had none of the objective clinical findings documented in the hospital medical record they use to validate bypass at the time of surgery.

Potential Risk   HIGH

In the wrong hands, bypass surgery can be one of the most dangerous operations. While techniques have improved and the number of potentially serious complications has declined, the risks still include the possibilities of heart attack, stroke, and death. Those risks are low in good hospitals with good doctors if you are otherwise in good health. But in some hospitals, one of every five patients dies. Most patients never ask the questions that would prevent them from checking in to such a hospital.

What It Is

Bypass surgery is performed when the main coronary arteries become narrowed by heart disease, restricting the flow of blood to the heart. The operation creates a new route for the blood, circumventing the blockages and enabling an adequate supply of oxygen to reach heart muscles once again. In one frequently used technique, the surgeon removes a vein from a leg, then grafts a section into place above and below the blockage, forming a conduit for the blood. In another method, the surgeon bisects a healthy artery in the chest cavity and stitches one end to the diseased coronary artery beyond the point of blockage. In several follow-up studies a decade later, researchers found that 90% of the grafts that involved chest arteries remained open, compared to only 65% of those that used leg veins.

You will want a surgeon who has been trained and is skilled in both techniques. While the statistics alone would indicate that chest arteries are preferable to vein grafts, that is not always the case. When multiple bypasses are being contemplated, the surgeon will have to weigh a number of factors—the extent of the disease and the location of the blockage, among others—in deciding whether to use chest arteries, veins, or a combination of the two. Sometimes the decision can be made only after the surgeon has begun the operation.

Step 1. Make Sure You Need the Surgery

There is a long and complex list of indications published by the American College of Cardiology, but the list requires a sophisticated medical background to use. This chapter outlines the following basic rules of thumb. Most are provided by the research company Value Health Sciences or have been presented in the *Journal of the American Medical Association.*

Appropriate Procedure

Not all of the following conditions need to be present; one alone may be reason enough to justify surgery.

■ Major blockages in all three main coronary arteries, and the operation can extend your life expectancy.

■ A blockage in the left main coronary artery, which could cause sudden death or a massive heart attack.

■ Symptoms of coronary artery disease that interfere with day-to-day life and can't be controlled with medications or other procedures, such as angioplasty.

Not an Appropriate Procedure

■ You have not yet exhausted everything that medical therapy can do for you. Many patients and their doctors opt for the quick fix. But since bypass surgery can be dangerous, the experts would rather you vigorously pursue medical treatment before you consider surgery.

- Blockages in your coronary arteries not severe enough to require surgery.

- Blockages in your arteries that cannot be bypassed (for instance, if they extend for the entire length of the vessel).

- Poor odds of surviving surgery.

Step 2. Consider an Alternative

This operation shouldn't be considered a quick fix for heart disease. Some doctors and their patients rush into bypass surgery before they have exhausted all available medical treatments. Patients may be helped by simple behavioral changes such as low-cholesterol diet, exercise, weight loss, stress management, and not smoking. Sometimes patients can be treated more safely and effectively through angioplasty, a procedure that unclogs blocked arteries with a balloon (see chapter on Angioplasty). You should know exactly what your doctor expects to achieve through surgery that can't be accomplished through other means. In the last few years a number of new drugs have been developed to treat heart disease. Used singly or in combination these drugs may control the symptoms enough so that surgery is not needed. They may slow or even reverse the actual progress of the disease, again eliminating the need for an operation. See the chapter on coronary artery disease for a complete rundown of all the available medical treatments.

Dr. Michael Horan, associate director for cardiology at the National Institute of Health's Heart, Lung and Blood Institute, reminds people, though, that it's important to know that the conservative route of going for pharmacologic therapy first is not always the best thing. It is an option. That is something you should consider when you go for a specialist's opinion.

Step 3. Get a Specialist's Opinion

WHEN YOU NEED ONE   You will need an expert opinion if your operation is not clearly indicated, you do not have a high chance of success, or you want to consider an alternative.

WHO TO GO TO   You have two choices. First is a board-certified cardiologist, who frequently performs or reviews presurgical angiograms that allow him or her to assess how likely you are to benefit from the operation. Second is a cardiac surgeon who will not be performing the actual operation but can advise on its technical feasibility.

WHAT TO DISCUSS   You should discuss the alternatives to bypass surgery, which include the alternative medical therapies listed under Step 2 and also angioplasty. You will want the doctor to carefully review your medical history and your medical tests and to be certain your condition is correctly diagnosed.

WHERE TO GO   You can go to one of the centers of excellence for bypass surgery listed just ahead under "Who to Call," one of the centers of excellence for cardiology listed under Step 4, or one of the teaching hospitals listed in the Appendix.

WHO TO CALL   If time, expense, or travel prohibit you from seeking a specialist's opinion, learn as much as you can by calling one of the centers of excellence or one of the organizations listed below. Make certain to ask these questions:

Do I need surgery?

Is there an alternative therapy?

How significant is the surgery?

What is the expected outcome?

Can you recommend an expert cardiologist or heart surgeon close to where I live?

Do I need to travel to a larger center?

Am I receiving state-of-the-art care, according to the available information?

Here are some organizations that can help you.

American Heart Association   Your local chapter can recommend physicians. These centers may not distinguish among physicians other than by their basic qualifications. The national headquarters can send you booklets and may be helpful in securing a local phone number.

7320 Greenville Ave
Dallas, TX 75231
214/373-6300

American College of Cardiology   This medical specialty society publishes guidelines and other information about cardiac care.

9111 Old Georgetown Rd
Bethesda, MD 20814
800/253-4643

American College of Surgeons   This group offers the names of fellows in your geographic area.

55 E Erie St
Chicago, IL 60611
312/664-4050

Coronary Club   This club publishes a monthly newsletter, "Heartline." There are also 10 local chapters in the United States.

Cleveland Clinic Foundation
9500 Euclid Ave, Rm E4-15
Cleveland, OH 44195
216/444-3690

Mended Hearts   With more than 200 chapters and 22,000 members nation-wide, this organization is an excellent source of information about bypass surgery and other heart operations. Members visit heart patients before and after surgery.

7320 Greenville Ave
Dallas, TX 75231
214/932-1427

NIH CRISP System
301/496-7543

University-Affiliated Teaching Hospitals   See Appendix.

Step 4. Choose a Hospital

Experience

RELATION BETWEEN CASE VOLUME AND RESULTS   There is a strong relationship between a hospital's volume of cases and the quality of its care. If practice doesn't make perfect, it dramatically improves the outcomes for patients. This has been amply demonstrated in numerous studies of cardiac care. Patients who underwent heart operations at the nation's busiest hospitals were far more likely to survive than those who had the surgery performed elsewhere. For instance, at the Cleveland Clinic, one of the leading centers of cardiac care, surgeons performed nearly 2,000 operations in 1990 and had correspondingly high success rates. The clinic's mortality rate was less than 1% for young patients with relatively straight-forward cases. Even among older patients who had some complications, the mortality rate was a modest 2.8%.

A number of medical groups have established criteria for the minimum annual number of open heart surgeries considered necessary for a hospital to maintain proficiency, ranging from the American College of Surgeon's 150 operations a year to the American College of Cardiology's 300 operations a year. Despite the differences in these standards, one thing is consistent: The number of deaths rises as the hospital's annual frequency of surgery falls. You should know the number of bypass operations performed each year at the hospitals you are considering for your surgery. Although bypass surgery can be a routine operation, you can run an extraordinarily and unnecessarily high risk of complications or death at the wrong hospital.

The following chart gives some indication of the relationship between the volume of surgery and the mortality rate for all patients.

NUMBER OF OPERATIONS PER YEAR	MORTALITY RATE
350	4.3%
200 to 350	5.2%
100 to 200	6.8%

Other Measures of Excellence

QUALITY OF SURGICAL TEAM   While volume is an important indicator of quality, it is not the only one. You should know, too, who will be on your surgical team and the hospital staff that will be available to manage your care during recovery. Your heart surgeon should be assisted by a team that has been with him or her for at least a year. That team should include an anesthesiologist trained in the special needs of heart patients, experienced "pump" technicians, and a radiologist trained in cardiovascular medicine.

QUALITY OF POST-OP CARE   Most deaths, however, do not occur in the operating room. After your surgery, cardiologists should be readily available, 24 hours a day, in a fully staffed and certified coronary care unit. They are the specialists best qualified to treat potentially fatal irregular heart rhythms. You should also look for programs with a full-time thoracic-surgery training program. If you develop complications at 4 a.m., you want a surgeon familiar with your case to be available.

Centers of Excellence for Cardiology

Emergency bypass operations can have an extremely high mortality rate. If you're a man over 50 or a woman over 60 who could conceivably need bypass surgery in an emergency, you should be aware of the local hospitals that meet these standards.

The following list of hospitals is provided only as a convenient starting place in your search for excellence. These hospitals are recommended on the basis of reputation, not experience and results. The list is not an endorsement. There may be hospitals just as excellent that have been omitted. You should apply the guidelines for experience, results, and other measures of excellence to any hospital you choose, whether or not it is on this list. Although hospitals from different sources have been combined into one list, the compilation in no way implies that one source has endorsed the hospital list of another source.

CALIFORNIA
Cedars-Sinai Medical Center   EX
8700 Beverly Blvd
Los Angeles, CA 90048

Stanford University School
    of Medicine   US
300 Pasteur Dr
Stanford, CA 94305

GEORGIA
Emory University Hospital   US
1364 Clifton Rd NE
Atlanta, GA 30322

MARYLAND
Johns Hopkins Hospital   US
600 N Wolfe St
Baltimore, MD 21205

MASSACHUSETTS
Brigham and Women's Hospital   US
75 Francis St
Boston, MA 02115

Lown Cardiovascular Center   EX
21 Longwood Ave
Brookline, MA 02146
(for second opinions)

Massachusetts General Hospital   US
55 Fruit St
Boston, MA 02114

MINNESOTA
Mayo Clinic   US
200 First St SW
Rochester, MN 55905

NEW YORK
New York Hospital–Cornell
    Medical Center   EX
525 E 68th St
New York, NY 10021

New York University
    Medical Center   EX
Tisch Hospital
560 First Ave
New York, NY 10016

NORTH CAROLINA
Duke University Hospital   US
Box 3708
Durham, NC 27710

OHIO
Cleveland Clinic Foundation   US/EX
One Clinic Center
9500 Euclid Ave
Cleveland, OH 44195

PENNSYLVANIA
Allegheny General Hospital   EX
320 E North Ave
Pittsburgh, PA 15212

TEXAS
St Luke's Episcopal Hospital   US
Texas Heart Institute
1101 Bates St
Houston, TX 77030

SOURCES

EX   indicates those hospitals recommended by experts interviewed.

US   indicates those hospitals recommended by *U.S. News & World Report.*

Centers of Excellence Rated by Experience and Results

In several years a book will be published that lists the best hospitals in the country for every major surgery, based on good, hard data, not opinion. That book will look very much like the list shown in Table 1. Since comparable data is not available for most other surgeries and procedures, only this chapter and the one on angioplasty have this information. Data was generated for Table 1 by Lexecon Health Service. This is very much a look into the future.

With the following qualifications, these hospitals are the best hospitals in the country for bypass surgery based on experience and results. These cases did not include the following patients:

Those suffering a heart attack

Those having a bypass redone after the first had failed

Those who had balloon angioplasty that failed

Those who had a cardiac arrest

Is it possible that hospitals with very low surgical rates operated on exceptionally healthy patients, some of whom didn't need the surgery at all? There is the possibility that some of those patients are included in the data and could make it look very good. Future lists will be able to account for that as well. However, the hospitals listed here do include some pretty sick patients, including some with congestive heart failure and very poor heart function. Every patient was over 65.

Here's how to read the chart.

Volume   This column shows the number of bypass surgeries performed each year at each hospital. To qualify for this list, each hospital must have performed at least 150 operations a year for Medicare patients during the previous two years.

Death Rate   This shows the percentage of those operated on who died. To qualify for this list, the hospital must have had a death rate of 4% or less for Medicare patients during the previous two years.

Hospital Charges   This represents the in-hospital cost of the procedure (without cardiac catheterization).

Length of Stay   This is the average number of days a patient stayed in the hospital (not including the angiogram).

How do you pick and choose? All these hospitals have excellent results. You can just choose one close to your home. To look for the best of the best, look at a hospital with a high volume and very low death rate. Some of the hospitals had *no* deaths! In your final decision-making process, look at other measures of excellence and ask if they can break out results for your subgroup of patients. For example, if you have congestive heart failure, ask to see results for other patients with congestive heart failure.

TABLE 1. Multiple-Data Chart for the Best-Rated Bypass Surgery Hospitals

Hospital Name	City, State	Volume	Death Rate	Hospital Charges	Length of Stay (days)
AMI Brookwood Medical Center	Birmingham, AL	172	3.2%	$50,989	13.0
Humana Hospital Montgomery	Montgomery, AL	199	3.4%	$43,087	12.4
Mesa Lutheran Hospital	Mesa, AZ	158	3.4%	$47,815	13.0
Humana Hospital Phoenix	Phoenix, AZ	157	0.0%	$38,894	11.0
Baptist Medical Center	Little Rock, AR	672	1.6%	$21,076	11.2
Springdale Memorial Hospital	Springdale, AR	165	1.0%	$18,857	9.8
Mt. Diablo Hospital Medical Center	Concord, CA	212	2.8%	$47,744	9.2
Seton Medical Center	Daly City, CA	173	2.9%	$48,463	13.4
St. Helena Hospital & Health Center	Deer Park, CA	156	2.7%	$29,823	10.1
St. Agnes Medical Center	Fresno, CA	231	1.2%	$45,567	9.7
Scripps Memorial Hospital La Jolla	La Jolla, CA	154	2.7%	$50,571	9.1
Cedars-Sinai Medical Center	Los Angeles, CA	247	2.9%	$67,311	14.8
Hospital of the Good Samaritan	Los Angeles, CA	344	4.0%	$41,089	9.6
Kaiser Foundation Hospital	Los Angeles, CA	225	1.0%	$31,555	12.0
St. Vincent Medical Center	Los Angeles, CA	168	4.0%	$42,348	11.3
Doctors Medical Center	Modesto, CA	283	2.8%	$65,490	9.9
Eisenhower Memorial Hospital	Rancho Mirage, CA	189	0.0%	$33,403	7.7
Sequoia Hospital	Redwood City, CA	163	1.1%	$35,852	10.0
Mercy General Hospital	Sacramento, CA	433	0.6%	$47,751	10.1
Sutter Memorial Hospital	Sacramento, CA	429	2.0%	$56,380	10.8
Alvarado Hospital Medical Center	San Diego, CA	194	1.4%	$62,885	11.8
Kaiser Foundation Hospital	San Francisco, CA	160	0.7%	$9,237	10.2
St. Mary's Hospital Medical Center	San Francisco, CA	311	2.7%	$39,955	10.4
St. Francis Hospital & Medical Center	Hartford, CT	504	2.6%	$26,995	14.4
Medical Center of Delaware	Wilmington, DE	268	3.9%	$34,571	11.3
Washington Hospital Center	Washington, DC	532	2.2%	$43,415	12.4
Delray Community Hospital	Delray Beach, FL	224	1.6%	$47,029	12.3
AMI North Ridge Medical Center	Fort Lauderdale, FL	425	1.6%	$32,784	11.8

Hospital Name	City, State	Volume	Death Rate	Hospital Charges	Length of Stay (days)
Holy Cross Hospital	Fort Lauderdale, FL	160	2.7%	$37,162	12.4
S.W. Florida Regional Medical Center	Fort Myers, FL	555	1.3%	$29,613	9.6
HCA North Florida Regional Hospital	Gainesville, FL	174	1.6%	$34,679	11.8
Memorial Med. Center of Jacksonville	Jacksonville, FL	151	3.6%	$32,275	11.7
St. Vincent's Medical Center	Jacksonville, FL	273	3.1%	$26,951	12.6
Largo Medical Center Hospital	Largo, FL	214	3.0%	$40,321	12.2
Holmes Regional Medical Center	Melbourne, FL	186	3.1%	$29,599	13.4
Miami Heart Institute	Miami Beach, FL	177	3.4%	$43,610	14.8
Florida Hospital	Orlando, FL	730	3.6%	$31,850	11.0
Ormond Beach Memorial Hospital	Ormond Beach, FL	181	4.0%	$26,225	11.9
West Florida Regional Medical Center	Pensacola, FL	155	2.6%	$29,058	10.3
St. Joseph's Hospital	Tampa, FL	256	3.6%	$32,564	10.9
Crawford Long Hospital	Atlanta, GA	155	3.8%	$33,758	10.6
Emory University Hospital	Atlanta, GA	513	3.8%	$30,558	12.3
St. Joseph's Hospital of Atlanta	Atlanta, GA	552	3.3%	$28,460	11.2
Medical Center of Central Georgia	Macon, GA	251	1.5%	$29,457	11.1
Memorial Medical Center	Savannah, GA	187	1.9%	$30,564	8.1
St. Luke's Regional Medical Center	Boise, ID	243	0.0%	$23,378	11.2
St. Francis Hospital & Health Center	Blue Island, IL	157	0.0%	$24,488	12.8
Good Samaritan Hospital	Downers Grove, IL	159	0.0%	$32,570	10.7
Christ Hospital & Medical Center	Oak Lawn, IL	193	0.9%	$33,758	12.2
Lutheran General Hospital	Park Ridge, IL	157	2.8%	$37,120	14.8
St. Francis Medical Center	Peoria, IL	184	3.2%	$34,525	14.1
St. John's Hospital	Springfield, IL	383	3.5%	$20,766	11.1
St. Francis Hospital Center	Beech Grove, IN	173	2.3%	$27,413	10.6
Parkview Memorial Hospital Inc.	Fort Wayne, IN	169	0.0%	$23,085	9.5
Methodist Hospital of Indiana Inc.	Indianapolis, IN	324	2.9%	$29,643	12.0
St. Vincent Hospital & Health Center	Indianapolis, IN	501	3.9%	$26,870	12.7
St. Joseph's Medical Center	South Bend, IN	187	0.7%	$28,223	8.3
St. Luke's Hospital	Cedar Rapids, IA	226	2.4%	$15,945	9.4
St. Luke's Hospital	Davenport, IA	225	4.0%	$28,629	13.9
Mercy Hospital Medical Center	Des Moines, IA	205	0.7%	$25,458	13.8

Hospital Name	City, State	Volume	Death Rate	Hospital Charges	Length of Stay (days)
University of Iowa Hospital & Clinic	Iowa City, IA	193	3.0%	$21,060	12.7
St. Francis Regional Medical Center	Wichita, KS	431	1.1%	$29,729	9.5
St. Elizabeth Medical Center	Covington, KY	187	2.3%	$23,326	10.2
St. Joseph Hosp.	Lexington, KY	328	1.4%	$20,387	10.6
Schumpert Medical Center	Shreveport, LA	194	1.5%	$25,836	10.6
Eastern Maine Medical Center	Bangor, ME	160	1.4%	$24,756	10.7
Johns Hopkins Hosp.	Baltimore, MD	338	3.8%	$24,269	14.9
Massachusetts General Hospital	Boston, MA	378	2.0%	$30,279	15.6
New England Medical Center Hospital	Boston, MA	271	1.6%	$27,674	11.2
Catherine McCauley Health Center	Ann Arbor, MI	270	1.7%	$36,749	12.0
Henry Ford Hospital	Detroit, MI	174	2.8%	$32,631	13.3
St. John Hospital	Detroit, MI	458	1.9%	$41,316	12.4
Blodgett Memorial Medical Center	Grand Rapids, MI	284	2.2%	$20,935	10.0
Borgess Medical Center	Kalamazoo, MI	237	2.1%	$27,061	9.3
Ingham Medical Center	Lansing, MI	278	2.2%	$25,852	10.6
William Beaumont Hospital	Royal Oak, MI	432	2.3%	$30,512	11.6
St. Mary's Medical Center	Saginaw, MI	510	2.8%	$27,503	11.5
Providence Hospital	Southfield, MI	156	2.8%	$47,642	15.4
Abbott-Northwestern Hospital	Minneapolis, MN	448	2.1%	$27,014	10.8
St. Mary's Hospital	Rochester, MN	370	2.2%	$21,294	11.2
Univ. of Missouri Hospital & Clinics	Columbia, MO	210	1.9%	$29,079	11.2
St. John's Regional Medical Center	Joplin, MO	187	2.0%	$25,746	11.2
Barnes Hospital	St. Louis, MO	254	1.2%	$34,698	12.7
Missouri Baptist Medical Center	St. Louis, MO	204	2.0%	$28,206	10.5
St. John's Regional Health Center	Springfield, MO	358	2.6%	$18,633	9.8
Deaconess Medical Center of Billings	Billings, MT	212	0.8%	$33,471	12.5
Deborah Heart & Lung Center	Browns Mills, NJ	415	4.0%	$27,871	13.5
Cooper Hospital/Univ. Medical Center	Camden, NJ	187	3.4%	$26,207	15.4
Morristown Memorial Hospital	Morristown, NJ	230	2.8%	$15,111	11.6
Presbyterian Hospital Center	Albuquerque, NM	269	0.5%	$27,265	10.4
Albany Medical Center	Albany, NY	304	2.7%	$23,607	12.4
St. Peter's Hospital	Albany, NY	179	2.3%	$19,197	11.0

Hospital Name	City, State	Volume	Death Rate	Hospital Charges	Length of Stay (days)
Buffalo General Hospital	Buffalo, NY	478	2.8%	$21,683	12.7
Millard Fillmore Hospital	Buffalo, NY	189	3.3%	$19,426	12.1
United Health Services	Johnson City, NY	181	0.0%	$17,590	10.2
Winthrop University Hospital	Mineola, NY	194	2.1%	$22,512	14.7
Long Island Jewish Medical Center	New Hyde Park, NY	187	0.0%	$14,887	11.5
Mt. Sinai Hospital	New York, NY	271	2.3%	$55,584	16.1
New York Hospital	New York, NY	417	2.7%	$32,926	16.7
Rochester General Hospital	Rochester, NY	401	0.3%	$13,242	10.6
St. Joseph's Hospital Health Center	Syracuse, NY	274	1.8%	$14,870	10.1
Charlotte Mem. Hospital & Med. Center	Charlotte, NC	396	2.2%	$34,412	13.6
Presbyterian Hospital	Charlotte, NC	245	0.0%	$18,463	8.4
The Moses H. Cone Memorial Hospital	Greensboro, NC	226	2.3%	$33,236	14.9
Pitt County Memorial Hospital	Greenville, NC	291	3.0%	$29,834	10.0
Wake County Hospital System	Raleigh, NC	472	2.5%	$30,276	14.1
St. Luke's Hospitals	Fargo, ND	200	2.4%	$25,310	10.5
Akron City Hospital	Akron, OH	168	1.7%	$26,951	11.9
Akron General Medical Center	Akron, OH	320	2.0%	$21,384	9.8
Cleveland Clinic Hospital	Cleveland, OH	780	1.7%	$29,711	12.0
St. Vincent Charity Hospital	Cleveland, OH	260	4.0%	$26,619	11.7
Good Samaritan Hosp. & Health Center	Dayton, OH	352	1.4%	$30,929	14.2
St. Vincent's Medical Center	Toledo, OH	178	0.0%	$30,854	11.8
St. Elizabeth Hospital	Youngstown, OH	286	2.4%	$43,115	14.9
St. Anthony Hospital	Oklahoma City, OK	155	3.2%	$24,699	12.9
St. John Medical Center Inc.	Tulsa, OK	182	3.7%	$33,029	13.0
Sacred Heart General Hospital	Eugene, OR	251	2.7%	$21,546	10.1
Rogue Valley Medical Center	Medford, OR	212	3.4%	$15,818	8.1
Good Samaritan Hospital & Med. Center	Portland, OR	293	0.5%	$29,513	9.3
St. Vincent Hospital & Medical Center	Portland, OR	363	1.3%	$24,351	10.5
Lehigh Valley Hospital Center	Allentown, PA	533	2.7%	$31,452	12.7
Altoona Hospital	Altoona, PA	155	0.7%	$24,052	8.6
St. Luke's Hospital of Bethlehem	Bethlehem, PA	173	1.9%	$29,393	13.2
Bryn Mawr Hospital	Bryn Mawr, PA	167	3.0%	$45,001	12.1
Geisinger Medical Center	Danville, PA	155	2.1%	$27,098	12.5
Hamot Medical Center	Erie, PA	233	3.2%	$30,540	12.1

Hospital Name	City, State	Volume	Death Rate	Hospital Charges	Length of Stay (days)
Polyclinic Medical Center	Harrisburg, PA	177	2.1%	$33,031	11.4
Lancaster General Hospital	Lancaster, PA	386	1.1%	$19,287	9.8
Albert Einstein Medical Center	Philadelphia, PA	324	2.7%	$61,577	11.6
Presbyterian-Univ. of PA Medical Center	Philadelphia, PA	222	3.8%	$35,466	11.7
Allegheny General Hospital	Pittsburgh, PA	578	2.3%	$42,650	13.7
Central Med. Ctr. Hosp.	Pittsburgh, PA	178	2.5%	$47,380	12.7
Mercy Hospital—Pittsburgh	Pittsburgh, PA	384	2.1%	$40,315	13.2
Shadyside Hospital	Pittsburgh, PA	440	3.3%	$55,391	14.3
Reading Hospital Medical Center	Reading, PA	302	3.8%	$19,623	11.0
Robert Packer Hosp.	Sayre, PA	198	1.4%	$19,577	10.9
San Pablo Hospital	Bayamon, PR	316	1.0%	$21,819	10.3
Rhode Island Hospital	Providence, RI	252	2.7%	$19,212	11.0
Providence Hospital	Columbia, SC	290	1.3%	$25,293	11.7
Greenville Memorial Medical Center	Greenville, SC	235	1.7%	$34,174	12.2
Sioux Valley Hospital	Sioux Falls, SD	284	2.3%	$18,168	11.6
Holston Valley Hospital Med. Center	Kingsport, TN	200	3.0%	$32,971	12.6
East Tennessee Baptist Hospital	Knoxville, TN	162	0.8%	$32,950	10.2
University of Tennessee Mem. Hospital	Knoxville, TN	156	2.6%	$29,442	11.3
Baptist Memorial Hospital	Memphis, TN	442	3.7%	$34,134	16.8
Methodist Hospitals of Memphis	Memphis, TN	504	2.7%	$38,577	20.6
Baptist Hospital	Nashville, TN	160	2.3%	$28,942	12.7
Centennial Medical Ctr.	Nashville, TN	225	2.4%	$32,534	11.9
St. Thomas Hospital	Nashville, TN	628	3.2%	$25,528	12.7
Humana Hospital Abilene	Abilene, TX	153	3.1%	$46,255	13.7
Seton Medical Center	Austin, TX	169	1.9%	$20,161	13.1
Baylor University Medical Center	Dallas, TX	317	2.6%	$30,500	10.4
Humana Hospital Medical City Dallas	Dallas, TX	315	0.9%	$34,456	10.7
Harris Methodist Fort Worth	Fort Worth, TX	225	1.6%	$20,575	9.3
St. Luke's Episcopal Hospital	Houston, TX	570	2.5%	$19,032	12.6
McKay-Dee Hospital Center	Ogden, UT	150	0.0%	$22,207	10.7
Latter-Day Saints Hospital	Salt Lake City, UT	334	1.3%	$20,669	10.0
Fairfax Hospital	Falls Church, VA	281	2.0%	$30,290	13.0
HCA Chippenham Hospital	Richmond, VA	159	1.0%	$37,454	12.0
Henrico Doctors Hospital	Richmond, VA	285	0.6%	$56,515	14.4
Roanoke Memorial Hospitals	Roanoke, VA	343	1.5%	$25,788	10.2
General Hospital Medical Center	Everett, WA	198	0.7%	$22,823	8.7

Hospital Name	City, State	Volume	Death Rate	Hospital Charges	Length of Stay (days)
Providence Medical Center	Seattle, WA	447	3.3%	$25,062	9.3
Sacred Heart Medical Center	Spokane, WA	380	0.0%	$22,962	10.9
Charleston Area Medical Center	Charleston, WV	589	1.7%	$32,238	12.7
Appleton Medical Center	Appleton, WI	174	2.3%	$19,160	10.8
La Crosse Lutheran Hospital	La Crosse, WI	205	3.2%	$24,925	13.0
St. Joseph's Hospital	Milwaukee, WI	195	1.8%	$26,018	12.7
St. Luke's Medical Center Inc.	Milwaukee, WI	787	3.3%	$20,874	12.8
Theda Clark Memorial Hospital	Neenah, WI	160	0.9%	$17,787	10.6

Step 5. Choose a Doctor

Experience

If you decide on the operation, you will want to select a surgeon who is certified by the American Board of Thoracic Surgery and who is experienced in cardiovascular surgery. How much experience? At the very least the surgeon and his or her assistants should perform 100–150 operations, primarily bypass surgeries, a year. Yet as many as 80% of surgeons who do bypass surgery don't meet that minimum standard. The American College of Cardiology and the American Heart Association, have agreed that this figure is a good indication of a surgeon's experience and competence. Busy heart surgeons average 160 operations a year and many perform far more.

Results

You will want to know which bypass techniques the surgeon prefers and what his or her mortality rate is. A good surgeon is likely to have a mortality rate below 2% in uncomplicated cases among young patients.

But the mortality rate among surgeons can vary widely. A study of 11 hospitals in northern New England, reported in the *Journal of the American Medical Association* in 1991, found that, while mortality rates ranged from 3.1–6.3% among hospitals, there was a far larger variation among surgeons. Their mortality rate ranged from a low of 2% in young patients to a high of 9.2% in the more complicated cases. In short, unless you also inquire about the surgeon's mortality rate, you could find yourself in the right hospital but with the wrong doctor performing the operation.

EXPERT SOURCES

Although dozens of experts were interviewed for these chapters, these physicians are acknowledged for their significant contributions to this section.

Dr. Jeffrey S. Borer, Gladys and Roland Harriman Professor of Cardiovascular Medicine, New York Hospital–Cornell Medical Center, New York, NY

Dr. Delos M. Cosgrove, Chairman, Department of Thoracic and Cardiovascular Surgery, The Cleveland Clinic, Cleveland, OH

Dr. Thomas B. Graboys, Director, Lown Cardiovascular Center, Harvard Medical School, Boston, MA

REFERENCES AND SUGGESTED READING

ACC/AHA Guidelines and Indications for Coronary Artery Bypass Graft Surgery. *Journal of the American College of Cardiology,* Vol. 17, No. 3 (March 1, 1991), pp. 543–589.

Booth, D. C., and others. Quality of Life After Bypass Surgery for Unstable Angina: 5-Year Follow-Up Results of a Veterans Administration Cooperative Study. *Circulation,* Vol. 83 (1991), pp. 87–95.

Brook, R. H., and others. Diagnosis and Treatment of Coronary Disease: Comparison of Doctors' Attitudes in the USA and UK. *Lancet,* Vol. 1 (1988), pp. 750–754.

CASS. Coronary Artery Surgery Study: A Randomized Trial of Coronary Artery Bypass Graft Surgery: Survival Data. *Circulation,* Vol. 68 (1983), pp. 939–950.

CASS. Myocardial Infarction and Mortality in the Coronary Artery Surgery Study (CASS): Randomized Trial. *New England Journal of Medicine,* Vol. 310 (1984), pp. 750–758.

Commentary: A New Role for Radiologists in the Development of Cardiac Surgery. *American Journal of Roentgenology,* Vol. 157, No. 6 (Dec. 1991), pp. 1295–1296.

Graboys, T. B., and others. Results of a Second-Opinion Program for Coronary Artery Bypass Graft Surgery. *Journal of the American Medical Association,* Vol. 258, No. 12 (Sept. 1987), pp. 1611–1614.

Hannan, E. L., and others. Investigation of the Relationship Between Volume and Mortality for Surgical Procedures Performed in New York State Hospitals. *Journal of the American Medical Association,* Vol. 262 (1989), pp. 503–510.

Hise, Joseph H., and others. Stroke Associated with Coronary Artery Bypass Surgery. *American Journal of Roentgenology,* Vol. 157, No. 6 (Dec. 1991), pp. 1291–1294.

Hochberg, M. S., and others. Coronary Angioplasty Versus Coronary Bypass. Three-Year Follow-Up of a Matched Series of 250 Patients. *Journal of Thoracic and Cardiovascular Surgery,* Vol. 97 (1989), pp. 496–503.

Johnson, W. D., and others. Factors Influencing Long-Term (10-Year to 15-Year) Survival After a Successful Coronary Artery Bypass Operation. *Annals of Thoracic Surgery,* Vol. 48 (1989), pp. 19–25.

King, Kathleen B., and others. Patterns of Referral and Recovery in Women and Men Undergoing Coronary Artery Bypass Grafting. *American Journal of Cardiology,* Vol. 69, No. 3 (Jan. 15, 1992), pp. 179–182.

Krueger, Hans, and others. Coronary Artery Bypass Grafting: How Much Does It Cost? *Canadian Medical Association Journal*, Vol. 146, No. 2 (Jan. 15, 1992), pp. 163–168.

Lazar, Harold L., and others. Changing Profiles of Failed Coronary Angioplasty Patients: Impact on Surgical Results. *Annals of Thoracic Surgery*, Vol. 53, No. 2 (Feb. 1992), pp. 269–273.

Loop, F. D., and others. Coronary Artery Bypass Graft Surgery in the Elderly: Indications and Outcome. *Cleveland Clinical Journal of Medicine*, Vol. 55 (1988), pp. 23–24.

Loop, F. D., and others. Reoperation for Coronary Atherosclerosis: Changing Practice in 2509 Consecutive Patients. *Annals of Surgery*, Vol. 212 (1990), pp. 378–386.

MacRae, C. A., and others. Need for Invasive Cardiological Assessment and Intervention: A Ten-Year Review. *British Heart Journal*, Vol. 67, No. 2 (Feb. 1992), pp. 200–203.

Manolio, Teri A., and Furberg, Curt D. Age as a Predictor of Outcome: What Role Does It Play? [editorial] *American Journal of Medicine*, Vol. 92, No. 1 (Jan. 1992), pp. 1–6.

O'Connor, G. T., and Plume, S. K. A Regional Prospective Study of In-Hospital Mortality Associated with Coronary Artery Bypass Grafting. *Journal of the American Medical Association*, Vol. 266, No. 6 (Aug. 1991), pp. 803–809.

Passamani, E., and others. A Randomized Trial of Coronary Artery Bypass Surgery: Survival of Patients with a Low Ejection Fraction. *New England Journal of Medicine*, Vol. 312 (1985), pp. 1665–1671.

Poses, Roy M., and others. Is There Sex Bias in the Management of Coronary Artery Disease? [letter] *New England Journal of Medicine*, Vol. 326, No. 8 (Feb. 1992), pp. 570–572.

Schweiger, Marc J., and others. Treatment of Patients Following Bypass Surgery: A Dilemma for the 1990s [editorials]. *American Heart Journal*, Vol. 123, No. 1 (Jan. 1992), pp. 268–272.

Showstack, J. A., and others. Association of Volume with Outcome of Coronary Artery Bypass Surgery. *Journal of the American Medical Association*, Vol. 257 (1987), pp. 785–789.

Solomon, N. W., and others. Coronary Artery Bypass Grafting in Elderly Patients: Comparative Results in a Consecutive Series of 469 Patients Older than 75 Years. *Journal of Thoracic and Cardiovascular Surgery*, Vol. 101 (1991), pp. 209–218.

Ulicny, Karl S. Jr., and others. Twenty-Year Follow-Up of Saphenous Vein Aortocoronary Artery Bypass Grafting. *Annals of Thoracic Surgery*, Vol. 53, No. 2 (Feb. 1992), pp. 258–262.

Van Lierde, Johan, and others. Long-Term Prognosis of Male Patients with an Isolated Chronic Occlusion of the Left Anterior Descending Coronary Artery. *American Heart Journal*, Vol. 122, No. 6 (Dec. 1992), pp. 1542–1547.

Winslow, C. M., and others. The Appropriateness of Performing Coronary Artery Bypass Surgery. *Journal of the American Medical Association*, Vol. 260, No. 4 (July 1988), pp. 505–509.

1989 DATA PA. Health Care Cost-Containment Council. *Wall Street Journal*, Jan. 22, 1992.

Angioplasty

Likelihood of Unnecessary Procedure HIGH

Angioplasty is frequently performed and often unnecessary. Experts estimate that 20% of the 300,000 angioplasties performed annually are inappropriate. This is alarming since angioplasty, while relieving symptoms of heart disease, has not been found to improve life expectancy on its own and, like all procedures, carries the risk of serious complications.

The research firm MediQual has the more conservative figure. In 1991 they reported that 10.16% of angioplasties they studied had none of the objective clinical findings documented in the hospital medical record they use to validate angioplasty at the time of the procedure. This report looked at single-vessel blockages only.

Potential Risk VERY HIGH

When angioplasty is performed well and appropriately, the results can be nearly miraculous. A patient who was crippled by heart disease can return to a normal life. But the possible side effects are so serious that you should be certain that the procedure is absolutely necessary and will be performed by the best possible team. These are the risks: death; abrupt closure of blood vessels, requiring emergency bypass surgery; nonfatal heart attack; reblockage of blood vessels within three to six months, requiring additional therapy; strong bleeding; and infection.

Angioplasty done on an emergency basis can have an exceptionally high mortality rate. To warrant an emergency procedure, you should be experiencing uncontrollable chest pain and decreased heart function or you should be in the midst of a heart attack.

What It Is

Angioplasty is an alternative to bypass surgery that can be performed without the risks associated with opening the chest and the general anesthesia that bypass surgery requires. The goals are to relieve chest pain, to improve the capacity for exercise, and to reduce the risk of death from heart attacks, although this has yet to be proven.

The procedure involves pushing aside partial blockages in the coronary arteries to improve blood flow to oxygen-starved heart muscles. An angiogram is performed first to locate the blockage. (See the chapter on Angiogram.) Then a long, narrow tube called a catheter is inserted into the body, usually from the femoral artery in the leg, and threaded through the circulatory system until it reaches the blockage. At that point a balloon near the tip of the catheter is inflated to push aside the blockage. There are other experimental techniques that operate on the same basic principle, including those using lasers and a new generation of mechanical "roto rooter"-like devices, but these are not yet in wide use.

Step 1. Make Sure You Need the Procedure

Because of the risks associated with the procedure, you should make sure it is clearly indicated before you consent. Check your diagnosis against the conditions listed just ahead under "Appropriate Procedure" (abbreviated from the American College of Cardiology guidelines). "Angioplasty is a modality to improve quality of life. There is no proof, yet, that your life expectancy will improve. It's a great device for making patients feel better," says Dr. Jeffrey Moses, Director of the Cardiac Catheterization Laboratory at Lenox Hill Hospital in New York City.

Appropriate Procedure

- Continuing chest pain after a heart attack

- Persistent chest pain that is not controllable by medication

- Cardiac arrest that cannot be attributed to a heart attack

- Before a high-risk noncardiac procedure such as vascular or hip-replacement surgery if there is angina or laboratory evidence of inadequate blood flow to the heart, if certain specific criteria are met

- Early during a heart attack (although this is currently the subject of intense investigation)

- Continuing chest pain, even if mild, if the patient wants to be active and not continue on medication

Probably Not an Appropriate Procedure

Most inappropriate procedures are performed on minor blockages before medical therapies have been exhausted.

- A blockage on an angiogram that measures as less than 50% of the artery

- After a heart attack if the blockages did not cause the attack

- Variant angina, a condition caused by a narrowing of the coronary artery, often because of a muscle spasm. In this case the chest pain is not the result of a blockage that can be pushed aside.

- No evidence of coronary artery disease found during an electrocardiogram (EKG) stress test (see chapter on Stress Test)

- Anticipated success rate less than 60% (see discussion of type C lesions under "Low Success Rate," just ahead)

Not an Appropriate Procedure

- Left main coronary artery obstruction (best corrected via surgery, since angioplasty could close off this artery, causing cardiac arrest)

- Severe blockages spread extensively through the involved vessels when diagnosed on an angiogram

- No accredited cardiac surgery program at the hospital (essential because of the possibility that you could need emergency bypass surgery)

- If abrupt vessel closure would result in cardiogenic shock (sudden loss of blood pressure) and probable death before immediate surgery could be performed

- Adequate trial of medical therapy not yet undertaken

- Multivessel disease of significant prognostic severity (bypass surgery is of value here)

Grade Your Chance of Success

Before you agree to angioplasty, you should ask your doctors to grade your chance of success based on the severity of the blockage. Even if the procedure is indicated, you should review your chance of success with the doctor who has been selected to offer an expert opinion.

Type A Blockage: High Success Rate (Greater than 85%)

Angioplasty is performed most successfully on blockages that are defined as type A, which have *all* of the following characteristics:

- Discrete, less than 10 mm in length

- Concentric, ringing the artery wall

- Smooth contour

- Little or no calcification (indicating the blockage has not been present long enough to harden)

- Readily accessible

- Not at a sharp turn in the artery (less than 45 degrees)

- Artery less than totally occluded

- No significant involvement of a major artery branch

- No blood clot

Type B Blockage: Medium Success Rate (60–85%)

Type B blockages have a medium success rate with angioplasty. They have the following characteristics:

- Tubular, about 10–20 mm long

- Eccentric (concentrated on one side of the artery)

- Irregular contour

- Moderate to heavy calcification

- Moderate tortuosity of first part of the artery (meaning twists and turns are present that can make maneuvering the catheter difficult)

- Located at a moderate turn in the artery (greater than 45 degrees but less than 90 degrees) *or* at the opening of an artery *or* at the point where an artery divides

- Total occlusions that are less than three months old (regular angiograms must be taken for this to be known)

- Some blood clot present

Type C Blockage: Low Success Rate (Less than 60%)

Angioplasty is least successful with type C blockages, which have the following characteristics:

- Degenerated vein grafts from bypass surgery or very rough contours

■ Total occlusion more than three months old, as seen on angiograms (meaning the blockage is older and harder)

■ Excessive tortuosity of first part of artery (too many twists and turns for the catheter to maneuver well)

■ A sharp (90-degree) turn in the artery (maneuvering the catheter becomes as difficult as threading a twisted coat hanger through a straw)

■ Inability to protect major side branches of the artery (which could shut down, thereby stopping the flow of blood to the heart if the procedure is unsuccessful)

Step 2. Consider an Alternative

Medical therapy has become very sophisticated. In the 1990s we find a variety of drugs on the market that can markedly improve your ability to function in a number of different ways, for instance, by improving the pumping function of the heart or by cutting down on dangerous, irregular heart beats.

Some drugs control the symptoms by decreasing the heart's need for oxygen through slowing the heart rate and the force of contractions without stopping the disease's progress. Your doctor may combine several of these drugs at low dosages to minimize side effects. They are described in the chapter on Coronary Artery Disease.

The conservative route of using drug therapy first is not always the best treatment. It is just an option. For some blockages, angioplasty or even bypass surgery can be a safer and more effective therapy. That is why you really need to seek an expert opinion.

Step 3. Get a Specialist's Opinion

You should discuss with any specialist the alternatives to angioplasty, which include the alternative medical therapies listed in Step 2 and bypass surgery. You will want the cardiologist to review your medical history carefully to be certain your diagnosis is correct. *A special precaution:* There is a tremendous opportunity to abuse angioplasty by "overreading" films. Some centers will read a 50% blockage as a 90% blockage and urge that you have an angioplasty.

WHEN YOU NEED ONE   You will need an expert opinion if your procedure is not clearly indicated, if the chance of success is not high, or if you wish to consider an alternative.

WHO TO GO TO   You have a choice between a noninvasive cardiologist, who may be more oriented toward conservative medical therapy, and an invasive cardiologist who performs angioplasties.

WHAT TO DISCUSS   You should discuss the alternatives to angioplasty, which include the medical therapies (see Step 2) and bypass surgery. You will want the doctor to carefully review your medical history and your medical tests and to be certain your condition is correctly diagnosed and your prognosis is properly evaluated.

WHERE TO GO   You can go to a center of excellence for angioplasty (see Step 4) or to a major teaching hospital (see Appendix).

WHO TO CALL   If time, expense, or travel prohibit you from seeking a specialist's opinion, learn as much as you can by calling one of the centers of excellence or one of the organizations listed below. Make certain to ask these questions:

Do I need angioplasty?

Is there an alternative therapy?

How significant is the procedure?

What is the expected outcome?

Can you recommend an expert cardiologist close to where I live?

Do I need to travel to a larger center?

Am I receiving state-of-the-art care, according to available information?

Here are some organizations that can help you.

American Heart Association   Your local chapter can recommend physicians. These centers may not distinguish among physicians except by their basic qualifications. The national headquarters can send you booklets and may be helpful in securing a local phone number.

7320 Greenville Ave
Dallas, TX 75231
214/373-6300

American College of Cardiology   This medical specialty society publishes guidelines and other information about cardiac care.

9111 Old Georgetown Rd
Bethesda, MD 20814
800/253-4643

American College of Surgeons   This group offers names of fellows in your geographic area.

55 E Erie St
Chicago, IL 60611
312/664-4050

Coronary Club   This club publishes a monthly newsletter, "Heartline." There are also ten local chapters in the United States.

Cleveland Clinic Foundation
9500 Euclid Ave, Rm E4-15
Cleveland, OH 44195
216/444-3690

Mended Hearts   With more than 200 chapters and 22,000 members nationwide, this organization is an excellent source of information about bypass surgery and other heart operations. Members visit heart patients before and after surgery.

7320 Greenville Ave
Dallas, TX 75231
214/932-1427

NIH CRISP System
301/496-7543

University-Affiliated Teaching Hospitals   See Appendix.

Step 4. Choose a Hospital

You should compare the results for the hospitals, quite literally using that information as a short, efficient shopping list. First, choose a hospital with a high volume of angioplasties. Then, of those with high volumes, choose the hospital that has the best results for your particular condition. If you are severely ill, for instance, you will want a hospital that has the best results for high-risk patients.

Experience

The hospital should perform an absolute minimum number of 200 angioplasties per year, since top-ranked hospitals do far more. For example, the Cleveland Clinic, one of the nation's leading cardiac centers, performed 1,270 angioplasties in 1990.

Results

Death Rate   Look for a death rate of 0.7% or less for a single vessel procedure. The average patient age was 68.6 years. This is for a single-vessel procedure. If the hospital has a mortality rate above 1%, most experts say you should definitely select another facility.

The following statistics are *averages*, not measures of excellence. The figures are provided by the American Heart Association, the American College of Cardiology, and the American College of Physicians. You should use them for comparison only.

Average Success Rate   Success rate with single blockage averages at 85%.

Other Complications (Averages) Reblockage within six months: 20%; Failure to open artery at all: 5%; Heart attack during procedure: 4.5%; and Emergency bypass surgery required: 3%.

Other Measures of Excellence

FOR SINGLE-VESSEL PROCEDURE

Average hospital charges: $12,496

Average length of stay: 4.8 days

Centers of Excellence for Angioplasty

The following is a list of hospitals recommended by experts interviewed. It is provided only as a convenient starting place in your search for excellence. These hospitals are recommended on the basis of reputation, not experience and results. The list is not an endorsement. There may be hospitals just as excellent that have been omitted. You should apply the guidelines for experience, results, and other measures of excellence to any hospital you choose, whether or not it is on this list.

CALIFORNIA
Cardiovascular Medicine and
    Coronary Intervention   EX
2940 Whipple Ave, Suite 10
Redwood City, CA 94062

Cedars-Sinai Medical Center   EX
8700 Beverly Blvd
Los Angeles, CA 90048

St. Mary's Hospital
    and Medical Center   EX
450 Stanyan St
San Francisco, CA 94117

Scripps Clinic and Research
    Foundation   EX
10666 N Torrey Pines Rd
La Jolla, CA 92037

Stanford University School
of Medicine   EX
300 Pasteur Dr
Stanford, CA 94305

DISTRICT OF COLUMBIA
Washington Hospital Center   EX
110 Irving St NW
Washington, DC 20010

GEORGIA
Emory University Hospital   EX
1364 Clifton Rd NE
Atlanta, GA 30322

St Joseph's Hospital   EX
5665 Peachtree Dunwoody Rd NE
Atlanta, GA 30342

LOUISIANA
Oschsner Foundation Hospital   EX
1516 Jefferson Hwy
New Orleans, LA 70121

MARYLAND
Johns Hopkins Hospital   EX
600 N Wolfe St
Baltimore, MD 21205

MASSACHUSETTS
Beth Israel Hospital   EX
330 Brookline Ave
Boston, MA 02215

Brigham and Women's Hospital   EX
75 Francis St
Boston, MA 02115

Lown Cardiovascular Center   EX
21 Longwood Ave
Brookline, MA 02146
(for second opinions)

Massachusetts General Hospital   EX
55 Fruit St
Boston, MA 02114

MICHIGAN
William Beaumont Hospital   EX
3601 W 13 Mile Rd
Royal Oak, MI 48073-6769

MINNESOTA
Mayo Clinic   EX
200 First St SW
Rochester, MN 55905

MISSOURI
St Luke's Hospital   EX
Mid America Heart Institute
44th St and Wornall Rd
Kansas City, MO 64111

NEW YORK
Lenox Hill Hospital   EX
100 E 77th St
New York, NY 10021

New York Hospital–
Cornell Medical Center   EX
525 E 68th St
New York, NY 10021

New York University Medical Center   EX
560 First Ave
New York, NY 10016

NORTH CAROLINA
Duke University Hospital   EX
Box 3708
Durham, NC 27710

OHIO
Cleveland Clinic Foundation   EX
One Clinic Center
9500 Euclid Ave
Cleveland, OH 44195

TEXAS
St Luke's Episcopal Hospital   EX
Texas Heart Institute
1101 Bates St
Houston, TX 77030

SOURCES

EX   indicates those hospitals recommended by experts interviewed.

Centers of Excellence Rated by Experience and Results

Table 2 presents hospitals rated best on a number of measures of excellence. Data for this table was generated by Lexecon Health Service. All patients covered were over age 65. Many of them were ill, but none required the procedure as an emergency due to a heart attack or cardiac arrest. Based on these qualifications, the listed hospitals rank as the best in the country for angioplasty. (See the chapter on Coronary Artery Bypass Surgery for more explanation of Lexecon's methodology.)
    Here's how to read the chart.

Volume   This column shows the number of angioplasties performed per year at each hospital. To qualify for this list, the hospital must do at least 150 procedures a year.

Complication Rate   This summarizes two complications: (1)emergency bypass surgery that is required because the blood vessel suddenly closed during angioplasty; and (2)death during or as a result of the procedure.

Hospital Charges   This represents the in-hospital cost of the procedure.

Length of Stay   This gives the average number of days a patient stayed in the hospital.

How do you pick and choose? All of these hospitals have excellent results. You can just choose one close to your home. To find the best of the best, look for a hospital with a high volume and very low complication rate. Some of the hospitals had *no* complications! In making your final decision, also check other measures of excellence and ask if the hospital can break out results for patients with your particular condition, for example, congestive heart failure.

TABLE 2. Multiple-Data Chart for the Best-Rated Bypass Angioplasty Hospitals

Hospital Name	City, State	Volume	Compli-cation Rate	Hospital Charges	Length of Stay (days)
Carraway Methodist Medical Center	Birmingham, AL	176	0.8%	$16,392	6.6
University of Alabama Hospital	Birmingham, AL	246	0.9%	$11,422	6.1
Humana Hospital Phoenix	Phoenix, AZ	192	0.6%	$26,696	4.4
Baptist Medical Center	Little Rock, AR	243	0.0%	$10,307	6.4
San Joaquin Community Hospital	Bakersfield, CA	179	0.0%	$12,061	2.9
St. Joseph Medical Center	Burbank, CA	173	0.9%	$15,242	4.4
Doctors' Medical Center	Modesto, CA	283	0.0%	$23,216	4.3

Hospital Name	City, State	Volume	Compli-cation Rate	Hospital Charges	Length of Stay (days)
Mercy General Hospital	Sacramento, CA	319	0.8%	$20,927	4.4
Sutter Memorial Hospital	Sacramento, CA	264	0.5%	$23,461	3.9
St. John's Hospital Health Center	Santa Monica, CA	156	0.0%	$16,871	4.0
Hartford Hospital	Hartford, CT	216	0.0%	$10,046	5.7
Hospital of St. Raphael	New Haven, CT	306	0.9%	$11,317	4.9
Medical Center of Delaware	Wilmington, DE	188	0.7%	$16,656	8.0
AMI Northridge Medical Center	Fort Lauderdale, FL	150	0.8%	$17,343	4.8
Florida Medical Center	Fort Lauderdale, FL	217	0.6%	$16,121	5.9
Holy Cross Hospital	Fort Lauderdale, FL	206	0.0%	$ 9,075	4.7
Holmes Regional Medical Center	Melbourne, FL	269	0.5%	$11,082	5.1
South Miami Hospital	Miami, FL	219	0.5%	$17,294	4.7
Munroe Regional Medical Center	Ocala, FL	226	0.7%	$12,859	6.2
Florida Hospital	Orlando, FL	780	0.3%	$15,758	4.9
Sarasota Memorial Hospital	Sarasota, FL	337	0.0%	$13,285	4.9
Tampa General Hospital	Tampa, FL	209	0.0%	$12,731	5.0
Crawford Long Hospital	Atlanta, GA	160	0.0%	$ 9,701	4.1
Georgia Baptist Medical Center	Atlanta, GA	216	0.5%	$12,894	4.3
University Hospital	Augusta, GA	325	0.4%	$13,778	5.2
St. Luke's Regional Medical Center	Boise, ID	198	0.6%	$ 8,851	4.4
St. Francis Hospital of Evanston	Evanston, IL	338	0.4%	$11,048	6.3
St. Francis Medical Center	Peoria, IL	167	0.8%	$11,686	5.4
Memorial Medical Center	Springfield, IL	172	0.0%	$10,955	6.8
St. Francis Hospital Center	Beech Grove, IN	180	0.8%	$10,229	5.0
Deaconess Hospital Inc.	Evansville, IN	156	0.0%	$15,792	6.5
Lutheran Hospital of Indiana Inc.	Fort Wayne, IN	161	0.9%	$10,680	5.6
Methodist Hospital of Indiana Inc.	Indianapolis, IN	357	0.4%	$ 9,068	4.8
St. Vincent Hospital & Health Center	Indianapolis, IN	705	0.9%	$12,549	5.4
The Community Hospital	Munster, IN	159	0.9%	$11,106	5.1
Iowa Methodist Medical Center	Des Moines, IA	209	0.8%	$ 9,391	4.5
St. Francis Regional Medical Center	Wichita, KS	392	0.0%	$14,682	5.3
Jewish Hosp.	Louisville, KY	374	0.9%	$10,656	4.2
Maine Medical Center	Portland, ME	338	0.4%	$ 9,824	7.2
St. Joseph Hospital	Baltimore, MD	174	0.7%	$ 7,524	3.7
Peninsula General Hospital	Salisbury, MD	157	0.9%	$ 7,556	5.7
Beth Israel Hospital	Boston, MA	202	0.7%	$16,960	8.5
New England Deaconess Hospital	Boston MA	298	0.4%	$15,592	5.9

Hospital Name	City, State	Volume	Compli-cation Rate	Hospital Charges	Length of Stay (days)
University Hospital	Boston, MA	166	0.7%	$12,906	6.5
Catherine McCauley Health Center	Ann Arbor, MI	264	0.0%	$11,549	3.9
University Hospital	Ann Arbor, MI	165	0.0%	$12,992	4.7
Oakwood Hospital	Dearborn, MI	153	0.0%	$10,451	3.8
St. John Hospital	Detroit, MI	194	0.0%	$15,643	5.2
Blodgett Memorial Medical Center	Grand Rapids, MI	222	0.6%	$ 7,383	3.1
Borgess Medical Center	Kalamazoo, MI	387	0.0%	$14,459	3.5
St. Mary's Medical Center	Saginaw, MI	289	0.0%	$ 9,827	4.2
Mercy Memorial Medical Center Inc.	St. Joseph, MI	156	0.9%	$11,555	3.8
Abbott–Northwestern Hospital	Minneapolis, MN	445	0.6%	$14,889	4.1
St. Mary's Hospital	Rochester, MN	269	0.5%	$ 8,891	5.5
St. Dominic Jackson Memorial Hospital	Jackson, MS	185	0.0%	$ 7,712	5.7
St. Luke's Hospital of Kansas City	Kansas City, MO	947	1.0%	$10,794	5.3
St. Louis University Medical Center	St. Louis, MO	252	0.6%	$14,074	5.0
St. John's Regional Health Center	Springfield, MO	534	0.7%	$ 7,621	5.0
St. Patrick Hospital	Missoula, MT	309	1.0%	$ 8,310	2.7
AMI St. Joseph Hospital	Omaha, NE	159	0.0%	$20,019	6.4
Desert Springs Hospital	Las Vegas, NV	180	0.9%	$13,910	4.3
Catholic Medical Center	Manchester, NH	174	0.0%	$11,006	4.0
Deborah Heart & Lung Center	Browns Mills, NJ	179	0.6%	$14,364	6.4
Hackensack Medical Center	Hackensack, NJ	281	0.5%	$ 8,186	6.3
Morristown Memorial Hospital	Morristown, NJ	190	0.6%	$ 8,058	5.9
Robert Wood Johnson Univ. Hosp.	New Brunswick, NJ	228	0.6%	$ 6,981	5.1
Presbyterian Hospital Center	Albuquerque, NM	282	0.5%	$11,723	4.7
St. Joseph's Hospital Health Center	Syracuse NY	203	0.6%	$ 5,631	4.2
Charlotte Mem. Hospital & Med. Center	Charlotte, NC	394	0.5%	$14,208	6.6
The Moses H. Cone Memorial Hospital	Greensboro, NC	214	0.8%	$14,107	6.2
North Carolina Baptist Hospitals	Winston-Salem, NC	158	1.0%	$10,761	6.8
Akron City Hospital	Akron, OH	203	0.0%	$ 8,828	4.3
Christ Hospital	Cincinnati, OH	310	0.4%	$11,763	6.5
Cleveland Clinic Hospital	Cleveland, OH	358	0.0%	$11,814	4.9
Riverside Methodist Hospital	Columbus, OH	512	0.3%	$11,920	5.2

Hospital Name	City, State	Volume	Compli-cation Rate	Hospital Charges	Length of Stay (days)
Good Samaritan Hosp. & Health Center	Dayton, OH	233	0.5%	$13,419	5.2
St. Francis Hospital Inc.	Tulsa, OK	246	0.0%	$11,281	5.2
St. John Medical Center Inc.	Tulsa, OK	219	0.7%	$12,843	7.0
St. Vincent Hospital & Medical Center	Portland, OR	318	0.4%	$ 9,563	3.0
Lehigh Valley Hospital Center	Allentown, PA	243	0.5%	$16,224	8.6
Hamot Medical Center	Erie, PA	150	0.0%	$12,983	5.4
Harrisburg Hospital	Harrisburg, PA	205	0.6%	$ 9,423	5.6
Lancaster General Hospital	Lancaster, PA	224	0.0%	$13,146	8.3
Albert Einstein Medical Center	Philadelphia, PA	348	0.7%	$25,245	10.2
Episcopal Hospital	Philadelphia, PA	177	0.6%	$16,859	6.3
Lankenau Hospital	Philadelphia, PA	203	0.6%	$20,821	8.5
Allegheny General Hospital	Pittsburgh, PA	526	0.9%	$15,884	5.8
Mercy Hospital–Pittsburgh	Pittsburgh, PA	253	0.5%	$ 8,911	3.7
Western Pennsylvania Hospital	Pittsburgh, PA	239	0.5%	$13,045	5.2
Reading Hospital Medical Center	Reading, PA	260	0.6%	$ 8,442	5.9
Rhode Island Hospital	Providence, RI	173	0.0%	$ 9,013	6.2
Greenville Memorial Medical Center	Greenville, SC	150	0.0%	$12,686	5.3
Sioux Valley Hospital	Sioux Falls, SD	271	0.0%	$12,936	6.4
East Tennessee Baptist Hospital	Knoxville, TN	186	0.8%	$13,752	5.9
Baptist Memorial Hospital	Memphis, TN	150	0.0%	$14,265	8.8
St. Thomas Hospital	Nashville, TN	287	0.6%	$ 9,853	5.5
Baylor University Medical Center	Dallas, TX	427	0.6%	$12,327	4.7
St. Luke's Episcopal Hospital	Houston, TX	425	0.6%	$11,675	4.9
The Methodist Hospital	Houston, TX	370	0.3%	$15,289	5.3
Methodist Hospital Lubbock	Lubbock, TX	304	0.4%	$14,830	6.8
Medical Center Hospital of Vermont	Burlington, VT	170	0.7%	$ 7,762	5.4
Henrico Doctors Hospital	Richmond, VA	211	0.6%	$17,242	6.9
Deaconess Medical Center	Spokane, WA	230	0.6%	$10,176	4.2
Sacred Heart Medical Center	Spokane, WA	195	0.8%	$ 9,499	3.9
St. Joseph Hospital Hlth. Care Center	Tacoma, WA	250	0.5%	$11,164	2.6
Appleton Medical Center	Appleton, WI	157	0.0%	$ 9,218	6.6
St. Joseph's Hospital	Milwaukee, WI	220	0.0%	$11,401	7.7

Step 5. Choose a Doctor

Experience

The doctor who performs your angioplasty should be a cardiologist certified by the American Board of Internal Medicine for Cardiovascular Diseases. In addition, the doctor should have completed one year of formal training in angioplasty. During that year he or she should have performed at least 125 procedures, 75 of them as the primary physician. Dr. Thomas B. Graboys, Director of the Lown Cardiovascular Center and a professor at Harvard Medical School, says there is a clearly identified learning curve with angioplasties. Patient risk of death or complication levels off after the doctor has performed the first 125. You want to avoid being number 70.

The doctor should perform a minimum of 75 procedures a year, according to the American Heart Association, American College of Cardiology, and American College of Physicians. The most experienced physicians have done 1,000 or more in their careers. Some doctors have done more than 7,000 angioplasties during their medical careers.

Results

Results should be equal to or better than hospital results (see Step 4).

EXPERT SOURCES

Although dozens of experts were interviewed for these chapters, these physicians are acknowledged for their significant contributions to this section.

Dr. Jeffrey S. Borer, Gladys and Roland Harriman Professor of Cardiovascular Medicine, New York Hospital–Cornell Medical Center, New York, NY

Dr. Thomas B. Graboys, Director, Lown Cardiovascular Center, Harvard Medical School, Boston, MA

Dr. Jeffrey W. Moses, Director, Cardiac Catheterization Laboratory, Lenox Hill Hospital, New York, NY

REFERENCES AND SUGGESTED READING

Banka, Vidya S., and others. Effectiveness of Decremental-Diameter Balloon Catheters (Tapered Balloon). *American Journal of Cardiology,* Vol. 69, No. 3 (Jan. 15, 1992), pp. 188–93.

Bourassa, M. G., and others. Completeness of Revascularization Early After Coronary Angioplasty (PTCA) in the NHLBI PTCA Registry (abstract). *Journal of the American College of Cardiology,* Vol. 9 (1987), p. 19A.

Clinical Competence in Percutaneous Transluminal Coronary Angioplasty. A Statement for Physicians from the ACP/ACC/AHA Task Force on Clinical Privileges in Cardiology. *Journal of the American College of Cardiology,* Vol. 15, No. 7 (June 1990), pp. 1469–1474.

de Cesare, Nicoletta B., and others. Establishing Comprehensive, Quantitative Criteria for Detection of Restenosis and Remodeling After Percutaneous Transluminal Coronary Angioplasty. *American Journal of Cardiology,* Vol. 69, No. 1 (Jan. 1, 1992), pp. 77–83.

de Jaegere, Peter, and others. Immediate and Long–Term Results of Percutaneous Coronary Angioplasty in Patients Aged 70 and Over. *British Heart Journal,* Vol. 67, No. 2 (Feb. 1992), pp. 138–143.

Ellis, S. G., and others. In-Hospital Cardiac Mortality After Acute Closure After Coronary Angioplasty: Analysis of Risk Factors from 8,207 Procedures. *Journal of the American College of Cardiology,* Vol. 11 (1988), pp. 211–216.

Goudreau, Evelyne, and others. Intracoronary Urokinase as an Adjunct to Percutaneous Transluminal Coronary Angioplasty in Patients with Complex Coronary Narrowings or Angioplasty-Induced Complications. *American Journal of Cardiology,* Vol. 69, No. 1 (Jan. 1, 1992), pp. 57–62.

Gruentzig, A. R., and others. Long-Term Follow-Up After Percutaneous Transluminal Coronary Angioplasty, the Early Zurich Experience. *New England Journal of Medicine,* Vol. 316 (1987), pp. 1127–1132.

Hermans, Walter R. M., and others. Postangioplasty Restenosis Rate Between Segments of the Major Coronary Arteries. *American Journal of Cardiology,* Vol. 69, No. 3 (Jan. 15, 1992), pp. 194–200.

Jawien, Arkadiusz, and others. Platelet-Derived Growth Factor Promotes Smooth Muscle Migration and Intimal Thickening in a Rat Model of Balloon Angioplasty. *Journal of Clinical Investigation,* Vol. 89, No. 2 (Feb. 1992), pp. 507–511.

Kent, K. M., and others. Percutaneous Transluminal Coronary Angioplasty in 1985–1986 and 1977–1981. The National Heart, Lung, and Blood Institute Registry. *New England Journal of Medicine,* Vol. 318 (1988), pp. 265–170.

Lazar, Harold L., and others. Changing Profiles of Failed Coronary Angioplasty Patients: Impact on Surgical Results. *Annals of Thoracic Surgery,* Vol. 53, No. 2 (Feb. 1992), pp. 269–273.

Lee, L., and others. Percutaneous Transluminal Coronary Angioplasty Improves Survival in Acute Myocardial Infarction Complicated by Cardiogenic Shock. *Circulation,* Vol. 78 (1988), pp. 1345–1351.

Leimgruber, P. P., and others. Restenosis After Successful Coronary Angioplasty in Patients with Single-Vessel Disease. *Circulation,* Vol. 73 (1986), pp. 710–717.

O'Keefe, J. H., and others. Procedural Risk and Long-Term Effectiveness of Multivessel Coronary Angioplasty—1980–1989 (abstract). *Journal of the American College of Cardiology,* Vol. 15 (1990), p. 205A.

O'Keefe, James H. Jr., and others. Myocardial Salvage with Direct Coronary Angioplasty for Acute Infarction. *American Heart Journal,* Vol. 123, No. 1 (Jan. 1992), pp. 1–6.

Potkin, Benjamin N., and others. Late, Out-of-Laboratory, Abrupt Closure After Angiographically Successful Directional Coronary Atherectomy. *American Journal of Cardiology,* Vol. 69, No. 3 (Jan. 15, 1992), pp. 263–265.

Reeder, G. S., and others. Degree of Revascularization in Patients with Multivessel Disease: A Report from the National Heart, Lung, and Blood Institute Percutaneous Transluminal Coronary Angioplasty Registry. *Circulation,* Vol. 77 (1988), pp. 638–644.

Roubin, G., and others. Event-Free Survival After Successful Angioplasty in Multivessel Coronary Artery Disease (abstract). *Journal of the American College of Cardiology,* Vol. 9 (1987), p. 15A.

Ruocco, Nicholas A. Jr., and others. Results of Coronary Angioplasty of Chronic Total Occlusions (the National Heart, Lung, and Blood Institute 1985–1986 Percutaneous Transluminal Angioplasty Registry). *American Journal of Cardiology,* Vol. 69, No. 1 (Jan. 1992), pp. 69–76.

Talley, J. D., and others. Clinical Outcome 5 Years After Attempted Percutaneous Coronary Angioplasty in 427 Patients. *Circulation,* Vol. 77 (1988), pp. 820–829.

Stress Test

Likelihood of Unnecessary Procedure   HIGH

Up to 20% of stress tests are done unnecessarily, according to expert estimates. Sometimes the procedure is performed, not because the risk of heart disease is high in the particular case, but because it is extremely profitable for the businesses engaged in testing. You will want to avoid unnecessary testing for a number of reasons: You may be misled by a false positive test, which inaccurately suggests the presence of heart disease. Often, individuals with false positive tests become "cardiac cripples," needlessly curtailing their lifestyle and suffering psychological distress. With a false positive, you also may be encouraged to undergo more hazardous tests. Other individuals are reassured by a false negative test, which fails to detect existing heart disease. They may not take the proper precautions or preventive measures.

Potential Risk   LOW

If you are not fit, the stress test may push the limits of your ability to exercise. If coronary artery disease exists, you run the risk of a heart attack or sudden death. The estimated risk is one death and two nonfatal complications per 10,000 tests. A skilled physician can minimize the risk by selecting patients carefully and monitoring for signs of trouble during the test. A poorly monitored test can be dangerous if you suffer chest pain, an irregular heart rhythm, or heart attack and proper resuscitation equipment and trained medical personnel are not available.

What It Is

The stress test is used to diagnose coronary artery disease by establishing the relationship between discomfort in the chest and the typical electrocardiogram (EKG) signs of insufficient blood supply to the heart. Before the test begins, EKG electrodes will be attached to your body. Then you will be asked to exercise, usually on a treadmill or bicycle, at a slowly increasing pace. The doctor will look for evidence on the EKG that your heart muscle is not getting enough oxygen. The test is discontinued when *one or more* of the following signs appears:

- Chest discomfort

- Severe shortness of breath

- Dizziness

- Fatigue

- Certain specific changes in the EKG

- A fall in systolic blood pressure (the higher number drops more than 15 points)

- Development of an irregular heart rate, called a ventricular tachyarrhythmia

Step 1. Make Sure You Need the Procedure

Since there is a relatively high risk of unnecessary testing, you should consider first your overall state of health and then if one of the following categories fits you. These guidelines are available from the American College of Cardiology's *Guidelines for Exercise Testing*.

Diagnosis: You Have No Known Coronary Artery Disease and Are Considered Healthy

Appropriate Test

If you are healthy and have no symptoms, there is no universally accepted reason to test.

Uncertain If Test Is Appropriate

- Male over age 40 or female over 55 who has no symptoms of heart disease and is in an occupation such as airline pilot, firefighter, police officer, bus or truck driver, or railroad engineer

- Male over age 40 with two or more of the following risk factors for coronary artery disease:

    Serum cholesterol over 240 mg/dl

    Blood pressure greater than 160/90

    Smokes cigarettes

    Diabetes

    Family history of heart disease before the age of 55

- Male over age 40 who is sedentary and plans to begin a vigorous exercise program

Not an Appropriate Test

- History of chest discomfort not thought to be of cardiac origin

- Overall good health

Diagnosis: Doctors Suspect You Have Coronary Artery Disease

Appropriate Test

- Male tentatively diagnosed with coronary artery disease but with atypical symptoms

- Symptoms of an irregular heart rate brought on by exercise, called exercise-induced cardiac arrhythmias

- Any other case in which coronary artery disease is suspected

Not an Appropriate Test

- Irregular heart rhythm, called a simple premature ventricular beat, but no other evidence of heart disease

- Coronary artery disease suspected plus have either Wolff-Parkinson-White syndrome or complete left bundle branch block, conditions that interfere with the heart's electrical pattern, making the EKG unreliable

Diagnosis: Doctors Know You Have Coronary Artery Disease

Appropriate Test

- Potential high risk for advanced coronary disease and/or dysfunction of the left ventricle, although heart scans are preferable

- Have had coronary artery bypass surgery or angioplasty, although most cardiologists prefer heart scans

- Exercise capacity or response to treatment being evaluated as part of monitoring of coronary artery disease

Not an Appropriate Test and Also Dangerous

- Chest pain of varying intensity and frequency that has not yet responded to medications (called unstable angina)

- Untreated, life-threatening, irregular heart rate (arrhythmias)

- Severe congestive heart failure

- Advanced heart block (known as atrioventricular heart block)

- Acute myocarditis (an infection of the heart muscle)

- Critical aortic stenosis (a narrowing of the heart's highest pressure valve)

Step 2. Consider an Alternative

If you have heart problems, other tests may be far better able to diagnose your condition. This is particularly true for women, since so many tests are false positive for women. These tests can create visual pictures of your heart through scans (known technically as radionucleide cineangiogram, thallium, and PET) or by electrocardiograms. They are described in the chapter on Coronary Artery Disease.

Step 3. Get a Specialist's Opinion

WHEN YOU NEED ONE   If the test is not clearly indicated, if your diagnosis is in doubt, or if another test is more appropriate, you may wish to get an expert opinion from a highly skilled cardiologist. That cardiologist should meet the criteria listed in Step 5.

WHO TO GO TO   Your best choice of a second-opinion doctor would be a highly skilled cardiologist who meets the same criteria as listed in Step 5.

WHAT TO DISCUSS   You should discuss the alternatives to EKG stress testing, which are listed in the chapter on Coronary Artery Disease. You will want the cardiologist to carefully review your medical history to be certain your diagnosis is correct.

WHERE TO CALL   Here are some organizations that can help you.

American Heart Association   This organization can provide educational literature that will help you to understand your disease.

7320 Greenville Ave
Dallas, TX 75231
214/373-6300

American College of Cardiology   This medical society publishes guidelines
and position papers on cardiac care.

9111 Old Georgetown Rd
Bethesda, MD 20814
800/253-4636

NIH CRISP System

301/496-7543

University-Affiliated Teaching Hospitals   See Appendix.

Step 4. Choose a Facility

Experience

It's not necessary to go to a major medical center for an EKG stress test, although
you should select a facility that is well prepared to handle emergencies. If you
decide on an alternative to the stress test, you may want to go to a specialty center
because the results can be difficult to interpret. The facility should have complete
advanced life support equipment and personnel trained in its use. Emergency
medical care should be nearby if the testing center is not in a hospital.

You can be assured that you are not at a stress test factory if you go to a hospital
with a good reputation for cardiology rather than a center that specializes in stress
tests. Remember, a stress test is part of an overall evaluation package.

Results

Any death rate is an indicator of poor quality. A center with a death rate of more
than 1 in 10,000 should be avoided.

Centers of Excellence for Cardiology

*The following list of hospitals is provided only as a convenient starting place in your search
for excellence. These hospitals are recommended on the basis of reputation, not experience
and results. The list is not an endorsement. There may be hospitals just as excellent that have
been omitted. You should apply the guidelines for experience, results, and other measures of
excellence to any hospital you choose, whether or not it is on this list. Although hospitals from*

different sources have been combined into one list, the compilation in no way implies that one source has endorsed the hospital list of another source.

ALABAMA
University of Alabama
    Medical Center   BIM
619 S 19th St
Birmingham, AL 35294

ARIZONA
University Medical Center   BIM
1501 N Campbell Ave
Tucson, AZ 85724

CALIFORNIA
Stanford University School
    of Medicine   BIM/US
300 Pasteur Dr
Stanford, CA 94305

COLORADO
University Hospital   BIM
4200 E Ninth Ave
Denver, CO 80262

CONNECTICUT
Yale–New Haven Hospital   BIM
20 York St
New Haven, CT 06504

DISTRICT OF COLUMBIA
Georgetown University School
    of Medicine   EX
3900 Reservoir Rd NW
Washington, DC 20007

FLORIDA
Jackson Memorial Hospital   BIM
1611 NW 12th Ave
Miami, FL 33136

Miami Heart Institute   BIM
4701 Meridian Ave
Miami Beach, FL 33140

GEORGIA
Emory University Hospital   BIM/US
1364 Clifton Rd NE
Atlanta, GA 30322

ILLINOIS
Northwestern University
    Medical Center   BIM
250 E Superior St
Chicago, IL 60611

MARYLAND
Johns Hopkins Hospital   BIM/US
600 N Wolfe St
Baltimore, MD 21205

University of Maryland School
    of Medicine   EX
655 W Baltimore St
Baltimore, MD 21201

MASSACHUSETTS
Brigham and Women's Hospital   BIM/US
75 Francis St
Boston, MA 02115

Massachusetts General Hospital   BIM/US
55 Fruit St
Boston, MA 02114

MINNESOTA
Mayo Clinic   BIM/US
200 First St SW
Rochester, MN 55905

NEW YORK
New York Hospital–Cornell
    Medical Center   BIM
525 E 68th St
New York, NY 10021

NORTH CAROLINA
Duke University Medical Center   BIM
Box 3005
Durham, NC 27710

Duke University Hospital   US
Box 3708
Erwin Rd
Durham, NC 27710

OHIO

Cleveland Clinic Foundation   BIM/US
One Clinic Center
9500 Euclid Ave
Cleveland, OH 44195

PENNSYLVANIA

Hahnemann University Hospital   BIM
Broad and Vine Sts
Philadelphia, PA 19102

TENNESSEE

Vanderbilt University Medical
    Center   BIM
1211 22nd Ave S
Nashville, TN 37232

TEXAS

Baylor College of Medicine
    and Hospitals   BIM
One Baylor Plaza
Houston, TX 77030

St Luke's Episcopal Hospital   US
Texas Heart Institute
1101 Bates St
Houston, TX 77030

University of Texas   EX
Southwestern Medical Center at Dallas
Southwestern Medical School
5323 Harry Hines Blvd
Dallas, TX 75235

VIRGINIA

University of Virginia Hospital   BIM
Jefferson Park Ave
Charlottesville, VA 22908

WASHINGTON

University of Washington
    Medical Center   BIM
1959 NE Pacific St
Seattle, WA 98195

SOURCES

BIM   indicates those hospitals recommended by *The Best in Medicine.*

US   indicates those hospitals recommended by *U.S. News & World Report.*

EX   indicates those hospitals recommended by experts interviewed.

Step 5. Choose a Doctor

Experience

The doctor who performs the stress test should be board certified in internal medicine and cardiology with extensive training and recent experience in related tests such as heart scans and echocardiograms. Your doctor should perform a minimum of five stress tests a week.

Note: Physicians who only conduct stress tests may lack other clinical skills necessary for diagnosis and treatment.

EXPERT SOURCES

Though dozens of experts were interviewed for these chapters, the following physicians are acknowledged for their significant contributions to this section.

Dr. Jeffrey S. Borer, Gladys and Roland Harriman Professor of Cardiovascular Medicine, New York Hospital–Cornell Medical Center, New York, NY

Dr. Thomas B. Graboys, Director, Lown Cardiovascular Center, Harvard Medical School, Boston, MA

REFERENCES AND SUGGESTED READING

ACP/ACC/AHA Task Force on Clinical Privileges in Cardiology. Clinical Competence in Adult Echocardiography. *Journal of the American College of Cardiology,* Vol. 15, No. 7 (June 1990), pp. 1465–1468.

ACP/ACC/AHA Task Force. Clinical Competence in Exercise Testing. American College of Cardiology 1990. *Journal of the American College of Cardiology,* Vol. 16, No. 5 (Nov. 1, 1990), pp. 1601–1605.

American College of Cardiology/American Heart Association Task Force on Assessment of Diagnostic and Therapeutic Cardiovascular Procedures (Subcommittee on Exercise Testing). Guidelines for Exercise Testing. *Journal of the American College of Cardiology,* Vol. 8, No. 3 (Sept. 1986), pp. 725–738.

Detrano, R., and Froelicher, V. F. Exercise Testing: Uses and Limitations Considering Recent Studies. *Progress in Cardiovascular Diseases,* Vol. 31 (1988), pp. 173–204.

Efficacy of Exercise Thallium-201 Scintigraphy in the Diagnosis and Prognosis of Coronary Artery Disease. *Annals of Internal Medicine,* Vol. 113, No. 9 (Nov. 1990), pp. 703–704.

Hilton, Thomas C., and others. Prognostic Significance of Exercise Thallium-201 Testing in Patients Aged >=70 Years with Known or Suspected Coronary Artery Disease. *American Journal of Cardiology,* Vol. 69, No. 1 (Jan. 1, 1992), pp. 45–50.

Kotler, T. S., and Diamond, G. A. Exercise Thallium-201 Scintigraphy in the Diagnosis and Prognosis of Coronary Artery Disease. *Annals of Internal Medicine,* Vol. 113, No. 9 (Nov. 1990), pp. 684–702.

Martin, D., and others. The Utility and Safety of Exercise Testing in Octogenarians. Presented at the 46th Annual Scientific Meeting of the American Geriatrics Society, May 14, 1989, Boston, Massachusetts.

McInnis, Kyle J., and others. Comparison of Ischemic and Physiologic Responses During Exercise Tests in Men Using the Standard and Modified Bruce Protocols. *American Journal of Cardiology,* Vol. 69, No. 1 (Jan. 1, 1992), pp. 84–89.

Siscovick, D. S., and others. The Incidence of Primary Cardiac Arrest During Vigorous Exercise. *New England Journal of Medicine,* Vol. 311 (1984), pp. 874–877.

Sox, H. C. Jr., and others. The Role of Exercise Testing in Screening for Coronary Artery Disease. *Annals of Internal Medicine,* Vol. 110, No. 6 (Mar. 15, 1989), pp. 456–459.

Angiogram

Likelihood of Unnecessary Procedure   VERY HIGH

An angiogram that is performed unnecessarily carries two dangers: the risk of the procedure itself, and the risk that it will be followed by another inappropriate operation or procedure. I have seen this happen countless times. A patient goes to a doctor for a minor complaint. The doctor then orders a routine stress test. The result is equivocal. Without any classic signs or symptoms of heart disease, an angiogram is ordered. Almost out of the blue, major open-heart surgery is scheduled.

As you progress from your initial office visit through stress testing, then to an angiogram and a possible bypass operation, you will want to consider each successive step carefully to ensure that surgery does not become a self-fulfilling prophecy. In 1991, the research firm MediQual reported that 35.26% of coronary artery angiograms they studied had none of the objective clinical findings documented in the hospital medical record they use to validate an angiogram at the time it was performed.

Most inappropriate procedures are performed on patients who fail to undergo other diagnostic tests first. A good rule of thumb to remember is: Make sure your first elective test is not an angiogram.

Potential Risk   HIGH

You run a small but very real risk of stroke, heart attack, or death from an angiogram. The potential benefit should be significant before you take this risk. The test should be done only if it is essential for you and your doctor to determine the treatment that will be most effective in your case.

What It Is

The cardiologist makes a small, temporary hole in a major artery in your arm or leg. Into that hole he or she passes a long, thin tube called a catheter. The catheter is threaded up into a coronary artery. Once the catheter is in place, a liquid containing special material that an x-ray device can "see" is injected into the coronary artery being studied. A series of moving black-and-white images is made as the fluid flows through the artery. These images are usually recorded from several different angles so that extent of blockage can be fairly assessed.

An angiogram is the single most accurate test to assess the severity of coronary artery disease. It allows doctors to peer inside coronary arteries and locate blockages that may cause chest pain, heart attack, or death. Doctors can then decide if those blockages should be bypassed through surgery, pushed aside by angioplasty, or treated by other methods. (See the respective chapters on Coronary Artery Bypass Surgery and Angioplasty.) Dr. Carl J. Pepine, chair of the American College of Cardiology Committee on Guidelines for Angiograms, says, "There is nothing else that will let you know what the angiogram can tell you. An angiogram can tell you where to bypass and which arteries need dilating for angioplasty."

Doctors use angiograms to plot treatment strategy. Can they see a good clean stretch of artery into which to sew a new blood vessel during bypass surgery? Is there a solitary blockage that can be pushed aside using a dilating balloon device called an angioplasty catheter?

In addition, angiograms are used to evaluate the following:

- Poorly functioning heart muscles

- Diseased or damaged heart valves

- Congenital heart defects

- Coronary artery bypass grafts

- Abnormal openings between an artery and a vein (called an arteriovenous fistula) or between different sides of the heart (known as septal defects). Such openings usually are a congenital problem but may develop after a major heart attack.

Step 1. Make Sure You Need the Procedure

Appropriate Procedure

The following list of diagnoses, based on guidelines from the American College of Cardiology, shows the circumstances that justify an angiogram. While it's pretty detailed, I've stripped it of medical jargon. You should scan the list to see if it contains your diagnosis. If it doesn't, remember, by undergoing an angiogram you could launch a whole sequence of events, from balloon angioplasty to surgery. Let's say you go to the doctor because of chest pain or an occasional irregular heartbeat. Despite the lack of risk factors for heart disease and overall good health, you may have a stress test with results that are not completely normal. Should additional tests also have ambiguous results, that would be the time to take a careful look at your treatment plan. Your next move would be to seek an expert second opinion, *not* to consent to the angiogram. Though there may be a legitimate reason for the angiogram, you need to be certain first.

Diagnosis: Doctors Suspect You Have Coronary Artery Disease

Although you have no physical symptoms of heart disease, a stress test indicates the existence of coronary artery disease. But since stress tests are notoriously inaccurate, additional tests should strongly confirm the diagnosis before you agree to an angiogram (see Step 2.)

In certain occupations, such as airline pilot, bus or truck driver, air traffic controller, firefighter, and athlete, you may be required to have an angiogram in order to prove that heart disease is not present. This happens most often because of the unreliability of stress tests. Airline pilots frequently find themselves in this situation. If a stress test, required by the Federal Aviation Administration, suggests coronary artery disease, the pilot may have to undergo an angiogram and eliminate the possibility of heart disease if he or she wants to continue to fly. An athlete with unexplained symptoms also may be urged by team doctors to have an angiogram. If you are in this category, you should exhaust all other diagnostic tests, including a reevaluation at a top cardiac teaching hospital, before agreeing to an angiogram.

Diagnosis: You Have Known Coronary Heart Disease

If you have coronary artery disease and are facing heart surgery, your doctor should order an angiogram in these situations:

■ Before major vascular surgery if there is intermittent chest pain (angina pectoris) or disruptions in the supply of blood to the heart (myocardial ischemia)

■ If your surgical risk can't be assessed by alternative methods because of other diseases

Diagnosis: You Have Atypical Chest Pain of Uncertain Origin

An angiogram may be performed if your doctor suspects that the pain is caused by coronary artery spasm or abnormal functioning of the left ventricle, the heart's main pumping chamber. This may be the case if congestive heart failure exists.

Diagnosis: You've Just Had a Heart Attack

Angiograms may be necessary after a heart attack if chest pain continues or if there was major damage to the heart structure.

Not an Appropriate Procedure

An angiogram should not be done under the following conditions:

■ As a diagnostic test for coronary artery disease, unless stress and other screening tests have been performed first

■ After bypass surgery or angioplasty, unless there are indications that the heart isn't getting enough oxygen

■ Terminal cancer, lung, kidney, or liver disease

■ Recent stroke

■ Increasing loss of kidney function

■ Bleeding in the stomach or intestine

■ Fever whose possible cause is an infection

■ In the presence of an active infection

■ Severe anemia

■ Uncontrolled high blood pressure

■ A serious noncardiac illness with an uncertain prognosis

■ Psychosis that makes patient's condition unstable during the procedure

■ Over age 80 unless medical therapy is absolutely failing

■ When no treatment will be undertaken even if results show a problem

■ Overall unstable condition when no cardiac surgical team is available in the hospital (If you are that unstable, get transferred to a center of excellence.)

■ Overdose of the drug digitalis

■ Documented allergies, called anaphylactic reactions, to the contrast fluid used in an angiogram (still can be premedicated with steroids to undergo procedure if problem is life-threatening)

■ Extremely poor heart function with no physical symptoms of heart disease, unless there are real surgical alternatives, such as transplant

■ Irregular heartbeat without other symptoms, and with good stress test results and no suggestion of an aneurysm

■ Mild chest pain that is not worsening

■ Atypical chest pain without clear-cut signs of insufficient blood supply to the heart and with an earlier, normal angiogram

Factors That Increase Risk Even if an Angiogram Is Appropriate

A number of conditions can increase the risks of the procedure. You should be very selective in your choice of doctor and hospital if the following conditions are present, because of the risk involved.

■ Abnormal blood pressure or sharp EKG changes during a stress test at a relatively low heart rate

■ Critical narrowing of left main coronary artery detected on one or more diagnostic tests

■ 90% blockages in the three main coronary arteries

■ Several diseased arteries and the heart's pumping capacity reduced to 35% of normal

■ Critical narrowing (stenosis) of the aortic valve

Step 2. Consider an Alternative

Before you have an angiogram, a heart scan should show strong evidence of heart disease. Although scans can't show the actual arteries, they can determine if your heart is pumping adequately and can indicate the parts of the heart muscle that aren't getting enough blood. A scan is like a photograph of a river delta taken from outer space. You may not be able to see the river, but if the surrounding area is green and thriving, you can assume that water is reaching the surrounding fields; if it is brown, the area is dry and fallow.

As scans have improved technically, they have been able to provide increasingly well-defined studies of the heart. Medical centers tend to specialize in one type of scan or another as their expertise develops. These are described in the chapter on Coronary Artery Disease.

Step 3. Get a Specialist's Opinion

WHEN YOU NEED ONE   You will need an expert opinion if your angiogram is not clearly indicated, if you do not have a high chance of success, or if you want to consider an alternative.

WHO TO GO TO   See a board-certified cardiologist. You have a choice between an invasive cardiologist who actually performs angiograms and a cardiologist who specializes in the noninvasive approaches such as stress tests and cardiac scans (see chapter on Coronary Artery Disease for a complete list).

WHAT TO DISCUSS   Discuss the alternatives to an angiogram. You will want the doctor to carefully review your medical history and your medical tests and to be certain your condition is correctly diagnosed.

WHERE TO GO   You can go to a center of excellence for cardiology (see Step 4) or to a teaching hospital listed in the Appendix.

WHO TO CALL   If time, expense, or travel prohibit you from seeking a specialist's opinion, learn as much as you can by calling one of the centers of excellence (see Step 4) or one of the following organizations.

American Heart Association   Your local chapter can recommend physicians. These centers may not distinguish among physicians other than by their basic qualifications. The national headquarters can send you booklets and may be helpful in securing a local phone number.

7320 Greenville Ave
Dallas, TX 75231
214/373-6300

American College of Cardiology   This medical specialty society publishes guidelines and other information about cardiac care.

9111 Old Georgetown Rd
Bethesda, MD 20814
800/253-4643

Coronary Club   This club publishes a monthly newsletter, "Heartline." There are also ten local chapters in the United States.

Cleveland Clinic Foundation
9500 Euclid Ave, Rm E4-15
Cleveland, OH 44195
216/444-3690

Mended Hearts   With more than 200 chapters and 22,000 members nationwide, this organization is an excellent source of information about bypass surgery and other heart operations. Members visit heart patients before and after surgery.

7320 Greenville Ave
Dallas, TX 75231
214/932-1427

NIH CRISP System

301/496-7543

University-Affiliated Hospitals   See Appendix.

Step 4. Choose a Hospital

An angiogram should be performed in a hospital. While there are independent laboratories, neither the American College of Cardiology nor the American Hospital Association approves of their use for angiograms. If complications develop, you could need immediate open-heart surgery that can only be done in a hospital. If the procedure is being performed on a child, it should be done in a center that specializes in pediatric cardiology with surgeons on staff who limit their practices to children in a similar age range with congenital heart disease.

An angiogram should be performed in an emergency only if it's a prelude to surgery or angioplasty. For that reason you should be admitted to the hospital where surgery will be performed. I was involved in a recent case where the patient, a woman with unstable angina, was admitted to a small hospital. The angiogram was scheduled for several days later. If it revealed blockages, she would have to be transferred to a center that specializes in cardiovascular disease. I advised the family to make the transfer even before the angiogram was done. At the Cleveland Clinic, a center of excellence for cardiology, the angiogram showed a large blockage in a main coronary artery. Angioplasty pushed aside the blockage and relieved her chest pain. The principle is simple: At the earliest hint of trouble, put yourself into the care of the best possible medical center where *all* the options can be covered. In medicine, always prepare for the unexpected.

Experience

The hospital should perform a minimum of 300 angiograms a year. The Cleveland Clinic, a leading cardiac care center, does nearly 4,600 a year. Select the hospital in your area that has the most experience in angiograms, because complications, though infrequent, can be very serious.

Results

DEATH RATE   According to the American College of Cardiology, the mortality rate should not exceed 0.13%. At centers of excellence the figure will be significantly less. The Cleveland Clinic's mortality rate for angiograms is 0.02%.

COMPLICATION RATE   The complication rate from stroke, heart attack, or hemorrhaging should be no greater than 0.5%.

Other Measures of Excellence

- No specific team is required, though there should be adequate medical backup.

- An in-house cardiac surgery team, meeting the criteria discussed in the chapter on Coronary Artery Bypass Surgery, should be available.

- A 20% rate of coronaries found to be normal after angiogram is an acceptable measure of excellence.

Centers of Excellence for Cardiology

The following list of hospitals is provided only as a convenient starting place in your search for excellence. These hospitals are recommended on the basis of reputation, not experience and results. The list is not an endorsement. There may be hospitals just as excellent that have been omitted. You should apply the guidelines for experience, results, and other measures of excellence to any hospital you choose, whether or not it is on this list. Although hospitals from different sources have been combined into one list, the compilation in no way implies that one source has endorsed the hospital list of another source.

CALIFORNIA
Stanford University School
 of Medicine   US
300 Pasteur Dr
Stanford, CA 94305

GEORGIA
Emory University Hospital   US
1364 Clifton Rd NE
Atlanta, GA 30322

MARYLAND
Johns Hopkins Hospital   US
600 N Wolfe St
Baltimore, MD 21205

MASSACHUSETTS
Brigham and Women's Hospital   US
75 Francis St
Boston, MA 02115

Massachusetts General Hospital   US
55 Fruit St
Boston, MA 02114

MINNESOTA
Mayo Clinic   US
200 First St SW
Rochester, MN 55905

NORTH CAROLINA
Duke University Hospital   US
Box 3708
Durham, NC 27710

OHIO
Cleveland Clinic Foundation   US
One Clinic Center
9500 Euclid Ave
Cleveland, OH 44195

TEXAS
St Luke's Episcopal Hospital   US
Texas Heart Institute
1101 Bates St
Houston, TX 77030

SOURCES

US   indicates those hospitals recommended by *U.S. News & World Report.*

Step 5. Choose a Doctor

Your doctor should be a board-certified cardiologist who has completed a three-year fellowship in the field that includes a year in a catheterization lab. The doctor should have performed a minimum of 300 catheterizations to ensure competency, with 200 of those as the primary operator. Not all cardiology fellowships emphasize proficiency in cardiac catheterizations. In fact, the majority of fellows will not perform 300 procedures. Your doctor should have been trained in a program that emphasizes cardiac catheterizations.

You also should look for the following.

Experience

The doctor should perform a minimum of three catheterizations a week, or about 150 a year. At the Cleveland Clinic one cardiologist performed 534 in 1990, and the clinic doctors average 320 annually. But a doctor can do too many angiograms. If the cardiologist is performing more than 1,000 a year, that's too many—the doctor isn't spending enough time on patient care.

Pediatric cardiologists need perform fewer angiograms a year to maintain their skills. About 50–100 is sufficient.

Results

DEATH RATE   The death rate should be about 0.13%, which is the average. Your doctor's results should compare favorably.

COMPLICATION RATE   The complication rate from stroke, heart attack, or death within 48 hours of the procedure should be less than 0.2%. Death, stroke, and heart attack are the top serious complications for angiogram.

Other Measures of Excellence

You should inquire about the number of patients who need the angiogram to be repeated. This may occur because the studies were inadequate or because the equipment is technically inferior. If it happens even once, it is too often. Ask your doctor, "If I have an angiogram here, what is the likelihood that it will be repeated?"

EXPERT SOURCES

Although dozens of experts were interviewed for these chapters, the following physicians are acknowledged for their significant contributions to this section.

Dr. Thomas B. Graboys, Director, Lown Cardiovascular Center, Harvard Medical School, Boston, MA

Dr. Jeffrey S. Borer, Gladys and Roland Harriman Professor of Cardiovascular Medicine, New York Hospital–Cornell Medical Center, New York, NY

Dr. Jeffrey W. Moses, Director, Cardiac Catheterization Laboratory, Lenox Hill Hospital, New York, NY

REFERENCES AND SUGGESTED READING

Chassin, M. R., and others. How Coronary Angiography Is Used. Clinical Determinants of Appropriateness. *Journal of the American Medical Association,* Vol. 258, No. 18 (Nov. 13, 1987), pp. 2543–2547.

Eigler, N., and others. The Role of Digital Angiography in the Evaluation of Coronary Artery Disease. *International Journal of Cardiology,* Vol. 10 (1986), pp. 3–13.

Guidelines for Coronary Angiography. *Journal of the American College of Cardiology,* Vol. 10, No. 4 (Oct. 1987), pp. 935–950.

Kennedy, J. W., and others. Complications Associated with Cardiac Catheterization and Angiography. *Catheterization and Cardiovascular Diagnosis,* Vol. 8 (1982), pp. 5–11.

MacRae, C. A., and others. Need for Invasive Cardiological Assessment and Intervention: A Ten-Year Review. *British Heart Journal,* Vol. 67, No. 2 (Feb. 1992), pp. 200–203.

Optimal Resources for Examination of the Heart and Lungs: Cardiac Catheterization and Radiographic Facilities. *Circulation,* Vol. 63 (1983), pp. 893A–930A.

Peduzzi, P., and others. Veterans Administration Cooperative Study of Medical Versus Surgical Treatment for Stable Angina—Progress Report 8. Prognostic Value of Baseline Exercise Tests. *Progress in Cardiovascular Diseases,* Vol. 28 (1986), pp. 285–292.

White, C. W., and others. Does Visual Interpretation of the Coronary Arteriogram Predict the Physiologic Importance of a Coronary Stenosis? *New England Journal of Medicine,* Vol. 310 (1984), pp. 819–824.

Cesarean Section

Likelihood of Unnecessary Surgery   EXTREMELY HIGH

The cesarean section, abbreviated c-section, is both the most overused procedure in the United States and the most common. Dr. Sidney Wolfe, director of the Public Citizen Health Research Group in Washington, D.C., and author of a study on the subject, states that 50% of the 967,000 c-sections performed in 1988 were unnecessary. In 1991 the research firm MediQual reported that 49.32% of c-sections they studied had none of the objective clinical findings documented in the hospital medical record they use to validate a c-section at the time of surgery.

Fear of a malpractice suit is a major reason for this overutilization. Since c-sections allow a much wider margin of error in a difficult delivery, many women are often moved into the operating room at the first sign of trouble. Moreover, doctors are performing c-sections at a much earlier stage of labor than they did before the current malpractice crisis. It's difficult to blame obstetricians. In many hospitals every single obstetrician has been sued at least once. Most lawsuits are filed, not because the delivery was mishandled, but because the parents hold the doctor responsible for *any* birth defects, even those completely unrelated to the delivery. To protect themselves, doctors are doing nearly five times as many c-sections as they did just 20 years ago:

YEAR	C-SECTIONS AS PERCENTAGE OF LIVE BIRTHS
1970	5.5%
1986	24.1
1987	24.4
1988	24.7

The likelihood that you will have a c-section depends in part on where you live and deliver. C-sections account for a far larger proportion of births in some geographic areas than in others. According to the Public Citizen Health group, statewide averages range from a low of 17.9% to a high of 30.3%! The kind of hospital at which you deliver can also make a difference. For-profit hospitals lead the pack with an average 24.6% cesarean births, while military and public health service hospitals average only 15%.

Your health coverage also may influence your chances of having a c-section. The more your insurer can pay, the more likely you are to have a c-section: Under private insurance, you have the greatest chance; as a member of a *large* HMO or if you are uninsured, you have the smallest chance. The chances of a member of a *small* health maintenance organization or one covered through the Medicaid program fall in between.

Potential Risk   MODERATE

These are the major risks of a c-section:

- Injury to infant in about 0.4% of cases

- Twice as much blood loss as with vaginal birth

- Blood clot in the lung or pulmonary embolus (rare)

- Infection of the urinary tract or surgical wound in about 1–7% of cases

- Infection of the womb in about 5–18% of deliveries

- Increased risk of abnormal blood clotting in the extremities

- Injury to surrounding organs such as bladder, ureter, and bowel in 0.1–0.3% of cases

- Higher incidence of trauma, plus a likelihood of future c-section because of scarring

- Increased infertility (from 2.2% in normal deliveries to 6.4% following a c-section)

- Increased maternal death rate (laboring mother estimated four to five times more likely to die during abdominal birth than during vaginal birth)

What It Is

A c-section is the surgical delivery of a baby through an incision in the uterus and is usually performed to save the baby or the mother from serious complications or death. The doctor makes an incision across the lower abdomen and into the uterus, removes the infant and placenta, and closes the incision.

Step 1. Make Sure You Need the Surgery

If your doctor recommends a c-section, you should consult the following lists, which give the conditions under which the procedure is considered appropriate and inappropriate.

Appropriate Procedure

■ Fetal distress, such as slowing of the heart rate, that fails to respond to treatment, especially if it occurs late in pregnancy and there is poor circulation as evidenced by high levels of acid in the blood

■ Lack of progress despite normal, active labor (including a cervix that fails to dilate after two or more hours of active labor, and a fetus that is not descending through the birth canal)

■ Obstructed labor because of uterine abnormalities such as pelvic cysts and fibroids

■ Prolonged labor because the baby's head is too large for the birth canal

■ Untreatable dysfunctional uterine activity

■ Bleeding from the placenta

■ Maternal risk where prompt vaginal delivery is not feasible, such as eclampsia (convulsions)

■ Transverse lie (fetus lying horizontally rather than longitudinally) that cannot easily be corrected

■ Low-birth-weight baby when vaginal delivery may be difficult and traumatic

■ Previous c-section for physical causes, for example, a small pelvis

■ Breech presentation in combination with a small pelvis, a big baby, or footling presentation

Not an Appropriate Procedure

REPEAT C-SECTION   In 1987, 35.3% of all c-sections performed in the United States were repeat c-sections. More important, they contributed 48% to the recent rise in c-section rates. The saying used to be "Once a c-section, always a c-section." But that is no longer true. The American College of Obstetrics and Gynecology believes that 50–80% of women who have had a previous cesarean can deliver vaginally. Most experts agree that c-sections should not be done routinely. With newer c-section incisions there is little chance that the uterus will rupture during labor. This fear of rupture had been the rationale for a repeat c-section. A recent alarming series of studies did report rupture of the uterus during vaginal delivery. However, the chance of such a rupture's occurring was still quite small, and adverse outcomes occurred only when the mother and fetus were not carefully monitored.

OVERRELIANCE ON ELECTRONIC FETAL MONITORING   High-tech monitoring devices can be notoriously misleading. In many cases, the medical staff is simply not trained adequately to interpret the readings. Experts fear that misinterpreted results on these high-tech monitoring devices account for much of the increased number of c-sections performed because of fetal distress such as an erratic heartbeat. Over a recent five-year period, the number of c-sections performed as a result of fetal distress rose 15%. But there was no concurrent decrease in fetal deaths. During those same five years, the reported incidence of fetal distress increased 225%. This means that new, sophisticated equipment is not saving babies' lives. A doctor properly trained in the use of electronic fetal monitoring makes fewer incorrect diagnoses and performs fewer unnecessary c-sections. But the devices often are unreliable. Even if the fetal monitor shows abnormal signs, there is only a one-in-four chance the infant is really in trouble.

MISDIAGNOSIS OF DYSTOCIA   Dystocia (abnormal uterine activity), often called the catchall diagnosis, is used as an "excuse" for c-section. A c-section often is performed when there are marginal indications of trouble or the established criteria are not met—for example, a baby's head is declared too large for the mother's pelvis although careful measurements don't confirm the diagnosis. Often, intravenous medications should be tried before the doctor resorts to a c-section. Although only 28% of c-sections are attributed to abnormal progression of labor, it has constituted a big chunk of the recent rise in c-sections.

OVERDUE DELIVERY   Passing a due date is no reason for performing a c-section. If pregnancy reaches its 41st week, tests should be done, before resorting to a c-section, to confirm that the child really needs to be delivered.

Step 2. Get a Specialist's Opinion

You can prevent an unnecessary c-section by doing your advance homework. Don't wait until you are already in labor in the hospital to realize you need an expert opinion. It's a little awkward to ask for one then.

You should consult an expert if you are scheduled for a c-section for an inappropriate reason, which most likely would be a repeat c-section. If a c-section is recommended early in pregnancy, you could ask your obstetrician for a consultation with another doctor. That doctor should be a highly skilled obstetrician at a hospital that performs a large number of deliveries and has a low rate of c-sections. Even after an otherwise perfect pregnancy, emergencies requiring a c-section can develop. That's why it is so important to have the right obstetrician from the start.

Compare statistics in Step 4.

American College of Obstetrics and Gynecology This group will send patient-education pamphlets and a list of local members. You should include a self-addressed stamped envelope.

409 12th St SW
Washington, DC 20024
202/638-5577

International Cesarean Awareness Network Inc. (I CAN) This organization holds monthly support group meetings, organizes symposia, and publishes a quarterly newsletter, "The Clairion." The national organization can refer you to a chapter in your area.

PO Box 152
Syracuse, NY 13210
315/424-1942

NIH CRISP System
301/496-7543

University-Affiliated Hospitals See Appendix.

Step 3. Choose a Hospital

The best way to avoid an inappropriate c-section is to deliver at a hospital that has a low rate of c-sections for the first and subsequent deliveries. You should make a list of the possible hospitals based on proximity, convenience, your physician's recommendations, and your personal preference. Include a university-affiliated teaching hospital as well as nearby community hospitals, then compare results. Your community hospital may be an excellent choice, as long as it compares favorably to the top-rated university center.

Some top university hospitals may have a higher-than-normal c-section rate because they accept referrals of high-risk women with problem deliveries. First look for a hospital with a high volume of normal deliveries. The hospital need not have a high number of c-sections. If the number is low, you are less likely to have one performed unnecessarily. Consider the overall quality of the obstetrical service and then the percentage of c-sections. You don't want to go to a second-rate hospital just because it performs few c-sections. Although many public hospitals have low c-section rates, some are just trying to save money. These public hospitals can wait too long to intervene, thus endangering mother and child.

Here are the performance figures you should look for.

Experience

Minimum: 1,500 live births a year

Ideal: More than 2,500 deliveries a year

Other Measures of Excellence

PERCENTAGE OF TOTAL DELIVERIES THAT ARE C-SECTIONS

University-Affiliated Hospital   The rate should be no higher than 17%, unless the hospital treats a large number of complicated cases or has a neonatal intensive care unit.

Medium-Sized Hospital   The rate should not exceed 10–12%. If it does, you should ask for an explanation.

Community Hospital   The rate should be no higher than 7%, because community hospitals see few high-risk patients.

PERCENTAGE OF REPEAT C-SECTIONS   You should also consider the rate of repeat c-sections that are performed, because that is a good indication that the procedure is used inappropriately. Ideally, the rate of repeat c-sections should be about 60–70%, though repeats are done in some hospitals more often than in others. Here is a general ranking of the percentage of repeat c-sections by hospital category.

RANK	HOSPITAL TYPE	PERCENTAGE
Highest	For-profit hospital	More than 95%
Very high	Private nonprofit hospital	92%
High	County hospitals	76%
Moderate	University-affiliated teaching hospital (based on a study of five facilities)	71%

Look for these other measures of excellence in your obstetrics unit of choice.

■ In-house training program for obstetrics

■ Board-certified anesthesiologist with wide experience in c-sections available in the hospital 24 hours a day

■ Neonatal pediatric specialists in the hospital 24 hours a day

■ Specially equipped and staffed nursery designated as "level II"

■ "Trial of labor" for patients who have had a previous c-section (if so, ask for the percentage of women who deliver vaginally)

- Fetal blood sampling or a fetal stimulation test, if electronic monitoring suggests the fetus is in trouble, for confirmation (at least one of these tests should be performed prior to a c-section, unless a serious emergency exists)

- Policy of requiring a second opinion before a nonemergency c-section (a second opinion has been shown to lower the number of c-sections)

- Specific policies to help prevent unnecessary c-sections

- Length of hospital stay: 4.5 days

- Average hospital charge: $4,771

There is, unfortunately, no list at present for centers of excellence for the *prevention* of c-sections.

Centers of Excellence for Gynecology

The following list of hospitals is provided only as a convenient starting place in your search for excellence. These hospitals are recommended on the basis of reputation, not experience and results. The list is not an endorsement. There may be hospitals just as excellent that have been omitted. You should apply the guidelines for experience, results, and other measures of excellence to any hospital you choose, whether or not it is on this list. Although hospitals from different sources have been combined into one list, the compilation in no way implies that one source has endorsed the hospital list of another source. Because none of the professional organizations or the doctors asked could provide a list of the best obstetrics hospitals, you may want to ask one of these hospitals where they recommend you go. To make your choice, apply the rules of thumb just presented.

ALABAMA
University of South Alabama
　　Medical Center BIM
2451 Fillingim St
Mobile, AL 36617
(Special interests: fertility
　　problems, endocrinology)

ARIZONA
University of Arizona Health
　　Sciences Center BIM
1501 N Campbell Ave
Tucson, AZ 85724

CALIFORNIA
Los Angeles County and University
　　of Southern California
　　Medical Center US
1200 State St
Los Angeles, CA 90033

University of California, Irvine,
　　Medical Center BIM
101 City Drive, S
Orange, CA 92668
(Special interests: fertility
　　problems, high-risk pregnancy,
　　cancer surgery)

University of California,
  Los Angeles, Medical Center   BIM/US
10833 Le Conte Ave
Los Angeles, CA 90024
(Special interests: fertility problems,
  high-risk pregnancy, cancer surgery)

CONNECTICUT
Yale–New Haven Hospital   BIM
333 Cedar St
New Haven, CT 06510
(Special interests: fertility
  problems, cancer surgery,
  high-risk pregnancy)

FLORIDA
University of Miami Affiliated
  Hospitals   BIM
1475 NW 12th Ave
Miami, FL 33136
(Special interests: high-risk
  pregnancy, cancer surgery,
  fertility programs)

ILLINOIS
Prentice Women's Hospital and
  Maternity Center   BIM
250 E Superior St
Chicago, IL 30311
(Special interests: high-risk
  pregnancy, surgical gynecology)

MARYLAND
Johns Hopkins Hospital   US
600 N Wolfe St
Baltimore, MD 21205

MASSACHUSETTS
Brigham and Women's Hospital   BIM/US
75 Francis St
Boston, MA 02115
(Special interests: fertility
  problems, high-risk pregnancy)

Massachusetts General Hospital   US
55 Fruit St
Boston, MA 02114

MICHIGAN
University of Michigan Hospitals   BIM
1500 E Medical Center Dr
Ann Arbor, MI 48109
(Special interests: fertility
  problems, cancer surgery)

MINNESOTA
Mayo Clinic   US
200 First St SW
Rochester, MN 55905

MISSISSIPPI
University Hospital   BIM
2500 N State St
Jackson, MS 39216
(Special interests: high-risk
  pregnancy, cancer surgery)

NEW YORK
Columbia-Presbyterian
  Medical Center   US
622 W 168th St
New York, NY 10032

Memorial Sloan-Kettering
  Cancer Center   US
1275 York Ave
New York, NY 10021

Mt. Sinai Hospital   BIM
One Gustav Levy Pl
New York, NY 10029
(Special interests: fertility
  problems, cancer surgery)

NORTH CAROLINA
Duke University Hospital   US
Box 3708
Durham, NC 27710

OHIO
Cleveland Clinic Foundation   US
One Clinic Center
9500 Euclid Ave
Cleveland, OH 44195

Ohio State University Hospitals   BIM
410 W Tenth Ave
Columbus, OH 43210
(Special interests: fertility
    problems, high-risk pregnancy)

PENNSYLVANIA
Hospital of the University
    of Pennsylvania   BIM
3400 Spruce St
Philadelphia, PA 19104
(Special interests: fertility
    problems, high-risk pregnancy,
    cancer surgery)

TENNESSEE
Vanderbilt University Hospital   BIM
1211 22nd Ave SW
Nashville, TN 37232
(Special interest: cancer surgery)

TEXAS
M. D. Anderson Cancer Center   US
University of Texas
1515 Holcombe Blvd
Houston, TX 77030

Parkland Memorial Hospital   BIM
5201 Harry Hines Blvd
Dallas, TX 75235
(Special interests: high-risk
    pregnancy, fertility problems)

VIRGINIA
University of Virginia Hospital   BIM
Jefferson Park Ave
Charlottesville, VA 22908
(Special interests: high-risk
    pregnancy, cancer surgery)

SOURCES
BIM   indicates those hospitals recommended in *The Best in Medicine.*
US   indicates those hospitals recommended in *U.S. News & World Report.*

Step 4. Choose a Doctor

Your doctor should be board-certified in obstetrics and gynecology, which means she or he has completed a four-year residency program in those fields and passed a national examination. Though for some procedures your doctor should have performed a certain volume to demonstrate proficiency, there is no absolute numerical requirement for c-sections. Although your doctor should have performed a high volume of c-sections, the overall percentage rate should be low, and in line with the previous figures for hospitals (see Step 3). If she or he has a low-risk community-based practice, the rate should be about 7%, with a high-risk practice it should be about 17%. These figures, provided by the Public Citizen Health Research Group, indicate a doctor who has wide experience but operates judiciously.

During your regular prenatal visits you also can ask about your doctor's views on appropriate indications for c-sections.

■ Does the doctor offer a "trial of labor" to women who have had a previous c-section? If so, what percentage deliver vaginally? It should be 60–70% or higher.

■ Does the doctor use fetal blood sampling or fetal stimulation techniques if electronic monitoring suggests fetal distress, prior to performing a c-section? Ideally both of these tests should be done. You can also inquire about the use of a fetoscope or strip monitoring as an alternative to electronic monitoring.

■ Does the doctor consider an independent second opinion for elective c-sections good medical practice?

■ Does the doctor perform external cephalic version (turning the baby) after 37 weeks if the baby lies in breech position?

■ Does the doctor have a set time for labor and second-stage pushing? Sometimes c-sections can be avoided if an epidural or other anesthesia that slows labor is allowed to wear off and the mother can resume pushing.

EXPERT SOURCES

Although dozens of experts were interviewed for these chapters, Dr. Edward J. Quilligan, Co-Editor in Chief of the *American Journal of Obstetrics and Gynecology,* Past Dean of the University of California, Irvine, School of Medicine, Professor of Obstetrics and Gynecology, University of California, Irvine, Medical Center, Irvine, CA, is acknowledged for his significant contribution to this section.

REFERENCES AND SUGGESTED READING

Benson, Michael D. *Obstetrical Pearls. A Practical Guide for the Efficient Resident.* Philadelphia: F. A. Davis Co., 1989.

Gabbe, S. G., and others (editors). *Obstetrics: Normal and Problem Pregnancies.* New York: Churchill Livingstone Press, 1991.

Hausknecht, R., and Heilman, J. R. *Having a Cesarean Baby: A Complete Guide for a Happy and Safe Cesarean Childbirth Experience.* New York: Plume Books, 1982.

Miller, J. Maternal and Neonatal Morbidity and Mortality in Cesarean Section. *Obstetrics and Gynecology Clinics of North America,* Vol. 15 (1988), p. 629.

Parnes, La Sala A., and Berkeley, A. Primary Cesarean Section and Subsequent Fertility. *American Journal of Obstetrics and Gynecology,* Vol. 157 (1987), p.379.

Petitti, D. B. Maternal Mortality and Morbidity in Cesarean Section. *Clinical Obstetrics and Gynecology,* Vol. 28 (1985), pp. 735–744.

Principles and Practice of Medical Therapy in Pregnancy. *Annals of Internal Medicine,* Vol.116, No. 5 (Mar. 1, 1992), p. 430.

Silver, Lynn, and Wolfe, Sidney M. *Unnecessary Cesarean Sections: How to Cure a National Epidemic.* Public Citizen Health Research Group, 1989.

Stafford, R. S. Alternative Strategies for Controlling Rising Cesarean Section Rates. *Journal of the American Medical Association,* Vol. 263, No. 5 (Feb. 2, 1990), pp. 683–687.

Taffel, S., and others. Trends in the United States Cesarean Section Rate and Reasons for the 1980–1985 Rise. *American Journal of Public Health,* Vol. 77 (1987), pp. 955–959.

Wolfe, Sidney M. *Women's Health Alert.* Reading, Mass.: Addison-Wesley, 1991.

Hysterectomy

Likelihood of Unnecessary Surgery **EXTREMELY HIGH**

Hysterectomy is the second most frequently performed operation in the United States. (Cesarean section ranks first.) The National Center for Health Statistics calculated that 591,000 were performed in 1990. The American College of Obstetrics and Gynecology estimates that one in three women will have a hysterectomy by age 60.

Critics claim that far too many hysterectomies are unnecessary. The estimate of unnecessary hysterectomies varies tremendously. The Public Citizen Health Research Group in Washington, D.C., contends that 25% (150,000 hysterectomies) a year are inappropriate, accounting for the single biggest waste of dollars in the medical system. The research organization Value Health Sciences, in Santa Monica, Calif., estimates that between 25% and 30% are inappropriate. Hysterectomy Educational Resources and Services, an educational organization in Bala-Cynwyd, Penna., found that 98% of the 54,000 women who consulted them did not need the operation. Too many women decide quickly on a hysterectomy without adequate consideration of the alternatives.

In 1991, the research firm MediQual reported that 52.67% of hysterectomies they studied had none of the objective clinical findings documented in the hospital medical record they use to validate hysterectomy at the time of surgery. (These were subtotal abdominal hysterectomies.)

Dr. Francis L. Hutchins Jr., Director of Gynecology and Women's Services at the Graduate Hospital in Philadelphia, warns patients to beware of doctors who make a diagnosis of pelvic relaxation and then recommend surgery when no symptoms are present.

You are more likely to have an unnecessary hysterectomy if you live in certain regions of the country. For instance, 80% more hysterectomies are performed in the South than in the Northeast, Midwest, or West. (The lowest numbers are in the Northeast.) Large differences exist even among hospitals in the same state (300% difference in Vermont, for example), in the frequency of the operation.

Potential Risk **MODERATE**

Hysterectomy is major surgery with complications in up to half of all patients. Between 8% and 15% of patients require blood transfusions, which carry the small risk of contracting blood-borne diseases such as hepatitis and AIDS. Since this is virtually always an elective procedure, you should consider donating your own blood. It is estimated that repeat surgery for complications related to the original hysterectomy is necessary in as many as 15% of patients.

The other risks include:

- Damage to surrounding organs, such as the bowel and ureter

- Infection

- Persistent pain

- Psychological stress

- Bleeding

- Incontinence

- Diminished sexual response

- Complications of general anesthesia

- Death

Your chance of dying is directly related to your age, increasing from 1 in 1,000 before the age of 45 to 2 in 1,000 between ages 45 and 65 and to 20 in 1,000 after age 65. According to the American College of Obstetrics and Gynecology, 600 women a year die as a result of complications following hysterectomies.

Many doctors believe that the risks are far too serious to justify an operation that is not absolutely necessary—and hysterectomy rarely is when cancer is not involved. Dr. Hutchins warns: "Curing a pelvic disease with a hysterectomy is the equivalent of treating a mild headache with decapitation. Treat the disease, don't get rid of the organ."

What It Is

A hysterectomy is the surgical removal of the uterus or womb. A separate operation, called an oophorectomy, may be done at the same time to remove the ovaries. The two are performed simultaneously in about 41% of cases, according to the National Center for Health Statistics. After the operation a woman stops menstruating and is no longer capable of conceiving. If the ovaries are removed, the long-term risks increase for women who have not yet undergone menopause and are unable to take replacement estrogen therapy. These risks include osteoporosis and heart disease.

The Framingham Heart Study showed a three-fold increase in the risk of heart disease among premenopausal women who had the operation. Here's an intriguing reason why: The uterus produces prostacyclin, the most potent known inhibitor of blood clots. With that protection erased by removing the uterus, blood is more likely to clot and could be a factor in causing heart attack.

Step 1. Make Sure You Need the Surgery

A very good rule of thumb is that an operation should be performed only after nonsurgical treatments have failed and only if it can prolong life and has a reasonable chance of success. Hysterectomy does not usually meet these criteria. While nearly 200,000 hysterectomies were performed in 1987 to remove cancer, the remaining operations could not be considered truly life-saving. Fully 90% were intended to relieve symptoms, not to save lives. In short, if hysterectomy is suggested, you needn't rush to surgery. According to the American College of Obstetrics and Gynecology and the National Center for Health Statistics, the most common reasons for the operation were:

REASON	NUMBER OF HYSTERECTOMIES
Endometrial hyperplasia	114,000
Fibroids	593,000
Endometriosis	372,000
Prolapse	318,000
Other	372,000

Before you agree to a hysterectomy, see if your diagnosis matches the conditions in the following lists.

Appropriate Procedure

- Cancer of the uterus

- Very large fibroids that press on and injure other organs or are associated with recurrent hemorrhaging and anemia

- Severe prolapse of the uterus so that it extends out of the birth canal (seen in women who have given birth to many children)

Possibly an Appropriate Procedure After Failure of Other Treatment

- Fibroids

- Tumors

- Uterine prolapse

- Endometriosis

- Endometrial hyperplasia

- Abnormal bleeding that has not been controlled by other therapy

- Pain caused by conditions in the uterus

Probably Not an Appropriate Procedure

- Minimal or asymptomatic fibroids, especially if no previous therapy has been tried

Not an Appropriate Procedure

- No alternative medical treatments tried yet

- Vague symptoms

- Pain of uncertain origin (thirty percent of such patients will continue to experience pain after surgery, according to Dr. Francis L. Hutchins Jr)

- Asymptomatic fibroids

Step 2. Consider an Alternative

Before undergoing surgery you should try a number of alternative medical treatments. Many of those therapies are highly effective. The key to avoiding surgery is to see a physician who is knowledgeable about your problem. Here are some alternative therapies you should consider, for a sample of four conditions.

Condition: Fibroids

MEDICAL TREATMENT   Gonadotropin-releasing hormone (GnRh). (FDA approval pending.)

WHAT IT DOES   GnRh temporarily shuts down estrogen production, which can shrink fibroids by 50%. Patients take GnRh either by monthly injections or by twice-daily nasal spray. While the fibroids will grow back after treatment is discontinued, relief from the pain and other symptoms may be long-lasting.

ALTERNATIVE SURGICAL TREATMENT   Myomectomy, Endometrial Ablation.

WHAT IT DOES   Tumors are removed, leaving the uterus itself intact.

Condition: Endometriosis

MEDICAL TREATMENT   GnRh, progestins or synthetic progesterones, testosterone (male sex hormone), Danazol.

WHAT IT DOES   Each of these four medications temporarily reduces the level of estrogen hormones, which stimulate the growth of endometrial tissue, either by counteracting the estrogen in the body or suppressing ovarian function. Each has side effects.

ALTERNATIVE SURGICAL TREATMENT   Conservative surgery.

WHAT IT DOES   Removes only the tissue that is causing immediate symptoms, such as pain, and the uterus remains intact.

Condition: Bleeding

MEDICAL TREATMENT   Progesterone.

WHAT IT DOES   This drug can slow or stop bleeding without surgery.

ALTERNATIVE PROCEDURE   Endometrial ablation. Gynecologists view the inside of the uterus by using a special scope. They "burn away" the lining of the uterus. This is an outpatient procedure.

WHAT IT DOES   Removes sites of bleeding.

Condition: Prolapse of Uterus/Pelvic Relaxation

MEDICAL TREATMENT   Estrogen.

WHAT IT DOES   Estrogen can reduce pressure symptoms and incontinence and improve vaginal support.

CONSERVATIVE TREATMENT   Vaginal pessary.

WHAT IT DOES   Reduces pressure symptoms.

CONSERVATIVE TREATMENT   Biofeedback.

WHAT IT DOES   Manages incontinence related to pelvic relaxation.

CONSERVATIVE TREATMENT   Kegel exercise.

WHAT IT DOES   Improves vaginal support and reduces incontinence.

Step 3. Get a Specialist's Opinion

You will need an expert opinion if a hysterectomy has been recommended. You should seek a second opinion from a doctor who treats similar cases and is qualified to review that recommendation and your diagnosis. The best choice would be a gynecologist who fulfills these criteria:

- Board-certified in gynecology

- Specializes in your condition (for instance, a reproductive endocrinologist for endometriosis; a gynecological oncologist for cancer)

- On staff at a university-affiliated teaching hospital

- Performs pelvic surgeries several times a week—*not* hysterectomies (Pelvic surgery gives the surgeon the experience needed; if he or she does a large number of hysterectomies and is not a cancer surgeon, they may be inappropriate surgeries.)

It's possible that your insurer may be unwilling to pay for alternative therapy. For instance, an insurer may pay for a hysterectomy but not for a minor operation to remove fibroids. If that's the case, you must be prepared to fight for the treatment that is best for you. The following organizations can help you in that fight.

WHO TO CALL

Hysterectomy Educational Resources and Services (HERS) hotline　This group offers patient information about alternatives to surgery, emotional and psychological support, and doctor referrals. HERS has individual counselors available to discuss your case.

422 Bryn Mawr Ave
Bala-Cynwyd, PA 19004
215/387-6700

Endometriosis Association　This self-help organization, with crisis counselors on call, provides extensive information about hysterectomies.

8585 North 76th Pl
Milwaukee, WI 53223
800/992-3636　in the United States
800/426-2363　in Canada

Step 4. Choose a Hospital

Though you can have a hysterectomy at a community hospital, you should make sure it has a surgical intensive care unit and a physician available 24 hours a day to respond to emergencies. The surgical team should consist of surgeon, first assistant, anesthesiologist, scrub nurse, and circulating nurse. One of our experts warned: Beware of big-name hospitals and university-affiliated hospitals: You're just as likely to be gutted and filleted there as elsewhere.

Experience

This is one type of surgery in which you are not looking for a large number of operations, because so many are inappropriate. You do want to make sure the hospital you choose is experienced in pelvic surgery, performing at least several hundred pelvic operations a year. Since the most appropriate reason for a hysterectomy is cancer, you should seek a hospital with an excellent department of gynecological oncology or one that is a designated National Cancer Institute Center (see Centers of Excellence for Cancer in the Cancer chapter).

Results

DEATH RATE   For abdominal hysterectomy (11,238 cases) 0.2% is the average. Your hospital's results should compare favorably. For vaginal hysterectomy (4,124 cases) the average is 0.02%. Your hospital's results should compare favorably.

Other Measures of Excellence

LENGTH OF STAY   Patients should not need lengthy hospitalizations. The normal stay for uncomplicated hysterectomy should be three to five days. Make sure to ask your doctor how long his or her patients usually remain hospitalized. The following data, provided by MediQual, are averages.

	ABDOMINAL HYSTERECTOMY	VAGINAL HYSTERECTOMY
Length of stay	5 days	4.1 days
Charges	$5,888	$4,736

Centers of Excellence for Gynecology

The following list of hospitals is provided only as a convenient starting place in your search for excellence. These hospitals are recommended on the basis of reputation, not experience and results. The list is not an endorsement. There may be hospitals just as excellent that have been omitted. You should apply the guidelines for experience, results, and other measures of excellence to any hospital you choose, whether or not it is on this list. Although hospitals from different sources have been combined into one list, the compilation in no way implies that one source has endorsed the hospital list of another source.

ALABAMA

University of South Alabama
　Medical Center　　　　　　BIM
2451 Fillingim St
Mobile, AL 36617
(Special interests: fertility problems,
　endocrinology)

ARIZONA

University of Arizona Health
　Sciences Center　　　　　　BIM
1501 North Campbell Ave
Tucson, AZ 85724

CALIFORNIA

Los Angeles County and
　University of Southern
　California Medical Center　　US
1200 State St
Los Angeles, CA 90033

University of California, Irvine,
　Medical Center　　　　　　BIM
101 City Drive S
Orange, CA 92668
(Special interests: fertility problems,
　high-risk pregnancy, cancer surgery)

University of California, Los
　Angeles, Medical Center　　BIM/US
10833 Le Conte Ave
Los Angeles, CA 90024
(Special interests: fertility problems,
　high-risk pregnancy, cancer surgery)

CONNECTICUT

Yale–New Haven Hospital　　BIM
333 Cedar St
New Haven, CT 06510
(Special interests: fertility problems,
　cancer surgery, high-risk pregnancy)

FLORIDA

University of Miami Affiliated
　Hospitals　　　　　　　　BIM
1475 NW 12th Ave
Miami, FL 33136
(Special interests: high-risk pregnancy,
　cancer surgery, fertility programs)

ILLINOIS

Prentice Women's Hospital and
　Maternity Center　　　　　BIM
250 E Superior St
Chicago, IL 30311
(Special interests: high-risk pregnancy,
　surgical gynecology)

MARYLAND

Johns Hopkins Hospital　　　US
600 No Wolfe St
Baltimore, MD 21205

MASSACHUSETTS

Brigham and Women's
　Hospital　　　　　　　　BIM/US
75 Francis St
Boston, MA 02115
(Special interests: fertility problems.
　high-risk pregnancy)

Massachusetts General Hospital　US
55 Fruit St
Boston, MA 02114

MICHIGAN

University of Michigan Hospitals　BIM
1500 E Medical Center Dr
Ann Arbor, MI 48109
(Special interests: fertility problems,
　cancer surgery)

MINNESOTA us
Mayo Clinic
200 First St SW
Rochester, MN 55905

MISSISSIPPI
University Hospital BIM
2500 No State St
Jackson, MS 39216
(Special interests: high-risk
    pregnancy, cancer surgery)

NEW YORK
Columbia-Presbyterian
    Medical Center us
622 W 168th St
New York, NY 10032

Memorial Sloan-Kettering
    Cancer Center us
1275 York Ave
New York, NY 10021

Mt. Sinai Hospital BIM
One Gustav Levy Pl
New York, NY 10029
(Special interests: fertility
    problems, cancer surgery)

NORTH CAROLINA
Duke University Hospital us
Box 3708
Durham, NC 27710

OHIO
Cleveland Clinic Foundation us
One Clinic Center
9500 Euclid Ave
Cleveland, Ohio 44195

Ohio State University Hospitals BIM
410 W Tenth Ave
Columbus, OH 43210
(Special interests: fertility problems,
    high-risk pregnancy)

PENNSYLVANIA
Hospital of the University of
    Pennsylvania BIM
3400 Spruce St
Philadelphia, PA 19104
(Special interests: fertility
    problems, high-risk
    pregnancy, cancer surgery

TENNESSEE
Vanderbilt University Hospital BIM
1211 22nd Ave SW
Nashville, TN 37232
(Special interest: cancer surgery)

TEXAS
M. D. Anderson Cancer Center us
University of Texas
1515 Holcombe Blvd
Houston, TX 77030

Parkland Memorial Hospital BIM
5201 Harry Hines Blvd
Dallas, TX 75235
(Special interests: high-risk
    pregnancy, fertility problems)

VIRGINIA
University of Virginia Hospital BIM
Jefferson Park Ave
Charlottesville, VA 22908
(Special interests: high-risk
    pregnancy, cancer surgery)

SOURCES

BIM indicates those hospitals recommended in *The Best in Medicine.*
us indicates those hospitals recommended in *U.S. News & World Report.*

Step 5. Choose a Doctor

A hysterectomy should not be performed by a general surgeon. The doctor should be an experienced gynecological surgeon who has completed a four-year residency program and is board-certified in the field. In addition, look for the following.

Experience

The surgeon should perform pelvic or gynecological surgery several times a week.

Results

DEATH RATE   The mortality rate should not exceed one or two per 1,000, according to the National Center for Health Statistics.

EXPERT SOURCES

Although dozens of experts were interviewed for these chapters, Dr. Francis L. Hutchins Jr., Director, Division of Gynecology and Women's Services, Graduate Hospital, Philadelphia, PA, is acknowledged for his significant contributions to this section.

REFERENCES AND SUGGESTED READING

American College of Obstetricians and Gynecologists. *Quality Assurance in Obstetrics and Gynecology: Guidelines.* May 1989.

Ballweg, Mary Lou, and others. *Overcoming Endometriosis: New Help from the Endometriosis Association.* Chicago: Congdon & Weed, 1987.

Bloomfield, Thomas. Endometrial Resection or Abdominal Hysterectomy in Menorrhagia? [letter] *British Medical Journal,* Vol. 304, No. 6819 (Jan. 11, 1992), pp. 120–121.

Clisham, P. Ronald, and others. Long-Term Transdermal Estradiol Therapy: Effects on Endometrial Histology and Bleeding Patterns. *Obstetrics and Gynecology,* Vol. 79, No.2 (Feb. 1992), pp. 196–201.

Gabbe, S. G., and others (editors). *Obstetrics: Normal and Problem Pregnancies.* New York: Churchill Livingstone Press, 1991.

Gambone, J. C., and others. The Impact of a Quality Assurance Process on the Frequency and Confirmation Rate of Hysterectomy. *American Journal of Obstetrics and Gynecology,* Vol. 163 (1990), pp. 545–550.

Goldfarb, H. A., and Greif, J. *The No-Hysterectomy Option: Your Body—Your Choice.* New York: Wiley, 1990.

Massachusetts Medical Society. Hysterectomy Prevalence and Death Rates for Cervical Cancer—United States, 1965–1988. *Morbidity and Mortality Weekly Report (MMWR)*, Vol. 41, No. 2 (Jan. 17, 1992), pp. 17–20.

Miller, Karl E., and others. Office Procedures: Evaluation and Follow-Up of Abnormal Pap Smears. *American Family Physician*, Vol. 45, No. 1 (Jan. 1992), pp. 143–150.

Parazzini, Fabio, and others. Oral Contraceptive Use and Risk of Uterine Fibroids. *Obstetrics and Gynecology*, Vol. 79, No. 3 (Mar. 1992), pp. 430–433.

Pitkin, Roy M. Operative Laparoscopy: Surgical Advance or Technical Gimmick? *Obstetrics and Gynecology*, Vol. 79, No.3 (Mar. 1992) pp. 441–442.

Pokras, Robert. Hysterectomy: Past, Present, Future. *Statistical Bulletin*, Vol. 70, No. 4 (Oct.-Dec. 1989).

Rankin, G. L. S. Laparoscopically Assisted Vaginal Hysterectomy. [letter to the editor] *Lancet*, Vol. 339, No. 8791 (Feb. 22, 1992), p. 501.

Reiter, R. C., and Gambone, J. C. Demographic and Historic Variables in Women with Idiopathic Chronic Pelvic Pain. *Obstetrics and Gynecology*, Vol. 75 (1990), pp. 428–432.

Roos, N. P. Hysterectomies in One Canadian Province: A New Look at Risks and Benefits. *American Journal of Public Health*, Vol. 74 (1984), pp. 39–46.

Studd, John. The Change. Women, Ageing and the Menopause. [book review] *British Journal of Obstetrics and Gynecology*, Vol. 99, No. 1 (Jan. 1992), p. 86.

Wolfe, Sidney M. *Women's Health Alert*. Reading, Mass.: Addison-Wesley, 1991.

Wright, Thomas C., Jr., and others. Treatment of Cervical Intraepithelial Neoplasia Using the Loop Electrosurgical Excision Procedure. *Obstetrics and Gynecology*, Vol. 79, No. 2 (Feb. 1992), pp. 173–178.

Gallbladder Surgery

Likelihood of Unnecessary Surgery   MODERATE

In 1991 the research firm MediQual reported that 9.20% of cholecystectomies (surgical excisions of the gallbladder) they studied had none of the objective clinical findings documented in the hospital medical record they use to validate the operation at the time of surgery, meaning that neither gallstones nor evidence of gallbladder disease was found. But the paradox is that you may be more likely to have an inappropriate operation if you *do* have gallstones. Here's why: Lots of us have gallstones that cause us no harm and that don't require surgery. Then we develop another illness, completely unrelated to our gallbladders. When routine tests show gallstones, we have our gallbladders out, even though in reality the gallstones had nothing to do with our symptoms!

Potential Risk   MODERATE

Nearly 500,000 gallbladder operations are performed each year in the United States. Gallbladder removal is the "meat and potatoes" of most general surgeons. But a cholecystectomy is still major surgery, and major complications can result:

- Damage to the common bile duct or blood vessels in the bowel

- Infection

- Collapsed lung

Death occurs most frequently in patients who have cardiovascular disease. If you are over age 40, your doctor should take a careful medical history and order an electrocardiogram before surgery to check for the presence of heart disease.

The operation is more dangerous in patients who also have pancreatitis or diabetes. Doctors are still debating the relative increase in risk for people with diabetes, although many surgeons believe that all diabetic patients with symptoms of gallbladder disorder should undergo surgery, because the likelihood of serious complications from gallstones later on is substantial.

What It Is

During an open cholecystectomy the surgeon makes an incision under the rib cage on the right-hand side of the abdomen, and retracts the liver to expose the gallbladder. The surrounding membrane is cut so the cystic duct and the artery supplying the gallbladder are displayed. After the artery and the cystic duct are tied off and severed, the gallbladder is removed. In a patient who has jaundice, x-rays are taken to see if stones are present in the common bile duct. If so, they are removed also. Up to 10% of patients will have stones remaining in the bile ducts after such bile duct surgery. Drains may be inserted under the liver and in the bile duct, if necessary, before the abdominal incision is closed. The drains are removed two to ten days later.

Step 1. Make Sure You Need the Procedure

Between 10 and 20% of adults will develop gallstones during their lifetimes. Some people have an especially high risk for this condition.

Risk Factors

The risk factors include:

- Increasing age

- Being a female

- Native American or Mexican American background

- Obesity

- Use of clofibrate, estrogens, and certain other drugs

- Prolonged total parenteral nutrition (nutrition delivered entirely through an intravenous line)

- Ileal disease (for instance, Crohn's disease)

- Operations that resect or bypass parts of the small bowel

- Chronic red blood cell destruction

- Cirrhosis

Symptoms of Gallstones

Before surgery is recommended, your doctor should take a comprehensive medical history to determine if gallstones are present. The symptoms are fairly precise. Pain occurs in the right upper quadrant of the chest about 15–60 minutes after eating, particularly if the meal has included foods high in fat. The pain may be present also in the abdomen or precordium surrounding the heart and radiate around the back. About 75% of patients have intermittent pain. Nausea or vomiting may occur. Dyspeptic symptoms occur in 80% of patients.

TESTS TO DETECT GALLSTONES Your doctor may use one of the following tests to detect gallstones:

■ Ultrasound (98% accurate)

■ Oral cholecystography (generally 95% accurate, but unreliable in patients with acute abdominal illness or jaundice)

■ Plain x-rays (only 15% of gallstones are calcified and therefore visible)

■ Bilirubin (if elevated, common bile duct cholangiography should be performed intraoperatively)

■ IDA (imino diacetic acid) scan (images provide strong evidence for cystic duct obstruction; most helpful in cases of suspected acute cholecystitis (infection))

You should match your diagnosis against the most frequent reasons for the procedure given in the following list.

Appropriate Procedure

Emergencies These include accumulation of pus, perforation and emphysematous cholecystitis (a condition caused by gas-producing organisms that invade the gall bladder and often infiltrate the surrounding tissues).

Acute Cholecystitis This condition occurs when a stone lodges in the cystic duct and prevents the gallbladder from emptying, resulting in inflammation and the risk of bacterial infection. The usual symptoms are:

■ History of biliary colic (75% of cases)

■ Persistent pain, tenderness, and spasm in upper right quadrant

■ High white blood cell count (usual range: 12,000–15,000 or higher)

■ Nausea or vomiting (50% of cases)

■ Fever (38.5° C or higher)

■ Murphy's sign (doctor palpates upper right quadrant as patient takes deep breath; if acute cholecystitis present, the pain will cause patient to interrupt the deep breath)

■ Enlarged, tender gallbladder, sometimes visible (35% of cases)

- Mild jaundice (10% of cases)

- Gallstones (95% of cases)

- Mildly elevated bilirubin

- Possibly elevated serum amylase

PROPHYLACTIC CHOLECYSTECTOMY   Certain patients with an abnormally high risk for complications from gallstones benefit from prophylactic cholecystectomy. This may be recommended for:

- American Indians, who have a high rate of gallbladder cancer

- Diabetics

- Patients with large gallstones, multiple tiny stones, or calcified stones

- The elderly

- Patients at high risk for gallbladder cancer (who often have a calcified gallbladder)

Probably Not an Appropriate Procedure

Asymptomatic Patients   Only about 2% of patients with "silent" gallstones will develop actual symptoms. Since gallstones in themselves are not life-threatening and every operation carries the risk of death, most doctors feel the operation should not be performed in these cases—unless it can be done safely at the time of an operation for another condition.

Step 2. Consider an Alternative

Alternative Procedures

LAPAROSCOPIC CHOLECYSTECTOMY   This is the preferred alternative, since the gallbladder is removed without major abdominal surgery, lowering the risks and substantially shortening recovery time. Up to 80% of nonemergency gallbladder removal is accomplished laparoscopically. This is now the procedure of choice.

In emergencies, however, it is used only about 25% of the time, primarily because of the additional skill required. Since this surgery is considered state-of-the-art, your doctor should have a good reason for not recommending it. There are several reasons why it may not be suggested, including prior upper abdominal surgery and obesity, which make the procedure technically impossible. Only a few surgeons are able to perform the laparoscopic cholecystectomy when any of the following conditions is present:

- Acute cholecystitis (an acute gallbladder attack)

- Jaundice (yellowish skin color)

- CBD (common bile duct) stones

- Pancreatitis

- Thick gallbladder wall as determined on ultrasound

- Severe cardiac and respiratory insufficiency

If possible, the operation should be avoided entirely, according to Dr. Philip S. Barie, Director of the Surgical Intensive Care Unit, New York Hospital–Cornell Medical Center in New York City, by patients with these conditions:

- Cirrhosis

- Coagulopathy (bleeding disorder)

- Respiratory insufficiency

- Pregnancy

CHOLECYSTOSTOMY   This procedure drains infection and sometimes removes gallstones but not the gallbladder. It is usually done for the following conditions:

- Acute cholecystitis in an unstable patient

- During another operation when a diseased gallbladder is found

- Inflammation so severe that the gallbladder can't be located or safely removed

- Elderly and poor-risk patients

LITHOTRIPSY   In this alternative treatment, sound waves are used to break up the gallstones, with the fragments then passed in the feces. Medicine is prescribed afterwards to dissolve the stone fragments and to prevent the formation of new stones. Only about 6–15% of patients are eligible for this procedure; and an even smaller percentage actually opt for it. A number of factors limit its use, including infection and the type, size, and number of stones. This procedure has largely fallen out of favor.

ENDOSCOPIC PAPILLOTOMY   In this procedure an endoscope is inserted into the throat and through the stomach to the opening where the bile duct empties into the duodenum. The endoscope is used to widen this opening so that the stones have a better chance of passing into the intestinal tract and out of the body. Sometimes a wire basket or snare attached to the end of the endoscope is employed to grab the stones and pull them into the intestine. This procedure is useful only for removing stones in the bile ducts. Since it can't help remove stones from the gallbladder, the procedure is not a true alternative to open cholecystectomy.

Little research has been done on its effectiveness. Some doctors believe the treatment can help for only a few weeks. But it can buy time for some individuals, for instance, an 89-year-old patient with pancreatitis and a heart attack who needs the surgery but is too fragile to survive.

Medications

Medications are a reasonable choice for those who must avoid surgery for medical reasons. An older individual with severe heart and lung disease, for example, may pose too high an operative risk.

URSODEOXYCHOLIC ACID   This oral medication acts to dissolve stones. It has an overall 35% success rate, with numerous stones reforming within two to three years. It can't be prescribed if any of these following conditions hold:

- Pigment stones

- Cystic duct obstruction

- Large, calcified, common duct stones

- Severe symptoms

- Pregnancy, actual or planned

CHENODIOL   This drug allows the normal cholesterol-dissolving mechanisms in the bile to act on the cholesterol gallstones. It is recommended for patients not healthy enough to undergo surgery, primarily the elderly with significant symptoms. Treatment can take two or more years, can cause side effects, and is not always effective. Stones recur in up to 50% of patients. The drug is very toxic, with a 10% risk of liver damage. It is not considered the standard treatment. Ursodeoxycholic acid is similar to chenodiol but less toxic. Now that ursodeoxycholic acid is available, few if any physicians prescribe chenodiol.

MONOOCTANOIN   This chemical solvent was approved in November 1985 by the Food and Drug Administration only for the treatment of cholesterol gallstones lodged in the bile duct. The drug is injected directly into the bile duct either with an endoscope inserted through the digestive tract into the duct or through a

T-tube left in place after surgery. Small amounts of the chemical are flushed continuously into the bile duct to dissolve the stones slowly. Monooctanoin does not enjoy a great reputation among experts I spoke to. Not many patients can use it, and it is known to cause liver failure in animals.

METHYL TERT BUTYL ETHER (MTBE)   This treatment involves puncturing the gallbladder and infusing it with ether.

Step 3. Get a Specialist's Opinion

You will need a specialist's opinion if your procedure is not clearly indicated or lacks a high chance of success or if the potential complication rate is particularly high. The best doctor to consult is a highly skilled general surgeon who meets the criteria in Step 5. If you are having an alternate procedure, you will want to see a doctor who can estimate your chance of success based on her or his experience. It is especially important to have an expert opinion when state-of-the-art laparoscopic cholecystectomy has *not* been recommended. You will want this procedure if at all possible.

WHO TO CALL

American College of Surgeons   They will offer you names of fellows in your geographic area.

55 E Erie St
Chicago, IL 60611
312/664-4050

NIH CRISP System
301/496-7543

University-Affiliated Teaching Hospitals   See Appendix.

Step 4. Choose a Hospital

Gallbladder operations are a standard general surgery procedure that can be performed at any hospital, from a major university teaching center to a small rural hospital. Just make sure the hospital you choose has a 24-hour recovery room and a qualified anesthesiologist. In addition to the surgeon, the medical team should include one or two assistants, a scrub nurse, and a circulating nurse.

The hospital's mortality and complication rates are less important than the surgeon's rates. Those rates can be found in Step 5.

Centers of Excellence for Gastroenterology

There is no available list of centers of excellence for abdominal surgery. What follows is a list of centers of excellence for gastroenterology. Many of them have excellent surgical programs to back up their medical expertise. This list is provided only as a convenient starting place in your search for excellence. These hospitals are recommended on the basis of reputation, not experience and results. The list is not an endorsement. There may be hospitals just as excellent that have been omitted. You should apply the guidelines for experience, results, and other measures of excellence to any hospital you choose, whether or not it is on this list. Although hospitals from different sources have been combined into one list, the compilation in no way implies that one source has endorsed the hospital list of another source.

CALIFORNIA
Stanford University School
of Medicine   NIH
Digestive Disease Center
300 Pasteur Dr
Stanford, CA 94305

University of California, Los
Angeles, School of Medicine   EX/NIH/US
Center for Ulcer Education
10833 LeConte Ave
Los Angeles, CA 90024

University of California, San
Diego, Medical Center   EX
225 W Dickinson St
San Diego, CA 92103

University of California, San
Francisco, Medical Center   EX/NIH
505 Parnassus Ave
San Francisco, CA 94143

COLORADO
University Hospital   NIH
Hepatobiliary Research Center
4200 E Ninth Ave
Denver, CO 80262

CONNECTICUT
Yale Liver Research Center   NIH
333 Cedar St
PO Box 3333
New Haven, CT 06510

FLORIDA
Shands Hospital   EX
University of Florida
1600 SW Archer Rd
Gainesville, FL 32610

University of Miami   EX
1600 NW 10th Ave
PO Box 016099 (R59)
Miami, FL 33101

ILLINOIS
Northwestern University
School of Medicine   EX
303 E Chicago Ave
Chicago, IL 60611-3008

University of Chicago Hospitals EX/NIH/US
5841 S Maryland Ave
Chicago, IL 60637

MARYLAND
Johns Hopkins Hospital   EX/US
600 N Wolfe St
Baltimore, MD 21205

MASSACHUSETTS

Beth Israel Hospital   EX
330 Brookline Ave
Boston, MA 02215

Tufts University   NIH
Center for Gastrointestinal
    Research on Absorptive and
    Secretory Processes
136 Harrison Ave
Boston, MA 02111

Lahey Clinic Foundation   EX
41 Mall Rd
Burlington, MA 01805

Massachusetts General Hospital   EX/NIH/US
Center for the Study of
    Inflammatory Disease
55 Fruit St
Boston, MA 02114

MICHIGAN

University of Michigan   NIH
Gastrointestinal Peptide
    Research Center
1301 Catherine Rd
Ann Arbor, MI 48109-0624

MINNESOTA

Mayo Clinic   EX/US
200 First St SW
Rochester, MN 55905

University of Minnesota
    Hospital and Clinic   EX
Harvard St at E River Rd
Minneapolis, MN 55455

MISSOURI

Barnes Hospital   EX
One Barnes Hospital Plaza
St Louis, MO 63110

University Hospital and Clinics   EX
One Hospital Dr
Columbia, MO 65212

NEW YORK

Albert Einstein Liver Research
    Center   NIH
1300 Morris Park Ave
Bronx, NY 10461

Columbia Presbyterian
    Medical Center   EX
622 W 168th St
New York, NY 10032

Memorial Sloan-Kettering
    Cancer Center   EX
1275 York Ave
New York, NY 10021

Mount Sinai Medical Center   EX/US
One Gustave Levy Pl
New York, NY 10029

New York Hospital–Cornell
    Medical Center   EX
525 E 68th St
New York, NY 10021-4885

NORTH CAROLINA

University of North Carolina   NIH
Center for Gastrointestinal
    Biology and Disease
Chapel Hill School of Medicine
Chapel Hill, NC 27599

OHIO

Cleveland Clinic Foundation   EX/US
One Clinic Center
9500 Euclid Ave
Cleveland, OH 44106

PENNSYLVANIA

Hospital of the University of
    Pennsylvania   EX
3400 Spruce St
Philadelphia, PA 19104

Presbyterian-University
    Hospital   EX
Desoto and O'Hara Sts
Pittsburgh, PA 15213

TENNESSEE
Vanderbilt University Medical
    Center   EX
1161 21st Ave S
Nashville, TN 37232

VIRGINIA
Medical College of Virginia
    Hospital   EX
401 N 12th St
Richmond, VA 23219

TEXAS
M.D. Anderson Hospital and
    Tumor Institute   EX
6723 Bertner Dr
Houston, TX 77030

WASHINGTON
University of Washington
    Medical Center   EX
1959 NE Pacific St
Seattle, WA 98195

University of Texas Southwestern
    Medical Center   EX
5323 Harry Hines Blvd
Dallas, TX 75235

SOURCES

US   indicates those hospitals recommended in *U.S. News & World Report.*
EX   indicates those hospitals recommended by experts interviewed.
NIH   indicates those centers funded by the National Institutes of Health's National
      Institute of Diabetes and Digestive and Kidney Diseases.

Step 5. Choose a Doctor

A general surgeon who has completed a five-year training program should be capable of performing this operation. Since it is one of the most common surgical procedures, the surgeon should have received sufficient experience during residency.

Experience

The surgeon should perform at least two operations a month to maintain skills. That number is bound to decrease as the laparoscopic cholecystectomy becomes the standard procedure. If you can't have the procedure of choice, the laparoscopic cholecystectomy, make certain your surgeon does enough of the old-fashioned kind.

If you choose laparoscopic cholecystectomy, look for a surgeon who has been properly qualified in the procedure and is also able to perform open gallbladder surgery. The surgeon should have done a minimum of 50–75 operations and should perform at least two a month, preferably four. A surgeon's skill improves notably after the first 10 procedures. Only doctors who have the skills to perform biliary-tract surgical procedures are able to determine the best method and to treat complications.

Results

DEATH RATE   The average for total cholecystectomy without overall common duct exploration and without complications is 0.3%. This is the most common scenario, and was measured by the research corporation MediQual for 7,953 patients with an average age of 46 years.

Research shows that the mortality rate drops as the number of laparoscopic procedures rises. During a surgeon's first 13 procedures, mortality was 1–2%, then declined. Death rate does vary with the kind of operation you are having. The following rates are averages. Your doctor's results should compare favorably:

Total cholecystectomy with common duct exploration, with complications: Death rate = 1.97%

Total cholecystectomy with common duct exploration, without complications, under age 50: Death rate = 0.08%

Total cholecystectomy without common duct exploration, with complications: Death rate = 1.21%

Reliable statistics are not currently available for the laparoscopic cholecystectomy. Since it is advocated as a safer, less taxing procedure, you should look for mortality rates, complications, hospital charges, and hospital stays that are less than those for an open surgical procedure.

OTHER COMPLICATIONS (for total cholecystectomy)

- Bleeding (1% on the average)

- Damage to the bile duct (Although this should never occur in theory, the actual incidence is 1 case in 10,000. One woman had damage so severe she eventually required a liver transplant. One expert told us this is so rare that it would be sensationalist to include it here and would only scare the reader. Then we asked a senior surgeon at Massachusetts General Hospital about bile duct damage and the laparoscopic procedure. He said, "I thought I'd no longer be able to teach my residents how to repair damaged bile ducts once laparoscopic cholecystectomies became common. I no longer have that fear." Enough damage is done to keep his residents quite busy.)

- Infection (under 2% on the average)

- Pulmonary atelectasis (collapse of part of the lung) (20% on the average)

Other Measures of Excellence

Figures for a total cholecystectomy without common duct exploration and without complications (most common) are:

Hospital charges: $5,252

Length of stay: 4.6 days

EXPERT SOURCES

Although dozens of experts were interviewed for these chapters, Dr. Philip S. Barie, Director, Surgical Intensive Care Unit, New York Hospital–Cornell Medical Center, New York, NY, is acknowledged for his significant contributions to this section.

REFERENCES AND SUGGESTED READING

Baxter, J. N., and O'Dwyer, P. J. For Debate: Laparoscopic or Minilaparotomy Cholecystectomy? *British Medical Journal* Vol. 304, No. 6826 (Feb. 29, 1992), pp. 559–560.

Bose, Bireswar, and others. Are General Surgeons a Dying Breed? [letter] *Canadian Medical Association Journal,* Vol. 146, No. 1 (Jan. 1, 1992), pp. 11–12, 14.

Diagnostic and Therapeutic Technology Assessment (DATTA) American Medical Association Technology Assessment. *Journal of the American Medical Association,* Vol. 265, No. 12 (Mar. 27, 1991), pp. 1585–1587.

Dubois, F., and others. Coelioscopic Cholecystectomy. *Annals of Surgery,* Vol. 211 (1990), pp. 60–62.

Goodman, Greg R., and Hunter, John G. Results of Laparoscopic Cholecystectomy in a University Hospital. *American Journal of Surgery,* Vol. 162, No. 6 (Dec. 1991), pp. 576–579.

Gracie, W. A., and Ransohoff, D. F. The Natural History of Silent Gallstones. The Innocent Gallstone Is Not a Myth. *New England Journal of Medicine,* Vol. 307 (1982), p. 798.

Greenberger, N. J., and Moody, F. G. *Yearbook of Digestive Diseases: 1990.* St. Louis: Mosby, 1990.

Hay, D. J. A Simple Device for Open Laparoscopy. *British Journal of Surgery,* Vol. 79, No. 2 (Feb. 1992), p. 155.

Hieken, Tina J., and Birkett, Desmond H. Postoperative T-Tube Tract Choledochoscopy. *American Journal of Surgery,* Vol. 163, No. 1 (Jan. 1992), pp. 28–31.

Hunter, John G. Laparoscopic Transcystic Common Bile Duct Exploration. *American Journal of Surgery,* Vol. 163, No. 1 (Jan. 1992), pp. 53–58.

Marks, J. W., and others. Low-Dose Chenodiol to Prevent Gallstone Recurrence After Dissolution Therapy. *Annals of Internal Medicine,* Vol. 100 (1984), p. 376.

Meiser, G., and others. Aggressive Extracorporeal Shock Wave Lithotripsy of Gall Bladder Stones Within Wider Treatment Criteria: Fragmentation Rate and Early Results. *Gut,* Vol. 33, No. 2 (Feb. 1992), pp. 277–281.

Miller, Catchpole R. Laparoscopic Cholecystectomy. *Journal of the American Medical Association,* Vol. 265 (1991), pp. 1585–1587.

Peters, J. H., and others. Safety and Efficacy of Laparoscopic Cholecystectomy. *Annals of Surgery,* Vol. 213 (1991), pp. 3–12.

Reddick, E. J., and Olden, D. O. Laparoscopic Laser Cholecystectomy. *Surgical Endoscopy, Ultrasound and Intervention Techniques,* Vol. 3 (1989), pp. 131–133.

Rogers, A. L., and others. Incidence and Associated Mortality of Retained Common Bile Duct Stones. *American Journal of Surgery,* Vol. 150 (1985) p. 690.

Scott, Coombes David, and Thompson, Jeremy N. Bile Duct Stones and Laparoscopic Cholecystectomy. [letter] *British Medical Journal,* Vol. 304, No. 6821 (Jan. 25, 1992), p. 254.

Soravia, C., and others. Flushing Technique in the Management of Retained Common Bile Duct Stones with a T Tube in Situ. *British Journal of Surgery,* Vol. 79, No. 2 (Feb. 1992), pp. 149–151.

Spiro, Howard M. Diagnostic Laparoscopic Cholecystectomy. *Lancet,* Vol. 339, No. 8786 (Jan. 18, 1992), pp. 167–168.

Thompson, J. S., and others. Operative Management of Incidental Cholelithiasis. *American Journal of Surgery,* Vol. 148 (1984), p. 821.

Tulloh, B. R., and others. Bile Duct Stones and Laparoscopic Cholecystectomy. [letter] *British Medical Journal,* Vol. 303, No. 6816 (Dec. 14, 1991), p. 1547.

Walsh, T. N., and Russell, R. C. G. Cholecystectomy and Gallbladder Conservation. *British Journal of Surgery,* Vol. 79, No. 1 (Jan. 1992) pp. 4–5.

Ware, Russell E., and others. Laparoscopic Cholecystectomy in Young Patients with Sickle Hemoglobinopathies. *Journal of Pediatrics,* Vol. 120, No. 1 (Jan. 1992), pp. 58–61.

Wolfe, B. M., and others. Laparoscopic Cholecystectomy: A Remarkable Development. *Journal of the American Medical Association,* Vol. 265, No. 12 (Mar. 27, 1991), pp. 1573–1574.

Zucker, K. A., and others. Laparoscopic Cholecystectomy: A Plea for Cautious Enthusiasm. *American Journal of Surgery,* Vol. 161 (1991), pp. 36–44.

Flexible Sigmoidoscopy

Likelihood of Unnecessary Procedure LOW

Flexible sigmoidoscopy may be one of the few underutilized procedures in this book. Only 129,000 are performed annually. The American Cancer Society recommends that individuals over the age of 50 have a flexible sigmoidoscopy performed every three to five years as a screening test for cancer. Since 50% of the cancers of the colon can be reached by a sigmoidoscope, this is a very powerful preventive test. In fact, a sigmoidoscopy performed as infrequently as once every ten years reduced the risk of fatal colon cancer by 70% over those not screened. Colorectal carcinoma is the second most common systemic cancer in the United States, affecting one in 20 Americans. An estimated 150,000 new cases are diagnosed each year. Tragically, ten-year survival rates average at 40%, but with early screening those rates can exceed 95%.

Potential Risk LOW

The chief risks of sigmoidoscopy are perforation of the colon's thin fragile wall, which can cause infection, and bleeding. But in the hands of an experienced operator, such complications should be rare.

What It Is

The doctor inserts a long, flexible instrument called a flexible sigmoidoscope into the anus, where it is advanced by angling, rotating, and applying mild pressure to the shaft. The doctor examines the rectum and lower colon for cancer, polyps, source of bleeding, and other causes of bowel problems. He or she may remove a small piece of diseased tissue to be examined further under a microscope. In some circumstances, surgery might be avoided altogether when doctors use a sigmoidoscope to treat disease. For instance, small polyps may be removed.

Step 1. Make Sure You Need the Procedure

You should match your diagnosis with the following conditions to make sure the procedure is advisable.

Appropriate Procedure

■ Presence of any risk factors for colon cancer or polyps, even if no symptoms are present

■ Diseases in the colon suspected and a colonoscopy is not appropriate

■ Tumor or other mass has been found via barium enema x-rays

■ Possibility of recurrence of cancer in the lower colon

■ Rectal bleeding, unless colonoscopy is more appropriate

■ Colon symptoms such as acute or chronic diarrhea, rectal pain or spasm, and constipation

Not an Appropriate Procedure

■ Colonoscopy is necessary for proper diagnosis (for example, should an abnormality be found in the right colon via barium enema x-ray, the sigmoidoscope simply wouldn't reach that far (see chapter on Colonoscopy))

Not an Appropriate Procedure, and Also Dangerous

■ Possible perforation of internal organs

■ Severe acute inflammation of the diverticulum, the colon, or the lining of the abdomen

■ Sudden, intense onset of colitis

■ Dilation and hypertrophy of the colon associated with amebic or ulcerative colitis

■ Poorly prepared or uncooperative patient

Step 2. Consider an Alternative

BARIUM ENEMA X-RAYS   An x-ray can "see" barium. Once barium is inserted into the rectum and colon in the form of an enema, a series of x-rays is taken. These x-rays may show tumors, polyps, or other changes in the colon.

COLONOSCOPY   The colonoscope allows doctors to explore the entire colon, not just the bottom part. Colonoscopy—not flexible sigmoidoscopy—is generally indicated for the actual removal of polyps. That's because additional polyps above the reach of the sigmoidoscope can be ruled out or removed if present only with colonoscopy. See chapter on Colonoscopy for more details.

Step 3. Get a Specialist's Opinion

If you are over 50 when your doctor recommends a sigmoidoscopy, there is little need for a second opinion, since that is standard advice. If you have never had the procedure before, you should have it as a general screening test anyway. If you are under 50, you will need an expert opinion if:

- A sigmoidoscopy has been ordered and the diagnosis may be incorrect or does not appear on the list of conditions for which a sigmoidoscopy is considered appropriate (see Step 1).

- You are unsure of the technical skill of your medical team.

Your best choice for a second opinion would be a gastroenterologist or a colon and rectal surgeon who meets the criteria listed in Step 5. After the doctor has carefully reviewed your medical history, you should discuss the alternatives to sigmoidoscopy, which include barium enema x-rays.

WHO TO CALL

American Society for Gastrointestinal Endoscopy (ASGE)
13 Elm St
Manchester, MA 01944
508/526-8330

Society of American Gastrointestinal Endoscopic Surgeons (SAGE)
1271 Stoner Ave, Ste 409
Los Angeles, CA 90025
310/479-3249

NIH CRISP System
301/496-7543

University-Affiliated Teaching Hospitals   See Appendix.

Step 4. Choose a Facility

Experience

Sigmoidoscopies are performed in doctors' offices, clinics, emergency rooms, and hospitals. If your case appears routine, go on to Step 5 for information on how to choose a doctor. If you are concerned because the procedure entails some risk or demands a high level of technical proficiency, you may refer yourself to a national center of excellence (see upcoming list) or a university-affiliated teaching hospital with a highly rated department of gastroenterology (see Appendix). Be certain the hospital does not have an above-average complication rate.

Results

COMPLICATION RATE   Bowel perforation can occur as a result of direct trauma from overly forceful manipulation. The rate for this complication is estimated at one in 5,000.

Centers of Excellence for Gastroenterology

The following list of hospitals is provided only as a convenient starting place in your search for excellence. These hospitals are recommended on the basis of reputation, not experience and results. The list is not an endorsement. There may be hospitals just as excellent that have been omitted. You should apply the guidelines for experience, results, and other measures of excellence to any hospital you choose, whether or not it is on this list. Although hospitals from different sources have been combined into one list, the compilation in no way implies that one source has endorsed the hospital list of another source.

CALIFORNIA
California Pacific Medical
  Center   EX
2340 Clay St
San Francisco, CA 94115

Stanford University School of
  Medicine   NIH
Digestive Disease Center
300 Pasteur Dr
Stanford, CA 94305

University of California,
  Los Angeles, School of
  Medicine   EX/NIH/US
Center for Ulcer Education
10833 LeConte Ave
Los Angeles, CA 90024

University of California, San
  Diego, Medical Center   EX
225 W Dickinson St
San Diego, CA 92103

University of California, San
  Francisco, Medical Center   EX/NIH
505 Parnassus Ave
San Francisco, CA 94143

COLORADO
University Hospital   NIH
Hepatobiliary Research Center
4200 E Ninth Ave
Denver, CO 80262

CONNECTICUT
Yale Liver Research Center   NIH
333 Cedar St
PO Box 3333
New Haven, CT 06510

FLORIDA
Shands Hospital   EX
University of Florida
1600 SW Archer Rd
Gainesville, FL 32610

University of Miami   EX
1600 NW 10th Ave
PO Box 016099 (R59)
Miami, FL 33101

ILLINOIS
Northwestern University
    School of Medicine   EX
303 E Chicago Ave
Chicago, IL 60611-3008

University of Chicago
    Hospitals   EX/NIH/US
5841 S Maryland Ave
Chicago, IL 60637

MARYLAND
Johns Hopkins Hospital   EX/US
600 N Wolfe St
Baltimore, MD 21205

MASSACHUSETTS
Beth Israel Hospital   EX
330 Brookline Ave
Boston, MA 02215

Tufts University   NIH
Center for Gastrointestinal
    Research on Absorptive
    and Secretory Processes
136 Harrison Ave
Boston, MA 02111

Lahey Clinic Foundation   EX
41 Mall Rd
Burlington, MA 01805

Massachusetts General
    Hospital   EX/NIH/US
55 Fruit St
Boston, MA 02114

MICHIGAN
University of Michigan   NIH
Gastrointestinal Peptide
    Research Center
1301 Catherine Rd
Ann Arbor, Michigan 48109-0624

MINNESOTA
Mayo Clinic   EX/US
200 First St SW
Rochester, MN 55905

University of Minnesota
    Hospital and Clinic   EX
Harvard St at E River Rd
Minneapolis, MN 55455

MISSOURI
Barnes Hospital   EX
One Barnes Hospital Plaza
St Louis, MO 63110

University Hospital and
    Clinics   EX
One Hospital Dr
Columbia, MO 65212

NEW YORK
Albert Einstein Liver Research
    Center   NIH
1300 Morris Park Ave
Bronx, NY 10461

Columbia Presbyterian
    Medical Center   EX
622 W 168th St
New York, NY 10032

Memorial Sloan-Kettering
    Cancer Center   EX
1275 York Ave
New York, NY 10021

Mount Sinai Medical Center   EX/US
One Gustave Levy Pl
New York, NY 10029

New York Hospital–Cornell
    Medical Center   EX
525 E 68th St
New York, NY 10021-4885

NORTH CAROLINA
University of North Carolina   NIH
Center for Gastrointestinal
   Biology and Disease
Chapel Hill School of Medicine
Chapel Hill, NC 27599

OHIO
Cleveland Clinic Foundation   EX/US
One Clinic Center
9500 Euclid Ave
Cleveland, OH 44106

PENNSYLVANIA
Hospital of the University of
   Pennsylvania   EX
3400 Spruce St
Philadelphia, PA 19104

Presbyterian-University
   Hospital   EX
Desoto and O'Hara Sts
Pittsburgh, PA 15213

TENNESSEE
Vanderbilt University
   Medical Center   EX
1161 21st Ave S
Nashville, TN 37232

TEXAS
M.D. Anderson Hospital and
   Tumor Institute   EX
6723 Bertner Dr
Houston, TX 77030

University of Texas Southwestern Medical Center   EX
5323 Harry Hines Blvd
Dallas, TX 75235

VIRGINIA
Medical College of Virginia
   Hospital   EX
401 N 12th St
Richmond, VA 23219
(Special interest: cancer of the
   gastrointestinal tract)

WASHINGTON
University of Washington
   Medical Center   EX
1959 NE Pacific St
Seattle, WA 98195

SOURCES

US   indicates those hospitals recommended in *U.S. News & World Report.*
EX   indicates those hospitals recommended by experts interviewed.
NIH   indicates those centers funded by the National Institutes of Health's National
      Institute of Diabetes and Digestive and Kidney Diseases.

Step 5. Choose a Doctor

Most surgeons, internists, emergency room physicians, and family practitioners
have adequate experience to perform a flexible sigmoidoscopy. The best doctor,
however, will be board-certified in internal medicine with a subspecialty in gastroenterology or is a colon and rectal surgeon. Training courses in flexible
sigmoidoscopy have been offered by the American Academy of Family Practice

and the American Society for Gastrointestinal Endoscopy. Training typically consists of classroom instruction and practice sessions on rubber models. The American Society for Gastrointestinal Endoscopy recommends that a minimum of 25 supervised procedures be completed during training.

Those numbers, however, are not universally agreed on. Some endoscopists estimate that 25–50 supervised examinations are needed to teach nonspecialists the use of a 60-cm scope, thus precluding its use for general screening. They advocate a 35-cm flexible scope for the nonspecialist. However, this shorter scope is seldom used. Family physicians disputed these estimates of training time in a 1990 article in the *Journal of the American Medical Association,* contending that 10–20 supervised examinations are enough to establish competence with the 60-cm scope. Lack of skill can prevent finding cancers that are within reach of the scope. Even though the scope can reach 60 cm into the bowel, the average depth of insertion in many cases is 40–50 cm.

Experience

To maintain competency, the doctor should perform 25 procedures a year, according to a study published in the *Annals of Internal Medicine* in 1990.

Results

COMPLICATION RATE   If the flexible scope is manipulated with excessive force, the bowel can be perforated. The rate is estimated at one in 5,000, according to a report published in 1990 in the *Journal of the American Medical Association.*

You should ask about the doctor's complication rate and the circumstances in which they occurred. If the doctor is removing a polyp, for instance, you should be certain that he does this dozens of times a year with no serious complications.

EXPERT SOURCES

Although dozens of experts were interviewed for these chapters, Dr. Emmet B. Keeffe, Chief of Hepatology, California Pacific Medical Center, San Francisco, CA, is acknowledged for his significant contributions to this section.

REFERENCES

American College of Physicians. Clinical Competence in Colonoscopy. *Annals of Internal Medicine,* Vol. 107, No. 5 (Nov. 1987), pp. 772–774.

American College of Physicians. Clinical Competence in the Use of Flexible Sigmoidoscopy for Screening Purposes. *Annals of Internal Medicine,* Vol. 107, No. 4 (Oct. 1987), pp. 589–591.

American Medical Association. Diagnostic and Therapeutic Technology Assessment (DATTA). *Journal of the American Medical Association,* Vol. 264, No. 1 (July 4, 1990), pp. 89–92.

American Society for Gastrointestinal Endoscopy. *Appropriate Use of Gastrointestinal Endoscopy,* May 1989.

American Society for Gastrointestinal Endoscopy. *Gastrointestinal Endoscopy Diagnostic and Therapeutic Procedures. An Information Resource Manual,* 1988.

Gurwitz, Jerry H., and others. Barium Enemas in the Frail Elderly. *American Journal of Medicine,* Vol. 92, No. 1 (Jan. 1992), pp. 41–44.

Levin, Bernard. Screening Sigmoidoscopy for Colorectal Cancer [editorial]. *New England Journal of Medicine,* Vol. 326, No. 10 (Mar. 5, 1992), pp. 700–702.

Selby, Joe V., and others. A Case-Control Study of Screening Sigmoidoscopy and Mortality from Colorectal Cancer. *New England Journal of Medicine,* Vol. 326, No. 10 (Mar. 5, 1992), pp. 653–657.

Thun, Michael J., and others. Aspirin Use and Reduced Risk of Fatal Colon Cancer. *New England Journal of Medicine,* Vol. 325, No. 23 (Dec. 5, 1991), pp. 1593–1596.

Wagner, Judith L., and others. Cost Effectiveness of Colorectal Cancer Screening in the Elderly. *Annals of Internal Medicine,* Vol. 115, No. 10 (Nov. 15, 1991), pp. 807–817.

Wigton, R. S., and others. Procedural Skills of Practicing Gastroenterologists. A National Survey of 700 Members of the American College of Physicians. *Annals of Internal Medicine,* Vol. 113, No. 7 (Oct. 1990), pp. 540–546.

Wigton, R. S., and others. Procedural Skills of the General Internist. A Survey of 2,500 Physicians. *Annals of Internal Medicine,* Vol. III, No. 12 (1989), pp. 1023–1034.

Colonoscopy

Likelihood of Unnecessary Procedure   LOW

Colonoscopy is very rarely performed without a medically sufficient reason; perhaps only about 5% of the two million procedures a year are inappropriate, according to Value Health Sciences, a research organization. Patients who complain of vague abdominal pain and have no specific findings suggestive of serious disease are at the highest risk for an inappropriate procedure. Although patients may believe that colonoscopy is the standard procedure in these cases, other diagnostic tests may be better.

Potential Risk   MODERATE

The colon has a thin wall that may be ruptured by the colonoscope. If that happens, bacteria can escape from the colon into the abdominal cavity and cause infection. In addition, older patients may react adversely to medications that are administered prior to the procedure—in particular, causing problems of oversedation in patients with depression or breathing or heart problems. But, correctly performed by a skilled doctor, this is a safe and very useful procedure. Still, it should be undertaken only when clearly indicated.

What It Is

The doctor inserts a long, flexible instrument called a colonoscope into the anus, where it is advanced by angling and rotating the tip, using horizontal and vertical controls and applying pressure to the shaft. Experienced colonoscopists are able to advance the scope from the rectum around the entire colon in approximately 95% of the procedures.

The scope contains either fiberoptic or video equipment that allows the doctor to inspect visually the entire rectum and colon. The doctor may examine the colon for disease or remove a small piece of diseased tissue to be examined further under a microscope. President Ronald Reagan's doctor used this procedure to discover his colon cancer at a stage early enough for surgery to cure him. In some circumstances surgery may be avoided altogether when doctors use a colonoscope to treat disease. In some cases, for example, small polyps may be removed or bleeding stopped.

Step 1. Make Sure You Need the Procedure

To determine if it is necessary, you should match your diagnosis against the most frequent conditions for use of the procedure in the following list.

Appropriate Procedure

■ A tumor, a polyp, or some other colon abnormality is suspected from a barium enema x-ray of the large intestine

■ Polyps detected by barium enema x-ray (for their removal)

■ A cancerous polyp in the lower colon has been revealed via examination with a sigmoidoscope (a straight or flexible metal tube used to explore the rectum and lower colon—see chapter on Sigmoidoscopy)

■ Unexplained bleeding from the bowel

■ Iron-deficiency anemia revealed during a complete medical workup

■ Colon cancer, as follow-up exam

■ Colon polyps (for their removal in patients with treatable cancer)

■ Family history of colon cancer or polyposis

■ Chronic ulcerative colitis (to screen for cancer)

■ Chronic inflammatory bowel disease if procedure will alter treatment

■ Previous suspicious findings, as follow-up

■ Bleeding due to an ulcer, polyp, or some other cause (to control through the use of electrocoagulation, heater probe, laser, or injection therapy)

■ Markedly overinflated colon (to decompress it)

■ Strictures or narrowings of the colon (to dilate them)

■ Severe diarrhea

■ Narrowing or bleeding from treatment of cancer symptoms (to control through the use of lasers or electrocoagulation)

Not an Appropriate Procedure

■ Benign disease (as follow-up after healing)

■ Chronic, but stable, irritable bowel syndrome that is responding to therapy

- Minor diarrhea

- Inflammatory bowel disease (as routine follow-up)

- Metastatic cancer that is not causing symptoms in the bowel when the origin of the cancer is unknown and the procedure will not influence treatment

- No colon-related symptoms or disease (for preoperative examination of colon)

- Bleeding whose cause has already been identified

- Earlier colon cancer has been removed (to look for recurrence at the same site)

- Bright red bleeding from a noncancerous source in the rectum

- Known hyperplastic polyps (as follow-up)

Not an Appropriate Procedure, and Also Dangerous

- Sudden, intense colitis (inflammation of the colon) or acute, severe diverticulitis (inflammation of a diverticulum)

- Major internal organ (such as bowel or spleen) possibly perforated

Step 2. Consider an Alternative

SIGMOIDOSCOPY   The doctor inserts a long, flexible instrument called a flexible sigmoidoscope into the anus to examine the rectum and lower colon for cancer, polyps, source of bleeding, or other causes of bowel problems. This is a good alternative procedure if only the lower bowel and rectum need examination. It does not require sedation, whereas colonoscopy does (see chapter on Sigmoidoscopy).

BARIUM ENEMA X-RAY   An x-ray can "see" barium. Once barium is inserted into the rectum and colon in the form of an enema, a series of x-rays is taken. These x-rays may show tumors, polyps, or other changes in the colon.

Step 3. Get a Specialist's Opinion

You will need a specialist's opinion if:

- A colonoscopy has been ordered and the diagnosis is uncertain or does not appear on the list of conditions under which the procedure is appropriate (Step 1).

- You are unsure of your doctor's proficiency.

Your best choice for a second opinion would be a gastroenterologist, a colon and rectal surgeon, or a highly skilled colonoscopist who meets the criteria in Step 5. If you are exploring alternatives or your diagnosis is questionable, you need not see a colonoscopist; a well-trained gastroenterologist can offer excellent advice. You should discuss the alternatives to colonoscopy, which include the procedures described in Step 2.

WHO TO CALL

American Society for Gastrointestinal Endoscopy (ASGE)

13 Elm St
Manchester, MA 01944
508/526-8330

Society of American Gastrointestinal Endoscopic Surgeons (SAGE)

1271 Stoner Ave, Ste 409
Los Angeles, CA 90025
310/479-3249

NIH CRISP System

301/496-7543

University-Affiliated Teaching Hospitals   See Appendix.

Step 4. Choose a Facility

You should compile a list of facilities that perform a high volume of colonoscopies and then choose the facility that has the best results and the most experience with your condition. Colonoscopy is a rather routine procedure that can be performed successfully in hospitals, clinics, and doctors' offices. You need not travel to a top-rated facility unless you have a difficult medical problem. You must make sure the hospital has an endoscopy unit that will be staffed during the procedure. The more experienced and skilled the team, the greater the likelihood that it will perform the procedure successfully, avoid complications, and eliminate the need for later surgery.

Look for the following.

Experience

The facility should perform at least five colonoscopies per week per specialist.

Results

DEATH RATE   The death rate for colonoscopy is extremely low, only three in 10,000 patients. A doctor or team with a substantially higher rate should be avoided.

COMPLICATION RATE   Complication rates for colonoscopy vary, depending on whether the procedure is used for diagnosis or treatment. The average rates to look for are:

Diagnosis: 0.2%

Treatment: 0.5%

When the procedure is used for diagnosis, the most serious complication is perforation of the colon through excessive pressure by a loop formed along the shaft of the instrument or by a blowout of a small sac in the colon called a diverticulum. Bleeding, even after a biopsy, is rare. When polyps are removed, the bleeding occurs in no more than 2.5% of patients. More common complications include fainting, bacteremia, distention, and irregular heartbeat.

Other Measures of Excellence

During the procedure a doctor and at least one but preferably two gastrointestinal nurses should be present.

Centers of Excellence for Gastroenterology

The following list of hospitals is provided only as a convenient starting place in your search for excellence. These hospitals are recommended on the basis of reputation, not experience and results. The list is not an endorsement. There may be hospitals just as excellent that have been omitted. You should apply the guidelines for experience, results, and other measures of excellence to any hospital you choose, whether or not it is on this list. Although hospitals from different sources have been combined into one list, the compilation in no way implies that one source has endorsed the hospital list of another source.

CALIFORNIA

California Pacific Medical
   Center   EX
2340 Clay St
San Francisco, CA 94115

Stanford University School
   of Medicine   NIH
Digestive Disease Center
300 Pasteur Dr
Stanford, CA 94305

University of California, Los Angeles,
   School of Medicine   EX/NIH/US
Center for Ulcer Education
10833 LeConte Ave
Los Angeles, CA 90024

University of California, San
   Diego, Medical Center   EX
225 W Dickinson St
San Diego, CA 92103

University of California, San
    Francisco, Medical Center   EX/NIH
505 Parnassus Ave
San Francisco, CA 94143

COLORADO
University Hospital   NIH
Hepatobiliary Research Center
4200 E Ninth Ave
Denver, CO 80262

CONNECTICUT
Yale Liver Research Center   NIH
333 Cedar St
PO Box 3333
New Haven, CT 06510

FLORIDA
Shands Hospital   EX
University of Florida
1600 SW Archer Rd
Gainesville, FL 32610

University of Miami   EX
1600 NW 10th Ave
PO Box 016099 (R59)
Miami, FL 33101

ILLINOIS
Northwestern University
    School of Medicine   EX
303 E Chicago Ave
Chicago, IL 60611-3008

University of Chicago
    Hospitals   EX/NIH/US
5841 S Maryland Ave
Chicago, IL 60637

MARYLAND
Johns Hopkins Hospital   EX/US
600 N Wolfe St
Baltimore, MD 21205

MASSACHUSETTS
Beth Israel Hospital   EX
330 Brookline Ave
Boston, MA 02215

Tufts University   NIH
Center for Gastrointestinal
    Research on Absorptive and
    Secretory Processes
136 Harrison Ave
Boston, MA 02111

Lahey Clinic Foundation   EX
41 Mall Rd
Burlington, MA 01805

Massachusetts General
    Hospital   EX/NIH/US
55 Fruit St
Boston, MA 02114

MICHIGAN
University of Michigan   NIH
Gastrointestinal Peptide
    Research Center
1301 Catherine Rd
Ann Arbor, MI 48109-0624

MINNESOTA
Mayo Clinic   EX/US
200 First St SW
Rochester, MN 55905

University of Minnesota
    Hospital and Clinic   EX
Harvard St at E River Rd
Minneapolis, MN 55455

MISSOURI
Barnes Hospital   EX
One Barnes Hospital Plaza
St Louis, MO 63110

University Hospital and
    Clinics   EX
One Hospital Dr
Columbia, MO 65212

NEW YORK
Albert Einstein Liver Research
    Center   NIH
1300 Morris Park Ave
Bronx, NY 10461

Columbia Presbyterian
 Medical Center EX
622 W 168th St
New York, NY 10032

Memorial Sloan-Kettering
 Cancer Center EX
1275 York Ave
New York, NY 10021

Mount Sinai Medical Center EX/US
One Gustave Levy Pl
New York, NY 10029

New York Hospital–Cornell
 Medical Center EX
525 E 68th St
New York, NY 10021-4885

NORTH CAROLINA
University of North Carolina NIH
Center for Gastrointestinal
 Biology and Disease
Chapel Hill School of Medicine
Chapel Hill, NC 27599

OHIO
Cleveland Clinic Foundation EX/US
One Clinic Center
9500 Euclid Ave
Cleveland, OH 44106

PENNSYLVANIA
Hospital of the University of
 Pennsylvania EX
3400 Spruce St
Philadelphia, PA 19104

Presbyterian-University
 Hospital EX
Desoto and O'Hara Sts
Pittsburgh, PA 15213

TENNESSEE
Vanderbilt University Medical
 Center EX
1161 21st Ave S
Nashville, TN 37232

TEXAS
M.D. Anderson Hospital and
 Tumor Institute EX
6723 Bertner Dr
Houston, TX 77030

University of Texas Southwestern Medical Center EX
5323 Harry Hines Blvd
Dallas, TX 75235

VIRGINIA
Medical College of Virginia
 Hospital EX
401 N 12th St
Richmond, VA 23219

WASHINGTON
University of Washington
 Medical Center EX
1959 NE Pacific St
Seattle, WA 98195

SOURCES

US indicates those hospitals recommended in *U.S. News & World Report.*

EX indicates those hospitals recommended by experts interviewed.

NIH indicates those centers funded by the National Institutes of Health's National
 Institute of Diabetes and Digestive and Kidney Diseases.

Step 5. Choose a Doctor

While lab technicians and nurses can perform a colonoscopy, it is highly recommended that you select a physician board-certified in both internal medicine and the subspecialty of gastroenterology or in colon and rectal surgery. A doctor who specializes in internal medicine but has not been trained in the procedure lacks the necessary skill. According to Dr. Emmet B. Keeffe, Chair of the Standards and Practices Committee of the American Society for Gastrointestinal Endoscopy, the doctor who performs the procedure should be a gastroenterologist who completed training in the mid-1970s, when a mandatory two-year endoscopy training program began. During training the doctor should have performed about 200–400 colonoscopies. The minimum required for competence is usually about 100. Gastroenterologists who graduated earlier should have substantial ongoing experience with the procedure.

Experience

Two to three colonoscopies per week is the absolute minimum.

Results

The death rates and the rate for complications should be comparable to the facility statistics in Step 4.

Other Measures of Excellence

The colonoscopist should be able to reach the small intestine with the colonoscope.

EXPERT SOURCES

Although dozens of experts were interviewed for these chapters, Dr. Emmet B. Keeffe, California Pacific Medical Center, San Francisco, CA, is acknowledged for his significant contributions to this section.

REFERENCES AND SUGGESTED READING

American College of Physicians. Clinical Competence in Colonoscopy. *Annals of Internal Medicine*, Vol. 107, No. 5 (Nov. 1987), pp. 772–774.

American College of Physicians. Clinical Competence in the Use of Flexible Sigmoidoscopy for Screening Purposes. *Annals of Internal Medicine*, Vol. 107, No. 4 (Oct. 1987), pp. 589–591.

American Medical Association. Diagnostic and Therapeutic Technology Assessment (DATTA). *Journal of the American Medical Association*, Vol. 264, No. 1 (July 4, 1990), pp. 89–92.

American Society for Gastrointestinal Endoscopy. *Appropriate Use of Gastrointestinal Endoscopy*, May 1989.

American Society for Gastrointestinal Endoscopy. *Gastrointestinal Endoscopy Diagnostic and Therapeutic Procedures. An Information Resource Manual*, 1988.

Bramble, M. G. Open Access Endoscopy—A Nationwide Survey of Current Practice. *Gut*, Vol. 33, No. 2 (1992), pp. 282–285.

Hobbs, F. D. Richard, and others. Acceptability of Opportunistic Screening for Occult Gastrointestinal Blood Loss. *British Medical Journal*, Vol. 304, No. 6825 (1992), pp. 483–486.

Osborne, M. J., and others. Colon Perforation During Colonoscopy: Surgical Versus Conservative Management. [letter] *British Journal of Surgery*, Vol. 78, No. 11 (Nov. 1991), p. 1402.

Wigton, R. S., and others. Procedural Skills of Practicing Gastroenterologists. A National Survey of 700 Members of the American College of Physicians. *Annals of Internal Medicine*, Vol. 113, No. 7 (Oct. 1990), pp. 540–546.

Wigton, R. S., and others. Procedural Skills of the General Internist. A Survey of 2,500 Physicians. *Annals of Internal Medicine*, Vol. 111, No. 12 (1989), pp. 1023–1034.

Arthroscopy

Likelihood of Unnecessary Surgery   LOW

About 6–8% of arthroscopies are performed unnecessarily, according to Value Health Sciences, the research organization. Doctors may rush into an arthroscopy when simpler measures would be just as effective. While the arthroscope is a highly effective tool for the diagnosis and treatment of joint problems in the knee and elsewhere, it should not be a substitute for a careful history and clinical examination.

Potential Risk   MODERATE

Arthroscopy can be a simple, flawless technique that produces few complications. However, in a major study of 3,261 procedures reported in the *Journal of Bone and Joint Surgery* in 1986, researchers found complications, ranging from major to minor, in slightly over 8% of the cases.

Major Complications

■ Damage to the joint or cartilage, including injury caused by instrument breakage within the joint due to mishandling by the doctor

■ Damage resulting from the use of excessive force, such as nerve lesions or fracture of the thigh bone

■ Injury to the popliteal artery

■ Gas distention that causes fatal air embolisms and subcutaneous emphysema (when air enters the tissues)

■ Postoperative complications from anesthesia when general anesthesia is used

■ Infection

■ Septic knee (0.1% probability)

■ Blood clot in the leg, known as thrombophlebitis, and blood in the joint following surgery

■ Cardiovascular problems, including episodes of chest pain and venous thrombosis (blood clots deep in the leg vein)

- Neurological disorders such as postoperative pain and loss of sensation

- Effusion (fluid found in the knee joint within four weeks of surgery)

- Adhesions (bands that limit mobility)

- Instrument breakage that leaves retrievable or irretrievable parts inside the body

- Reflex sympathetic dystrophy, a condition causing diffuse pain, elevated temperature, and discolored skin in and around the knee and lasting from one to four months after surgery

Minor Complications

- Slow healing of wounds

- Ecchymosis (bruising of soft tissues not related to the healing of wounds)

What It Is

The surgeon injects either air or a saline solution into the joint to expand it, then inserts the endoscope, through a small incision in the skin, into the joint. This enables the surgeon to examine the joint, to check for damage by probing or lifting structures, and to operate if necessary.

The operation is usually performed on an outpatient basis, under general anesthesia, although a nerve block is used occasionally. Patients are discharged after recovering from the effects of the anesthesia. They are able to return to work and resume regular activities approximately six days after removal of the meniscus, tissue which acts like a shock absorber separating bone from bone. Patients should be seen by the arthroscopist at least once following the operation and by the referring physician within two weeks of the procedure.

Step 1. Make Sure You Need the Surgery

To make sure the surgery is necessary, you should match your diagnosis against the ones in the following lists.

Appropriate Procedure

- Damage to knee cartilage

- Partial ruptures of ligaments

- Blood in the joint

- Osteochondral fractures that extend through both bone and cartilage (often found on x-rays; surgery is indicated if the site of the osteochondral defect cannot be located or if arthroscopic removal of the fragment is contemplated)

- Suspected tears of the meniscus

- Persistent knee pains of uncertain origin after injury

- Partial ruptures of the cruciate ligament (This is the only technique that can determine rupture extent.)

- Acute locking of the knee joint (Since this is an emergency, arthroscopy is performed without further examination aside from the normal x-ray.)

- Rheumatic disease that does not respond to therapy

Possibly an Appropriate Procedure

- Chondromalacia of the patella (a condition in which the underside of the kneecap becomes roughened due to excess strain and softening of the cartilage) (Some orthopedic surgeons believe that arthroscopy is inappropriate for this condition, especially if the patella is to be "scraped," and should be considered only after extensive physical therapy and the use of antiinflammatory drugs.)

- Ligament reconstruction (Each year the frontiers of arthroscopy expand: More and more knee reconstructions can be done using an arthroscope. You will want an orthopedic surgeon who has lots of experience and excellent results repairing ligaments using an arthroscope.)

- Cartilage damage in the femoral-tibial joint (The decision as to further treatment depends on the arthroscopic findings.)

- Persistent pain after surgery for the removal of a meniscus, if the cause was not established during the initial operation

Probably Not an Appropriate Procedure

- Vague symptoms (For example, with a 45-year-old patient who has minor arthritis in a joint, the arthroscopist may be tempted to "clean it up." But arthroscopy won't solve the problem or eliminate the eventual need for replacement with an artificial joint.)

Not an Appropriate Procedure

- Ankylosis (loss of movement in a joint caused by degeneration and fusion of the bony surfaces)

- Infection or inflammation following a previous joint operation

- Bacterial contamination of lacerations or abrasions in the knee region (unless pus is present in the knee joint, in which case arthroscopy is indicated)

- The surgeon is going to operate anyway (For example, cartilage is badly torn and requires an operation. Then the indication for proceeding with an arthroscopy is doubtful.)

Step 2. Consider an Alternative

You should consider some of the following possible alternatives to arthroscopy.

MAGNETIC RESONANCE IMAGERY (MRI) SCANS   This completely noninvasive test is good for diagnosing many bone and joint problems and can be an excellent first step, especially if your surgeon suspects the condition doesn't require an operation or arthroscopy. Beware, however, that arthroscopy is not ordered simply on the basis of an MRI. A physical exam needs to concur with the findings of an MRI.

REEXAMINATION BY AN ORTHOPEDIC SUBSPECIALIST   Here's an example: A doctor schedules an arthroscopy for purely diagnostic purposes on a marathon runner. On the basis of an initial physical examination the doctor assumes, *incorrectly*, that the patient has a torn meniscus (the knee's main shock absorber). However, a sports medicine doctor who specializes in running injuries is able to make the diagnosis on the basis of history and examination alone.

OTHER SURGERY   In some cases, opening the joint is necessary to effect the best repair of the knee. You should explore the pros and cons of arthroscopy versus surgery.

PHYSICAL THERAPY   If the pain is chronic or due to an injury, the doctor should order physical therapy or try removing fluid from the knee.

MEDICATIONS   Nonsteroidal antiinflammatory drugs (NSAIDS) are the most likely first option. Advil, Motrin, Nuprin, and ibuprofen (the generic form) are names with which you may be familiar. As an example, should you have knee pain caused by a roughening of the underside of the kneecap, medication plus physical therapy is the recommended treatment.

Step 3. Get a Specialist's Opinion

If your operation is not clearly indicated, you will want to get an expert opinion. A highly skilled orthopedic surgeon who meets the same criteria as those in Step 5 is your best choice for a second opinion. You should discuss the alternatives to arthroscopy and have your medical history and clinical examination reviewed carefully to be certain your diagnosis is correct.

WHO TO CALL

Arthroscopy Association of North America   This organization can provide you with a list of three arthroscopists in your area. It is a professional organization but offers the public guidelines for arthroscopists and educational and informational materials on surgery.

2250 E Devon Ave, Ste 149
Des Plaines, IL 60618
708/299-9444

American Academy of Orthopedic Surgeons   This organization provides callers with educational information on various types of orthopedic surgery as well as academy guidelines and position papers.

222 S Prospect Ave
Park Ridge, IL 60068
708/823-7186

American Orthopedic Society for Sports Medicine   This group provides callers with a list of members in their area. It also may provide limited information or educational brochures on sports medicine.

2250 E Devon Ave, Ste 115
Des Plaines, IL 60018
708/803-8700

NIH CRISP System
301/496-7543

University-Affiliated Teaching Hospitals   See Appendix.

Step 4. Choose a Hospital

This operation can be performed safely at a hospital or an outpatient clinic, but it should *not* be done in your doctor's office. The medical team at the hospital should include the arthroscopist, an anesthesiologist, a scrub nurse, and a circulating nurse. A local or regional anesthesia is preferable to general anesthesia because the recovery is quicker and the complications fewer.

Experience/Results

Experience and results depend on the individual orthopedic surgeon. These are listed in Step 5. Most hospitals do not have available statistics on arthroscopy. Individual doctors should have their own rates.

Centers of Excellence for Orthopedics

The following list of hospitals is provided only as a convenient starting place in your search for excellence. They are recommended on the basis of reputation, not experience and results. The list is not an endorsement. There may be hospitals just as excellent that have been omitted. You should apply the guidelines for experience, results, and other measures of excellence to any hospital you choose, whether or not it is on this list. Although hospitals from different sources have been combined into one list, the compilation in no way implies that one source has endorsed the hospital list of another source.

CALIFORNIA

University of California, Los
   Angeles, School of Medicine   US
10833 LeConte Ave
Los Angeles, CA 90024

University of Southern California
   Medical Center   EX
1200 N State St
Los Angeles, CA 90033

ILLINOIS

Rush-Presbyterian-St. Luke's
   Medical Center   EX
1653 W Congress Pkwy
Chicago, IL 60612
(Special interest: joint replacement)

IOWA

University of Iowa Hospitals
   and Clinics   EX
650 Newton Rd
Iowa City, IA 52242
(Special interests: joint replacement,
   children's orthopedics, metabolic
   disorders, neuromuscular diseases)

MARYLAND

Johns Hopkins Hospital   EX
600 N Wolfe St
Baltimore, MD 21205
(Special interests: joint replacement)

MASSACHUSETTS

Brigham and Women's Hospital   US
75 Francis St
Boston, MA 02115

Massachusetts General Hospital   EX/US
55 Fruit St
Boston, MA 02114
(Special interests: fracture, trauma, joint
   replacement, children's orthopedics)

MINNESOTA

Mayo Clinic   EX/US
200 First St SW
Rochester, MN 55905
(Special interests: reconstructive surgery,
   joint replacement, children's
   orthopedics)

NEW YORK

Hospital for Special Surgery   EX/US
535 E 70th St
New York, NY 10021
(Special interests: joint replacement,
   reconstructive surgery; a multi-
   purpose arthritis center)

TENNESSEE

Campbell Clinic of the
   University of Tennessee   EX
869 Madison Ave
Memphis, TN 38104
(Special interests: joint replacement,
   arthritis surgery, children's orthopedics, fractures, and trauma)

SOURCES

US   indicates those hospitals recommended in *U.S. News & World Report.*

EX   indicates those hospitals recommended by experts interviewed.

Step 5. Choose a Doctor

Dr. David Altchek at the Hospital for Special Surgery in New York City recommends seeing an orthopedic surgeon who specializes in knee injuries or sports medicine. The doctor should have finished five years of surgical training and an additional one year fellowship in sports medicine. During that time the surgeon should also have performed 100–200 operations and assisted in another 1,000.

Experience

The surgeon should perform about 200 operations a year, according to Dr. Thomas L. Wickiewicz, Assistant Director of the Sports Medicine Performance and Research Center at the Hospital for Special Surgery. A minimum of 50–100 operations a year are needed to maintain competency.

Results

COMPLICATIONS   A recent study published in the *Journal of Bone and Joint Surgery* found that complications from arthroscopy are attributable to two main factors: the length of time that a tourniquet is used during the operation, and the age of the patient. The tourniquet is applied just as in any emergency to decrease the flow of blood. In this case, it makes the procedure easier because the surgeon does not have to deal with the bleeding that might otherwise occur. A tourniquet applied for more than 40 minutes poses a moderate risk of complications, while one in place for more than 60 minutes carries high risk. Age magnifies the projected risks as follows:

Average Complication Rates for Various Ages and Tourniquet Times

■ Under age 30, tourniquet time of less than 40 minutes: 3.2%

■ Over age 30, tourniquet time of less than 40 minutes, or under age 30 with tourniquet time 40–59 minutes: 5.2%

■ Over age 30, tourniquet time 40–59 minutes: 8.1%

■ Any age, tourniquet time over 60 minutes: 14.3%

Other Measures of Excellence

Ask about expertise in ligament reconstruction. This is a complex procedure. If the doctor also does these through an arthroscope, you can expect that he or she is exceptionally skillful.

EXPERT SOURCES

Although dozens of experts were interviewed for these chapters, Dr. David W. Altchek of the Hospital for Special Surgery, New York, NY, is acknowledged for his significant contributions to this chapter.

REFERENCES AND SUGGESTED READING

Bedford, A., and others. Arthroscopy: The First Hundred Are the Worst. *Journal of the Royal Society of Medicine,* Vol. 72 (1979), p. 6.

Brief, L. P. Arthroscopy, Self-Education and Humility. *Arthroscopy,* Vol. 2 (1986), pp. 88–89.

Carlsen, A. A Broken Telescope: A Complication of Arthroscopy. *Arthroscopy,* Vol. 2, (1986), pp. 182–183.

DeLee, J. C. Complications of Arthroscopy and Arthroscopic Surgery: Results of a National Survey. *Arthroscopy,* Vol. 1 (1985), pp. 214–220.

Driver-Jowitt, J. P. Arthroscopy—Expertise, Expedience and Expectation. *South African Medical Journal,* Vol. 70 (1986), p. 652.

Erisksoon, E., and others. Knee Arthroscopy with Local Anesthesia in Ambulatory Patients. Methods, Results and Patient Compliance. *Orthopedics,* Vol. 9 (1986), pp. 186–188.

Fullerton, L. R., Jr. Knee Arthroscopy in the Military Population: An Analysis of 600 Knee Arthroscopies. *Arthroscopy,* Vol. 2 (1986), pp. 259–261.

Geiringer, Steve R. Sports Injuries: Recognition and Management [book review]. *American Journal of Physical Medicine and Rehabilitation,* Vol. 70, No. 4 (Aug. 1991), p. 225.

Glinz, W. *Diagnostic and Operative Arthroscopy of the Knee Joint,* 2d ed. Toronto: Hogrefe & Huber, 1990.

Groh, Gordon I., and others. Results of Total Knee Arthroplasty Using the Posterior Stabilized Condylar Prosthesis: A Report of 137 Consecutive Cases. *Clinical Orthopaedics and Related Research,* Vol. 269 (Aug. 1991), pp. 58–62.

Hofmann, Aaron A., and others. Total Knee Arthroplasty Two- to Four-Year Experience Using an Asymmetric Tibial Tray and a Deep Trochlear-Grooved Femoral Component. *Clinical Orthopaedics and Related Research,* Vol. 269 (Aug. 1991), pp. 78–88.

Hughes, Sean. Operative Arthroscopy. *Lancet,* Vol. 338, No. 8764 (1991), p. 433.

Jackson, D. W. Videoarthroscopy: Present and Future Developments. *Arthroscopy,* Vol. 1 (1985), pp. 108–115.

Kujala, U. M., and others. Knee Injuries in Athletes. Review of Exertion Injuries and Retrospective Study of Outpatient Sports Clinic Material. *Sports Medicine,* Vol. 3 (1986), pp. 447–460.

Metcalf, R. W. Arthroscopic Knee Surgery. *Advances in Surgery,* Vol. 17 (1984), pp. 197–240.

Nielsen, Allan Buhl, and Yde, Johannes. Epidemiology of Acute Knee Injuries: A Prospective Hospital Investigation. *Journal of Trauma,* Vol. 31, No. 12 (Dec. 1991), pp. 1644–1648.

Older, J., and Cardoso, T. First Year's Experience of Day-Case Arthroscopy in Diagnosis and Management of Disorders of the Knee Joint. *Lancet,* Vol. 2 (1983), pp. 264–267.

Rand, James A. Bone Deficiency in Total Knee Arthroplasty Use of Metal Wedge Augmentation. *Clinical Orthopaedics and Related Research,* Vol. 271 (Oct. 1991), pp. 63–71.

Sherman, O. H., and others. Arthroscopy (No-Problem Surgery). An Analysis of Complications in 2640 Cases. *Journal of Bone and Joint Surgery,* Vol. 68-A (1986), pp. 256–265.

Small, N. C. Complications in Arthroscopy: The Knee and Other Joints. *Arthroscopy,* Vol. 2 (1986), pp. 253–258.

Smith, Ian, and others. Effects of Local Anesthesia on Recovery After Outpatient Arthroscopy. *Anesthesia and Analgesia,* Vol. 73, No. 5 (1991), pp. 536–539.

Herniated Disc Surgery

Likelihood of Unnecessary Surgery   **EXTREMELY HIGH**

Disc surgery (laminectomy) is near the top of the list of unnecessary operations. Of the 200,000 laminectomies performed each year, experts at the Rand Corporation, the research think tank, estimate that up to 40% or 80,000 operations, are unnecessary. In 1991 the research firm MediQual reported that 51.39% of laminectomies they studied had none of the objective clinical findings documented in the hospital medical record they use to validate laminectomy at the time of surgery. And researchers at Johns Hopkins University calculate that over half of patients they studied with continuing back pain did not need this operation. Those most likely to have an unnecessary operation had injured their backs at work or in a motor vehicle accident.

I originally believed that surgeons were not totally to blame for those numbers, and that patients, eager to rush into surgery to relieve pain, were also at fault. Senior surgeons who reviewed the manuscript for this book placed the blame back on the surgeon for acquiescing to patient demand. The operation is frequently a mistake. Up to 70% of patients with a herniated disc will improve without surgery. And, according to follow-up studies done up to ten years after back pain was first diagnosed, patients who had surgery fared no better than those treated medically.

You should be aware that there are tremendous regional differences in the treatment of back pain. A University of Wisconsin study found that this operation was performed seven times more frequently in some counties than in others. The areas of the country where you are most likely to find unnecessary operations are the South, the Midwest, and the West. Comparatively fewer operations are done unnecessarily in the East.

One last warning: Be very careful about the interpretation of your test results and the kind of tests you agree to take. I spoke with a senior surgeon who received referrals for back surgery based on x-ray and imaging studies. In 1991 he had 362 new patients referred for back surgery. Of these, 147 patients had scans or imaging studies that had been interpreted as showing discs requiring surgery. His correct reading, however, showed that *none* of these 147 actually required surgery. In fact, of the 362 patients referred, he found that tests were *not* really necessary, on the basis of the clinical exam, for 100 of the MRIs, 39 of the CAT scans, and eight of the myelograms. He also warned me that the discogram, held to be notoriously unreliable by neurosurgeons, is coming back into favor among some orthopedic surgeons. He was concerned enough to warn that, should a discogram be suggested, patients should look for another doctor!

Potential Risk   MODERATE

While back surgery is performed routinely and most surgeons have a high degree of competence, complications still occur. The most common are infection and damage or scarring around the nerves during the operation.

What It Is

Between vertebrae in your back there is a shock absorber called an intervertebral disc. Part of this disc can protrude from its normal position to compress a nerve as the nerve leaves the spine. The pressure on the nerve is what causes the pain. The polite term "herniation" is used to describe how the disc is squeezed out of position. Dr. William Fager, Chief of Neurosurgery at the Lahey Clinic in Burlington, Massachusetts, points out that the process is really much more violent. The disc actually ruptures. It's an important distinction, since many imaging studies show a benign bulging of the disc rather than an outright rupture.

The operative procedure is called a laminectomy. The surgeon removes the part of the disc that is squeezing the nerve and causing pain. The material they remove at surgery is called the nucleus.

Step 1. Make Sure You Need the Surgery

Doctors assess the chance of a successful operation based on clinical findings, x-ray tests, and other imaging studies. If you have a fragmented or protruding disc that is compressing a nerve and clearly causing the pain, your results are likely to be excellent, although you may still do just as well without surgery. If your case is ambiguous, the likelihood of success diminishes. Surgery could make you worse, not better. If your doctor recommends the operation, check your test and examination results against the ones in the following list.

Appropriate Procedure

EMERGENCY   The disc interferes with your ability to defecate and urinate and causes weakness or numbness in both legs. This is considered an emergency procedure because of the potential for permanent loss of bowel and bladder control. Only about 1–3% of all disc operations are considered true emergencies, however.

HERNIATED DISC   With *all* of the following findings, *after* conservative treatment is tried:

■ Magnetic resonance imaging (MRI) or CT myelogram showing disc has ruptured and is compressing nerve (be quite certain scan has been correctly interpreted as showing a real ruptured disc, not a bulge or artifact)

■ Pain radiating from back down past your knees

■ Loss of some neurologic function (for example, inability to stand on the toes or heel of one foot)

■ Inability to raise a leg without increasing discomfort and resistance (This test is often misinterpreted. The discomfort should increase pain in your leg, not in your back. A straight leg raise that causes pain in your back is *not* an indication for surgery. This test used to be performed with the patient on his or her back. It is now best performed with the patient sitting.)

About 95% of patients who meet these guidelines do quite well after surgery because the cause and effect are clearly linked. The diagnostic x-rays reveal a bulging disc compressing a nerve and causing pain and loss of function. This is like finding a burnt-out fuse for your refrigerator circuit and then confirming that the refrigerator is not running. But with the most difficult back cases, no such link can be found. The pain and loss of function can't be correlated with the x-rays. As a result, unnecessary operations are performed.

Probably an Appropriate Procedure

SITUATION 1: YOU *DO* HAVE

■ MRI or CT myelogram showing disc has ruptured and is compressing a nerve

■ Pain radiating from your back down past your knees

■ Loss of some neurologic function

■ An appropriate trial of conservative therapy

BUT YOU *DON'T* HAVE

■ Discomfort raising your legs while sitting or lying on your back on a table

SITUATION 2: YOU *DO* HAVE

■ MRI or CT myelogram showing disc has extruded and is compressing nerve

■ Pain radiating from your back down past your knees

■ An appropriate trial of conservative therapy

BUT YOU *DON'T* HAVE

- Loss of some neurologic function

Probably Not an Appropriate Procedure

YOU *DO* HAVE

- MRI or CT myelogram revealing a bulge in disc but no fragmentation or protrusion

- A positive discogram that reproduces the pain (considered a very unreliable test)

- Pain radiating in a straight line from your back to your feet

BUT YOU *DON'T* HAVE

- Loss of some neurologic function

- Discomfort raising your legs while lying on your back on a table

- A positive EMG (special test for the subtle loss of muscle function) showing no loss of function

Not an Appropriate Procedure

YOU *DO* HAVE

- Pain confined to the back, with no radiation down your leg

- Minor injury of back muscles or pain due to stress

BUT YOU *DON'T* HAVE

- Loss of some neurologic function

Patients who have simply injured the back muscles from sleeping positions or lifting the wrong way or who suffer back pain due to stress are unlikely to find relief through surgery. Many patients desperate for pain relief will "push their doctors to the wall" to "do something," but that "something" should not be surgery.

Step 2. Consider an Alternative

Percutaneous Discectomy

Percutaneous discectomy involves removal of portions of a damaged disc. In this procedure, a needle is introduced into the disc and disc material sucked out. This is a very controversial procedure. National experts I conferred with emphasized that procedures such as discectomy are not as effective as surgical resection, since they won't fix the problem. They say the disc material still remains around the affected nerve, leaving the problem unsolved.

Conservative Treatment

Patients frequently believe that conservative treatment of back pain isn't "doing anything." Yet study after study shows that, with time and conservative treatment, many cases are healed. You should take this kind of treatment seriously and not dismiss it as simply a temporary expedient prior to surgery. If you are disabled or lack motivation, you should consult a physical therapist.

STAGE ONE TREATMENT (for acute back pain)

- Bed rest, preferably for three days and up to a maximum of five

- Use of nonsteroidal antiinflammatory drugs

- Analgesics as needed

- Muscle relaxant if necessary

- Steroids injected directly into the spinal area (not all surgeons agree with this recommendation although it is frequently performed)

STAGE TWO TREATMENT (for rehabilitation and prevention of back injuries)   There are several forms of physical therapy that can help:

- Stretching exercises to build up flexibility

- Abdominal strengthening exercises that will reduce strain on the back

- Extension exercises to stretch and strengthen the back if you injured your muscles by bending

- Aerobic exercise that can increase the supply of blood to the nerve root, thus changing its metabolism and promoting healing and possibly preventing injuries as well

STAGE THREE TREATMENT (for prevention of back injuries)   You can help prevent back injuries with the following simple steps:

- Not smoking (by reducing the supply of blood to the back, smoking makes the discs less elastic and springy)

- Maintaining weight within 10% of that recommended for your height and build

- Taking nonsteroidal antiinflammatory drugs if prescribed by your doctor

Step 3. Get a Specialist's Opinion

You will want to consult an expert if your procedure is not clearly indicated or has a low probability of success. You can go to a neurologist, who can do an excellent diagnostic workup and will probably be a strong advocate for conservative therapy. When it's not an emergency, I often recommend a physical medicine doctor (specialist in rehabilitation medicine), who can help patients escape surgery. Be certain your doctor devotes the bulk of her or his practice to back surgery. If conservative therapy fails, see a highly skilled orthopedic surgeon or neurosurgeon who meets the criteria detailed in Step 5.

Make certain you discuss your chances of success Remember, doctors grade your chance of success based on your clinical findings and the x-ray tests. A fragmented disc or a ruptured disc that is compressing a nerve and clearly causing your pain and disability makes surgery a good option. The less clear-cut your case is though, the lower the likelihood that surgery will help, and it could even hurt. That is why you should give conservative therapy and alternative methods of pain relief the best possible shot you can.

WHO TO CALL

American College of Surgeons They will offer you names of fellows in your geographic area.

55 E Erie St
Chicago, IL 60611
312/664-4050

American Academy of Orthopedic Surgeons This organization can provide callers with educational information on various types of orthopedic surgery as well as academy guidelines and position papers.

222 S Prospect Ave
Park Ridge, IL 60068
708/823-7186

American Association of Neurological Surgeons Though this is a professional organization, callers can receive limited educational material.

22 S Washington St
Park Ridge, IL 60068
708/692-9500

NIH CRISP System
301/496-7543

University-Affiliated Teaching Hospitals See Appendix.

Step 4. Choose a Hospital

You should look for a hospital with a high volume of disc surgeries that also has excellent results for patients in your condition.

Experience

The hospital should do a minimum of 100–150 operations a year. The Mayo Clinic, with an excellent reputation for disc surgery, performs more than 800 annually.

Results

Here are the best-known results for disc surgery. Try to find a hospital that has comparable results.

Infection: Less than 1%

Nerve damage: Less than 1%

Successful relief of pain and disability: Greater than 95%

In a "virgin spine," that is, where no operation has ever been performed, complications should be 0.5% or less.

Other Measures of Excellence

■ An excellent rehabilitation program that can help strengthen your abdomen and lower back after the operation

■ A back school to teach you how to build a strong back and how to avoid injuries

■ A low ratio of surgery-referral patients to operations performed (For instance, at the Lahey Clinic in Massachusetts, 650 operations are performed each year out of a total of 6,500 patients referred.)

Centers of Excellence for Orthopedics

The following list of hospitals is provided only as a convenient starting place in your search for excellence. They are recommended on the basis of reputation, not experience and results. The list is not an endorsement. There may be hospitals just as excellent that have been omitted. You should apply the guidelines for experience, results, and other measures of excellence to any hospital you choose, whether or not it is on this list. Although hospitals from different sources have been combined into one list, the compilation in no way implies that one source has endorsed the hospital list of another source.

LAMINECTOMY PERFORMED BY NEUROSURGEONS

ARIZONA
Barrow Neurologic Institute   EX
350 W Thomas
Phoenix, AZ 85013

CALIFORNIA
University of California, Los Angeles,
    School of Medicine   EX
10833 LeConte Ave
Los Angeles, CA 90024

University of California, San
    Francisco, Medical Center   EX
505 Parnassus Ave
San Francisco, CA 94143

FLORIDA
University of Miami School
    of Medicine   EX
1600 NW 10th Ave
PO Box 016099 (R59)
Miami, FL 33101

ILLINOIS
Rush-Presbyterian St. Luke's
    Medical Center   EX
1653 W Congress Pkwy
Chicago, IL 60612

IOWA
University of Iowa College
    of Medicine   EX
200 Eckstein Medical Research Bldg
Iowa City, IA 52242

LOUISIANA
Alton Ochsner Medical Foundation   EX
1516 Jefferson Hwy
New Orleans, LA 70121

MASSACHUSETTS
Lahey Clinic   EX
41 Mall Rd
Burlington, MA 01803

MINNESOTA
Mayo Clinic   EX
200 First St SW
Rochester, MN 55905

OHIO
Case Western Reserve University
    School of Medicine   EX
2119 Abington Rd
Cleveland, OH 44106-2333

Mayfield Clinic   EX
University of Cincinnati College
    of Medicine
231 Bethesda Ave
Cincinnati, OH 45267-0555

Ohio State University College of
    Medicine   EX
200 Meiling Hall
370 W 9th Ave
Columbus, OH 43210

PENNSYLVANIA
Pennsylvania Hospital   EX
800 Spruce St
Philadelphia, PA 19107

WISCONSIN
Medical College of Wisconsin   EX
8701 Watertown Plank Rd
Milwaukee, WI 53226

LAMINECTOMY PERFORMED BY ORTHOPEDIC SURGEONS

CALIFORNIA
University of California, San Diego   EX
School of Medicine
La Jolla, CA 92093

University of California,
    San Francisco   EX
513 Parnassus Ave
San Francisco, CA 94143-0410

FLORIDA
University of Miami   EX
Jackson-Memorial Medical Center
1611 NW 12th Ave
Miami, FL 33136

MARYLAND
Johns Hopkins Hospital   EX
600 N Wolfe St
Baltimore, MD 21205

MASSACHUSETTS
Massachusetts General Hospital   EX
55 Fruit St
Boston, MA 02114

MINNESOTA
Mayo Clinic   EX
200 First St SW
Rochester, MN 55905

Minnesota Spine Center   EX
606 24th Ave S, Ste 602
Minneapolis, MN 55454

University of Minnesota   EX
UMHC Box 293
420 Delaware St SE
Minneapolis, MN 55455

NEW YORK
Hospital for Special Surgery   EX
535 E 70th St
New York, NY 10021

SOURCES

EX   indicates those hospitals recommended by experts interviewed.

Step 5. Choose a Doctor

Your doctor should be board-certified in neurosurgery or orthopedic surgery. An orthopedic surgeon should have completed a back fellowship.

Experience

The doctor should perform 100–150 back operations annually. These need not be disc operations.

Results

SUCCESS RATES   The doctor should have a success rate in relieving pain and restoring function of 95% or more.

COMPLICATION RATES   Complications should occur in less than 1% of cases.

EXPERT SOURCES

Although dozens of experts were interviewed for these chapters, these physicians are acknowledged for their significant contributions to this section.

Dr. William Fager, Chief of Neurosurgery, Lahey Clinic, Burlington, MA

Dr. Frank P. Cammisa Jr., The Hospital for Special Surgery, New York, NY

REFERENCES AND SUGGESTED READING

Bazzoli, Allan S. Chronic Back Pain: A Commonsense Approach. *American Journal of Physical Medicine and Rehabilitation,* Vol. 71, No. 1 (Feb. 1992), pp. 53–54.

Powell, Michael. Advances and Technical Standards in Neurosurgery [book review]. *Journal of Neurology, Neurosurgery and Psychiatry,* Vol. 55, No. 2 (Feb. 1992), p. 170.

Waugh, Douglas. Vista: Chiropractic Manipulation. *Canadian Medical Association Journal,* Vol. 146, No. 5 (Mar. 1, 1992), p. 762.

Carotid Endarterectomy

Likelihood of Unnecessary Surgery VERY HIGH

In 1987, a landmark study was published in the *Journal of the American Medical Association*. It reported that 32% of the 81,000 endarterectomies performed annually were unnecessary. Most unnecessary procedures are performed on patients whose carotid vessels are not narrowed enough to justify surgery. Since that study, there has been a national effort to decrease the number of unnecessary surgeries. Still, in 1991 the research firm MediQual reported that 28.65% of endarterectomies they studied had none of the objective clinical findings documented in the hospital medical record they use to validate endarterectomy at the time of surgery.

Potential Risk VERY HIGH

Carotid endarterectomies are extremely controversial because of a notorious tradeoff. You can risk a stroke or death by forgoing the operation or you can risk heart attack, stroke, or death during surgery. Even when the operation is indicated, it poses too great a risk if the death rate exceeds 5%, at which rate the risk of the operation exceeds the risk of doing nothing at all. The complication rate can reach 20%.

What It Is

Carotid endarterectomy is performed to remove blockages from the carotid arteries and to reduce the possibility of stroke. The carotids are two of the three main vessels supplying blood to the brain. Prime candidates for the operation have had early warnings signs of a stroke such as vision that blurred temporarily. This is one form of a transient ischemic attack (TIA). During the operation the surgeon opens the carotid artery in the neck and removes blood clots or other material obstructing the blood flow from the artery.

Step 1. Make Sure You Need the Surgery

Remember this rule of thumb: The patients who benefit the most from this operation are those whose carotid artery is blocked more than 70%. According to a study in the British medical journal *The Lancet* in 1991, strokes in such cases can be reduced six-fold. With less than 30% of the artery blocked the risks definitely outweighed the benefits. Between these two extremes the results were inconclusive. Another study, by the National Institutes of Health in 1991, found that in patients with a 70–90% narrowing of the carotid artery, surgery reduced the likelihood of stroke from more than 25% to less than 10%. In the 18 months after surgery, 24% of the patients treated medically but only 7% of the surgical patients had a stroke on the same side as the narrowed artery. During that same period, 12% of the medical patients, compared to 5% of the surgical patients, had a major or fatal stroke or died of any cause.

Dr. Henry J. M. Barnett, of the University of Western Ontario and Coordinator of the North American Symptomatic Carotid Endarterectomy Trial, says that a major problem with the operation is the absence of well-defined standards for determining the extent of blockage. In 1991 Barnett proposed a set of standards in the *New England Journal of Medicine.* Since some medical centers use criteria that are not demanding enough, you should make certain that your blockage has met the 70% guideline on the basis of precise measurements of an angiogram, not a doctor's "eyeball" estimate.

Before you agree to an endarterectomy, check to see if your diagnosis matches the conditions in the following lists.

Appropriate Procedure

- After a TIA or small stroke, if 70% or more of one artery is blocked on the same side as the stroke or TIA; and not a high surgical risk because of age, high blood pressure, diabetes, or other complications.

- After a TIA or small stroke, if 50% of the artery is blocked and the blockage is located near an ulcer in the artery (Stroke-producing blood clots are more likely to form around ulcers that occur in the artery.)

- After several transient ischemic attacks that have not responded to medical treatment, if most of the artery is blocked or an ulcer has formed in the artery and there is low to medium risk for surgery.

- TIAs that are increasing in intensity, if a large blockage or ulcer is present on the same side of the brain that produces the symptoms, for instance, sudden trouble speaking and the left artery is blocked (since speech is under the control of the left brain); surgical risk must be low to medium.

- Following a very minor stroke when a large blockage or ulcer is found in the artery on the same side as the symptoms have occurred (Surgery should be delayed one month to lower the risk of a subsequent stroke); surgical risk should be low to medium.

- No symptoms plus large blockages in both carotid arteries.

Uncertain If Procedure Is Appropriate

- Stroke-in-evolution that may have a dramatic response to surgery but where risk for complications is high

Not an Appropriate Procedure

- No substantial blockage of carotid artery

- Medical treatment for near-strokes is working

- Surgical risks are high because of severe heart disease or other conditions

- Artery is totally blocked and surgery will produce no benefits

- Symptoms from blocked arteries in the rear of the brain, called vertebrobasilar-distribution transient ischemic attacks

- Dementia from multiple strokes, and quality of life won't improve after surgery

- Following a stroke that has caused significant and lasting brain damage

- Severe brain damage from any cause

- Evidence of bleeding into the brain (another indication of stroke)

- After major stroke

- Being scheduled for major noncardiac surgery, and criteria noted under Appropriate Procedure are not met

Step 2. Consider an Alternative

Since carotid endarterectomy is considered a preventive measure, there are no clear alternatives. However, some doctors recommend aspirin because of studies that suggest it can be beneficial. Those studies compared aspirin alone to aspirin combined with surgery. The combination of aspirin and surgery was far more beneficial in the prevention of stroke and heart attack. Taking aspirin alone is a method of prevention, like eating a low-cholesterol diet and not smoking. Older studies found that the best benefits came in patients, especially those who had recently undergone surgery, who took four tablets a day. But studies published in 1991 suggest that a much lower dosage can produce just as good results. In one study, a mere 30 milligrams of aspirin—the standard tablet contains 325 milligrams—were sufficient to prevent stroke. The amount of aspirin doctors actually prescribe remains controversial. Ticlid was approved in 1991 as an alternative to aspirin for the prevention of strokes in those who cannot take aspirin. Since the drug suppresses the production of white blood cells in some patients, its use must be monitored carefully.

Step 3. Get a Specialist's Opinion

You'll want to discuss the various tradeoffs with your doctor—the risks of surgery versus the danger of waiting. For example, let's say doctors can hear a rumbling sound, called a bruit, when they listen to your carotid arteries with a stethoscope. While your chance of dying with that condition is 1.5% in any one year, you may have a substantially higher risk of complications during surgery. You'll want to get an expert opinion if your diagnosis is unclear, your angiogram does not show conclusively a 70% or greater blockage, or your surgery is not indicated or not clearly necessary.

For an expert opinion you can consult either a vascular surgeon or a neurosurgeon. There are no reliable statistics suggesting that you will have a better outcome with one or the other. It depends entirely on the skill of the individual doctor. In Europe and the United States, vascular surgeons performed this operation first. In Canada, neurosurgeons were the pioneers. The doctor you choose should meet the standards outlined in Step 5.

WHO TO CALL

A Major University-Affiliated Teaching Hospital or Stroke Center Contact the chief of neurology, the chief of neurosurgery, or the chief of cardiovascular thoracic surgery (see Appendix).

American Heart Association Call your local chapter or the following:

National Headquarters
7320 Greenville Ave
Dallas, TX 75231
214/373-6300

National Stroke Association This group provides educational brochures and information to stroke survivors, health care professionals, and caregivers. There are six chapters throughout the United States. A newsletter for stroke survivors, "Be Stroke Smart," is published quarterly; a newsletter for health care professionals, called "Stroke Clinical Updates," is also available.

300 E Hampden Ave, Ste 240
Englewood, CO 80110
303/762-9922

NIH CRISP System
301/496-7543

Step 4. Choose a Hospital

Too few community hospitals have a large enough caseload of endarterectomies to judge them properly. You are best served by choosing a hospital with a national or at least a regional reputation in this field. "There are good community hospitals but I'm certain it's a fact that morbidity and mortality is lower at the teaching hospitals," says Dr. James T. Robertson, Past President of the American Academy of Neurological Surgery.

Experience

This is one operation where a high volume of cases may not be the best indicator of quality. Since there are large numbers of unnecessary operations, the hospital may be operating on marginal cases or as an endarterectomy factory. High volume in such instances is not a measure of excellence, since it breeds higher death rates.

Results

DEATH RATE   The death rate should be no greater than 2% in the 30 days following surgery.

COMPLICATION RATE   Remember that an endarterectomy is a tradeoff: You risk death or complications from the procedure; you risk stroke or death by not having the operation. You and your physician need to weigh the risks of operating versus the risks of not. If the risk of operating is greater, *don't operate!* You should aim for an overall risk of complication that is no more than 3%. That figure includes preoperative tests, surgery, and recovery. If you have a very high risk of imminent stroke, you might accept a higher complication rate. That upper limit of risk should not exceed 5.8%.

Other Measures of Excellence

Length of stay: 6.9 days

Hospital charges: $10,440

Centers of Excellence for Cardiovascular Surgery

The following list of hospitals is provided only as a convenient starting place in your search for excellence. These hospitals are recommended on the basis of reputation, not experience and results. The list is not an endorsement. There may be hospitals just as excellent that have been omitted. You should apply the guidelines for experience, results, and other measures of excellence to any hospital you choose, whether or not it is on this list. Although hospitals from different sources have been combined into one list, the compilation in no way implies that one source has endorsed the hospital list of another source.

ARIZONA

Barrow Neurological Institute   SCE
St. Joseph's Hospital &
     Medical Center
350 W Thomas Rd
Phoenix, AZ 85013

CALIFORNIA

University of California, Los
     Angeles, School of Medicine   NIH/SCE
10833 LeConte Ave
Los Angeles, CA 90024-1682

University of California,
     San Diego   SCE
UCSD Stroke Center
225 Dickinson St
San Diego, CA 92103-1990

University of California, San
     Francisco, Medical Center   NIH
505 Parnassus Ave
San Francisco, CA 94143

University of Southern California
     School of Medicine   SCE
Dept of Neurology, Unit 1, Rm 5641
Los Angeles, CA 90073

CANADA

Roberts Research Institute   SCE
100 Perth Dr
P.O. Box 5015
London, Ontario N6A 5K8

FLORIDA

University of Miami School
     of Medicine   NIH/SCE
Department of Neurology, D 4-5
1501 NW 9th Ave
P.O. Box 016960
Miami, FL 33101

ILLINOIS

University of Illinois Hospital   SCE
912 So. Wood, 855N
Chicago, IL 60612

IOWA

University of Iowa Hospitals   NIH/SCE
Division of Neurology
Iowa City, IA 52242

MARYLAND

Johns Hopkins Hospital   NIH
600 No. Wolfe St
Baltimore, MD 21205

University of Maryland School
     of Medicine   NIH
22 So. Green St
Baltimore, MD 21201

MASSACHUSETTS

Beth Israel Hospital   SCE
Dept of Neurology
330 Brookline Ave
Boston, MA 02215

Boston University School
     of Medicine   SCE
Dept of Neurology, Ste 1105
720 Harrison Ave
Boston, MA 02118

Massachusetts General Hospital NIH
55 Fruit St
Boston, MA 02114

MICHIGAN
Henry Ford Hospital NIH
2799 W Grand Blvd
Detroit, MI 48302

MINNESOTA
Mayo Clinic NIH
200 First St SW
Rochester, MN 55901

University of Minnesota Hospital SCE
Dept of Neurosurgery
P.O. Box 96; B590 Mayo Mem. Bldg.
420 Delaware St SE
Minneapolis, MN 55455

MISSISSIPPI
University of Mississippi
 Medical Center SCE
Dept of Neurosurgery
2500 N. State St
Jackson, MS 39216-4505

MISSOURI
St. Louis University Medical Center SCE
Dept of Neurology
3660 Vista Ave
St. Louis, MO 63110

University of Missouri School of
 Medicine SCE
M741-Neurology
#1 Hospital Dr
Columbia, MO 65212

Washington University School of
 Medicine NIH
510 So. Kings Hwy
St. Louis, MO 63110

NEW HAMPSHIRE
Dartmouth-Hitchcock
 Medical Center SCE
Hitchcock Clinic
Dept of Neurology
2 Maynard St
Hanover, NH 03756

NEW MEXICO
University of New Mexico
 School of Medicine SCE
Dept of Neurosurgery
2211 Olamas NE
Albuquerque, NM 87131

NEW YORK
Albert Einstein/Montefiore
 Hospital SCE
Montefiore Medical Center, NW 7
111 E 210 St
Bronx, NY 10467

Columbia University
 Neurological Institute SCE
Dept of Neurology
710 W 168th St
New York, NY 10032

Cornell University
 Medical College NIH
1300 York Ave
New York, NY 10021

New York University
 Medical Center SCE
530 First Ave
New York, NY 10016

State University of New York SCE
Neurology Service
VAMC
800 Irving Ave
Syracuse, NY 13210

NORTH CAROLINA
Bowman Gray School
 of Medicine NIH
300 So. Hawthorne Rd
Winston-Salem, NC 24103

Duke University Medical Center   NIH
Box 3813
Durham, NC 27710

OHIO

Case Western Reserve University   SCE
2119 Abington Rd
Cleveland, OH 44106-2333

Good Samaritan Hospital   SCE
3217 Clifton Ave
Cincinnati, OH 45220-2489

Ohio State University   SCE
429 Means Hall
1655 Upham Dr
Columbus, OH 43210

OREGON

Comprehensive Stroke Center
of Oregon   NIH
University of Oregon Health
Sciences Center
3181 SW Sarn Jackson Park Rd
Portland, OR 97201

PENNSYLVANIA

Hospital of the University
of Pennsylvania   NIH
Johnson Pavilion (Gl), Rm 429
36th and Hamilton Walk
Philadelphia, PA 19104

Temple University Hospital   SCE
Dept of Neurosurgery
3401 No. Broad St
Philadelphia, PA 19140

University of Pittsburgh   SCE
Dept of Neurology
325 Scaife Hall
Pittsburgh, PA 15261

RHODE ISLAND

Rhode Island Hospital   SCE
110 Lockwood St
Providence, RI 02903

TENNESSEE

University of Tennessee Health
Science Center   SCE
Dept of Neurosurgery
956 Court Ave
Memphis, TN 38163

TEXAS

University of Texas Health
Science Center   SCE
Department of Medicine/Neurology
7703 Floyd Curl Dr
San Antonio, TX 78284

University of Texas Health
Science Center   NIH/SCE
Dept of Neurology, Rm 7044 MSB
6431 Fannin St
Houston, TX 77030

University of Texas Southwestern
Medical Center   SCE
Dept of Surgery, E7126
5323 Harry Hines Blvd
Dallas, TX 75235-9031

VIRGINIA

Virginia Commonwealth University   SCE
Division of Neuro-Ophthalmology
Richmond Eye & Ear Hospital
1001 E Marshall, Rm 403
Richmond, VA 23219

WISCONSIN

Marshfield Clinic   SCE
Dept of Neurology
1000 No. Oak Ave
Marshfield, WI 54491-5790

SOURCES

NIH indicates the Stroke Clinical Research Centers from the list maintained by the NIH.

SCE indicates those centers that were North American Symptomatic Carotid Endarterectomy Trial Hospitals.

Step 5. Choose a Doctor

You can have this operation performed by either a vascular surgeon or a neurosurgeon. Some experts say that neurosurgeons are better diagnosticians because they know the diseases of the brain. However, vascular surgeons, while lacking that background, are trained to repair and operate on arteries. If you decide on a vascular surgeon, it is a good idea to consult a neurosurgeon or neurologist also, just to make certain the carotid lesion is causing the problem.

Vascular Surgeon

The vascular surgeon should be board-certified in general surgery, with a subspecialty in cardiovascular surgery. Doctors who trained after 1984 should have completed a one- to two-year vascular fellowship.

Experience

The doctor should perform 50 vascular operations a year, including carotid endarterectomies.

Results

DEATH RATE   This figure should not exceed 2%.

Neurosurgeon

The neurosurgeon should have completed one year of general surgical training and five years of specialized neurosurgery, including 12 months as a senior resident. The doctor should have performed 12–15 operations during residency. Many neurosurgeons have finished longer training programs. About half of the hospitals in the United States with teaching programs in neurosurgery require six years of training. Others, including Massachusetts General Hospital, require seven years.

Experience

Dr. James T. Robertson, Past President of the American Academy of Neurological Surgery, states: "If you get the country thinking they can judge quality by numbers, what happens is you get a marginal operator feeling the pressure to perform more and more operations, some of which may be unnecessary, just to stay up to snuff. In other words, it can breed exactly that which you are trying to avoid, inappropriateness."

No study has found a correlation between doctor volume and risk of complications. Like the vascular surgeon, 50 vascular operations a year are a good indicator for experience, though some experts believe as few as 10 operations a year can still ensure competency.

Results

DEATH RATE   The measure of excellence established by MediQual based on 2,293 cases is a death rate of only 0.8%. The average patient age was 68.6 years. I recommend you make sure to choose a doctor for whom the death rate in the 30 days following surgery does not surpass 2%.

COMPLICATION RATE   Complications should occur in no more than 5.8% of cases. Since the danger of complications increases with the severity of the disease, you should also check the statistics for hospitals in Step 4. Your doctor should meet these standards as well.

Other Measures of Excellence

REGULAR CASE REVIEW   Experienced surgeons audit their work continuously. Typically they will review their last 100 consecutive cases for problems. When you ask a surgeon for death rates, she or he should know her or his own statistics from regular case review.

EXPERT SOURCES

Although dozens of experts were interviewed for these chapters, these physicians are acknowledged for their significant contributions to this section.

Dr. James T. Robertson, Chair, Department of Neurosurgery, University of Tennessee, Memphis, TN

Dr. Henry J. M. Barnett, Coordinator of North American Symptomatic Carotid Endarterectomy Trial, Robarts Research Institute, London, Ontario, Canada

REFERENCES AND SUGGESTED READING

American College of Physicians. Indications for Carotid Endarterectomy. Position Paper 1989. *Annals of Internal Medicine,* Vol. 111, No. 8 (Oct. 15, 1989), pp. 675–677.

American Heart Association. *1991 Heart and Stroke Facts.*

American Heart Association. Special Report: Assessing Risk Associated with Carotid Endarterectomy. *Circulation,* Vol. 79 (1989), pp. 472–473.

Donnan, Geoffrey A. Investigation of Patients with Stroke and Transient Ischaemic Attacks. *Lancet,* Vol. 339, No. 8791 (Feb. 22, 1992), pp. 473–477.

Dyken, M. L. Carotid Artery Surgery: Does the Benefit Outweigh the Risk? American Heart Association's Thirteenth Science Writers Forum, Sarasota, Fl., Jan. 12–15, 1986.

Landi, Gianluca. Clinical Diagnosis of Transient Ischaemic Attacks. *Lancet,* Vol. 339, No. 8790 (Feb. 15, 1992), pp. 402–405.

Nadeau, Stephen E., and others. Carotid Endarterectomy [letter]. *New England Journal of Medicine.* Vol. 326, No. 11 (Mar. 12, 1992), pp. 762–765.

National Stroke Association Carotid Endarterectomy: Stroke Prevention Surgery More Effective Than Previously Thought. *Be Stroke Smart,* Vol. 8, No. 1 (Spring 1991).

National Stroke Association. Indications for Carotid Endarterectomy: An Update. *Stroke Clinical Updates,* Vol. 2, No. 2 (July 1991).

North American Symptomatic Carotid Endarterectomy Trial (NASCET). North American Symptomatic Carotid Endarterectomy Trial: Methods, Patient Characteristics and Progress. *Stroke,* Vol. 22 (1991), pp. 711–720.

Pulsinelli, William. Pathophysiology of Acute Ischaemic Stroke. *Lancet,* Vol. 339, No. 8792 (Feb. 29, 1992), pp. 533–536.

Robertson, J. T. Bleeding Around the Brain. American Heart Association's Thirteenth Science Writers Forum, Sarasota, Fl., Jan. 12–15, 1986.

Surgery to Prevent Recurrence of Stroke. *Lancet,* May 25, 1991, p. 1235.

U.K. TIA Study Group. The United Kingdom Transient Ischaemic Attack (UK-TIA) Aspirin Trial: Final Results. *Journal of Neurology, Neurosurgery and Psychiatry,* Vol. 54, No. 12 (Dec. 1991), pp. 1044–1054.

U.S. Department of Health and Human Services. *Carotid Endarterectomy.* DHHS Publication No. (PHS) 91–3472, Dec. 1990.

Winslow, C. M., and others. The Appropriateness of Carotid Endarterectomy. *New England Journal of Medicine,* Vol. 318, No. 12 (Mar. 24, 1988), pp. 721–727.

Cataract Surgery

Likelihood of Unnecessary Surgery   MODERATE

This is the number-one surgical procedure performed on patients in the United States. There are, however, substantial regional variations in the frequency of the operation and in the surgical techniques used. Ophthalmologists also take different approaches to the care of patients before and after the operation. For example, some ophthalmologists regularly use ultrasound in their preoperative examinations, while others do not. As a result the cost of the operation varies considerably. Dr. Robert W. Dubois of the research organization Value Health Sciences says, "Cataract surgery is unlike many of the procedures discussed in this book. Cataract extraction is performed not to extend life or to prevent major morbidity. Rather the decision to operate is based upon quality-of-life issues. How much does the cataract interfere with my life? Thus, the decision to operate is based more on social rather than medical issues." Dr. Walter Stark, Director of the Cornea Service at Johns Hopkins Hospital, points out: "The diagnosis or presence of cataract is not by itself an indication for surgery. The cataract will not hurt one's eye and should not be equated with a cancer or a growth that will cause problems. The only indication for removal of a cataract is if the cataract reduces the patient's visual acuity to a level that interferes with a patient's activities, especially reading, driving, or occupation."

Potential Risk   MODERATE

Although risks have diminished as the operation has become more commonplace, they still exist. The most common include:

- Retinal detachment, which occurs in about 3% of cases

- Cystoid macular edema (accumulation of fluid within the portion of the retina that allows the eye to see fine detail), which occurs in less than 1% to nearly 3% of cases, depending on the type of replacement lens used

- Corneal edema, whose risk is 1% or less

- Low-grade, chronic inflammation, which may lead to glaucoma (implanted lens being responsible for inflammation); risk of less than 1%

■ Hemorrhage, which can result in loss of vision or severe infection; risk of less than 1%

■ Other problems: secondary glaucoma, hyphema, lens dislocation, and endophthalmitis; risk less than 1%

What It Is

A cataract is a clouding of the eye's normally transparent lens. As the lens becomes increasingly opaque, it is less able to focus light on the retina to produce a clear image. As a result, vision dims. The disease is characterized by the progressive, painless loss of vision and disturbances in the ability to distinguish among colors. It is the leading cause of blindness in the United States. Cataracts develop primarily as part of the aging process. Other causes include eye diseases, trauma, and endocrine and metabolic disorders, such as diabetes mellitus.

In cataract surgery, the clouded lens is removed and a clear lens implanted to restore vision.

Step 1. Make Sure You Need the Surgery

Before you have cataract surgery, your doctor should assess your overall health to identify other diseases that might influence the decision to operate or the techniques used in surgery. Bronchitis, obesity, heart disease, diabetes mellitus, and the use of medications such as immunosuppressive agents or anticoagulants may influence the surgery and need to be considered.

VISION TESTS TO DETERMINE SUITABILITY   Before the operation your doctor should check to see whether your glasses are the correct prescription. If she or he doesn't, then do not have the surgery—or anything else—done by that doctor. You also should be sure that the following tests are performed to determine if your operation is necessary:

■ Snellen visual acuity test, the most universally used exam for vision

■ Glare test

■ Reading vision test

■ Pinhole test, which can assess the likely improvement in vision after surgery

■ Glaucoma examination

- Examination of retina by dilating pupil

- Assessment of field of vision

If the doctor doesn't perform these tests before deciding on surgery, he or she has not done an adequate job. Some doctors feel that any ophthalmologist who has not ordered these tests shouldn't be operating.

Once these tests have been performed, you should match your diagnosis against the following list of conditions that warrant the procedure.

Appropriate Procedure

- Normal activities hampered by decreased vision

- Cataract-hampered diagnosis or treatment of other ocular diseases, such as diabetic retinopathy and potential intraocular malignancy

- Cataract-initiated eye diseases, such as uveitis and glaucoma

- Lens-centered diseases that threaten sight, such as phakomorphic glaucoma and phakolytic glaucoma

- Decreased visual acuity that interferes with normal activities (usually associated with Snellen acuity test or glare test visual acuity worse than 20/40; glare disability may reduce vision to 20/100 or worse)

- Need to visualize the fundus in an eye that has the potential for sight (In some diseases, doctors need to look through the lens into the back of the eye. For example, a patient who has diabetes with significant risk of reduced vision must have the fundus examined regularly so that when changes are seen, laser surgery can be performed to prevent the loss of vision. If doctors can't examine the fundus, the patient could lose his or her sight.)

Not an Appropriate Procedure

This operation should not be performed under the following circumstances:

- Glasses or visual aids offer satisfactory eyesight

- Surgery will not improve eyesight

- Patient is medically unfit

- Cataract is mild and causes no disability

Step 2. Consider an Alternative

Your doctor can determine if new glasses or contact lenses can restore your vision. Your prescription should be evaluated before you agree to surgery.

Step 3. Get a Specialist's Opinion

You will need an expert opinion if your procedure is not clearly indicated, if you do not have a high chance of success, if you question the need for the operation, or if the use of anesthesia carries more than minimal risk.

Your best choice for a specialist would be a highly skilled ophthalmologist expert in cataract surgery and in your type of eye disease. You should discuss the alternatives to cataract surgery and the appropriate timing for the operation. For instance, is it too early for you to benefit from surgery? Is a cataract really responsible for your visual problems? You will want the ophthalmologist to review your medical history to be certain your diagnosis is correct. The expert should meet the standards for doctors outlined in Step 5.

WHO TO CALL

American Academy of Ophthalmology   The academy will send you guidelines for ophthalmologists, position papers, and educational material.

P.O. Box 7424
San Francisco, CA 94120-7424
415/561-8500

American Society of Cataract and Refractory Surgeons   This organization can provide patient information and a list of members in your area who are cataract and refractory specialists.

3702 Pender Drive, Ste 250
Fairfax, VA 22030
703/591-2220

NIH CRISP System

301/496-7543

University-Affiliated Teaching Hospitals   See Appendix.

Step 4. Choose a Facility

You should evaluate a variety of hospitals and medical centers that perform a high volume of operations, and select the one that has the best results for your disease. In addition, you may want to consider free-standing surgical centers. Their quality depends very much on the skill of your surgeon. Since insurers will pay less for operations that are performed in such units, there is a temptation to cut costs. Just make certain it's not your care that is short-changed. You've really got to be able to count on the quality of your surgeon.

Experience

The hospital should perform several hundred operations a year.

Results

SUCCESS RATE   Final results depend on the health of the retina. Although surgery is done to restore sight, superb vision may not always be possible. According to a study of 50,000 patients by the Food and Drug Administration, 20/40 or better vision was found in 84.6% of cases one year after surgery with intraocular lens implants. Excluding patients who had additional problems such as glaucoma, vision was restored to 20/40 or better in 90–93% of cases. In seeking excellence, look for at least a 93% success rate in restoring vision to 20/40 or better.

Other Measures of Excellence

Since most cataract patients are older, the hospital needs to have an excellent department of anesthesia to deal with heart, lung, and other chronic diseases. Cataracts are not life-threatening, so the risk related to surgery should be extremely small.

Centers of Excellence for Ophthalmology

The following list of hospitals is provided only as a convenient starting place in your search for excellence. These hospitals are recommended on the basis of reputation, not experience and results. The list is not an endorsement. There may be hospitals just as excellent that have been omitted. You should apply the guidelines for experience, results, and other measures of excellence to any hospital you choose, whether or not it is on this list. Although hospitals from different sources have been combined into one list, the compilation in no way implies that one source has endorsed the hospital list of another source.

ALABAMA
University of Alabama at
   Birmingham   NIH
UAB Station
Birmingham, AL 35294

CALIFORNIA
Doheny Eye Institute   NIH
1355 San Pablo St
Los Angeles, CA 90033

University of California, Los
   Angeles, School of Medicine   US
Jules Stein Eye Institute
100 Stein Plaza
Los Angeles, CA 90024

Los Angeles County Harbor-
   UCLA Medical Center   NIH
1000 W Carson St
Torrance, CA 90509

Scripps Clinic and Research
   Foundation   NIH
10666 Torrey Pines Rd
San Diego, CA 92037

University of California, Davis   NIH
School of Medicine
Davis, CA 95616

University of California, Irvine   NIH
College of Medicine
Irvine, CA 92717

University of Southern California NIH
1975 Zonal Ave
Los Angeles, CA 90033

University of California,
   Santa Cruz   NIH
Cowell Student Health Center
Santa Cruz, CA 95064

CONNECTICUT
University of Connecticut
   Health Center   NIH
Farmington Ave
Farmington, CT 06032

FLORIDA
Applied Genetics Laboratories, Inc. NIH
1335 Gateway Dr, Ste 2001
Melbourne, FL 32901

Bascom Palmer Eye Institute   US
University of Miami
900 NW 17th St
Miami, FL 33136

GEORGIA
Emory University   NIH
Woodruff Health Sciences Center
   Administration Bldg
1440 Clifton Rd NE
Atlanta, GA 30322

Georgia Institute of Technology   NIH
225 North Ave NW
Atlanta, GA 30332

Medical College of Georgia   NIH
1120 Fifteenth St
Augusta, GA 30912

Morehouse School of Medicine   NIH
720 Westview Dr SW
Atlanta, GA 30310-1495

ILLINOIS
Northwestern University   NIH
303 E Chicago Ave
Chicago, IL 60611-3008

Northwestern University   NIH
1999 Sheridan Rd
Evanston, IL 60208

Rush-Presbyterian-St. Lukes
   Medical Center   NIH
1653 W Congress Pky
Chicago, IL 60612

INDIANA
Purdue University NIH
504 Northwestern Ave
West Lafayette, IN 47907

KANSAS
Kansas State University NIH
113 Eisenhower Hall
Manhattan, KS 66506

KENTUCKY
University of Louisville NIH
Health Sciences Center
Louisville, KY 40292

MARYLAND
Henry M. Jackson Foundation for
    Advanced Military Medicine NIH
1401 Rockville Pike
Bethesda, MD 20852

Johns Hopkins University NIH
600 No. Wolfe St
Baltimore, MD 21205

University of Maryland NIH
Baltimore Professional School
10 So. Pine St, Rm 5-00A
Baltimore, MD 21201

Wilmer Eye Institute US
Johns Hopkins Hospital
600 No. Wolfe St
Baltimore, MD 21205

MASSACHUSETTS
Boston Biomedical Research
    Institute NIH
20 Staniford St
Boston, MA 02114

Brigham and Women's Hospital NIH
75 Francis St
Boston, MA 02115

Harvard University NIH
25 Shattuck St
Boston, MA 02115

Massachusetts Eye and Ear
    Infirmary US
243 Charles St
Boston, MA 02114

Massachusetts Institute of
    Technology NIH
77 Massachusetts Ave.
Cambridge, MA 02139

Physical Sciences, Inc. NIH
20 New England Business Center
Andover, MA 01810

Tufts University NIH
136 Harrison Ave
Boston, MA 02111

MICHIGAN
Oakland University NIH
Dept of Biological Sciences
Rochester, MI 48309-4401

Wayne State University NIH
540 E Canfield
Detroit, MI 48201

MINNESOTA
Mankato State University NIH
P.O. Box 8400
Box 34
Mankato, MN 56002-8400

Mayo Clinic NIH
200 First St SW
Rochester, MN 55905

University of Minnesota of
    Minneapolis–St. Paul NIH
UMHC Box 293
420 Delaware St SE
Minneapolis, MN 55455

MISSOURI
Kirksville College of Osteopathic
    Medicine NIH
800 W Jefferson St
Kirksville, MO 63501

Missouri Lions Eye Research
Foundation   NIH
404 Portland St
Columbia, MO 65201

University of Missouri Columbia   NIH
MA204 Medical Sciences Bldg
One Hospital Dr
Columbia, MO 65203

Washington University   NIH
660 So. Euclid Ave
St. Louis, MO 63110

NEW JERSEY
University of Medicine &
Dentistry of New Jersey   NIH
New Jersey Medical School
185 So. Orange Ave
Newark, NJ 07103-2757

NEW YORK
Adelphi University   NIH
South Ave
Garden City, NY 11530

Albert Einstein Medical Center   NIH
1300 Morris Park Ave
Bronx, NY 10461

Columbia University   NIH
630 W 168th St
New York, NY 10032

Health Science Center at Syracuse   NIH
College of Medicine
750 E Adams St
Syracuse, NY 13210

Mount Sinai School of Medicine   NIH
One Gustave Levy Pl
New York, NY 10029

New York University   NIH
560 First Ave
New York, NY 10016

Rensselaer Polytechnic Institute   NIH
Center for Biophysics and Biology
Science Center
Troy, NY 12180-3590

State University New York
Binghamton   NIH
P.O. Box 6000
Binghamton, NY 13902-6000

State University of New York,
Stony Brook   NIH
Health Sciences Center
School of Medicine
Stony Brook, NY 11794

University of Rochester   NIH
601 Elmwood Ave
Rochester, NY 14642

NORTH CAROLINA
North Carolina State University   NIH
4700 Hillsborough St
Box 8401
Raleigh, NC 27695

University of North Carolina
Chapel Hill   NIH
School of Medicine
Chapel Hill, NC 27599

OHIO
Case Western Reserve University   NIH
2119 Abington Rd
Cleveland, OH 44106-2333

Children's Hospital Medical Center   NIH
Elland and Bethesda Aves
Cincinnati, OH 45229

OREGON
Oregon Health Sciences University   NIH
3181 SW Sam Jackson Park Rd
Portland, OR 97201-3098

PENNSYLVANIA
Fox Chase Cancer Center   NIH
7701 Burholme Ave
Philadelphia, PA 19111

University of Pennsylvania   NIH
36th and Hamilton Walk
Philadelphia, PA 19104-6015

Wills Eye Hospital   US
900 Walnut St
Philadelphia, PA 19107

TENNESSEE
University of Tennessee at
    Memphis   NIH
800 Madison Ave
Memphis, TN 38163

TEXAS
Baylor College of Medicine   NIH
One Baylor Plaza
Houston, TX 77030

Houston Biotechnology, Inc.   NIH
3608 Research Forest Dr
The Woodlands, TX 77380

Texas College of Osteopathic
    Medicine   NIH
3500 Camp Bowie Blvd
Fort Worth, TX 76107

University of Texas Medical
    Branch   NIH
301 University Blvd
Galveston, TX 77550

University of Texas Southwest
    Medical Center   NIH
Southwestern Medical School
5323 Harry Hines Blvd
Dallas, TX 75235

VIRGINIA
University of Virginia Medical
    Center   NIH
Box 395 McKim Hall
Charlottesville, VA 22908

WASHINGTON
University of Washington   NIH
School of Medicine
Seattle, WA 98195

WISCONSIN
University of Wisconsin Madison   NIH
1300 University Ave
Madison, WI 53706

SOURCES

NIH indicates the currently active centers funded by the National Institutes of Health's National Eye Institute.

US indicates those hospitals recommended in *U.S. News & World Report.*

Step 5. Choose a Doctor

The doctor who performs your operation should be board-certified in ophthalmology. He or she should have performed at least 50, and preferably 100, KPE (phacoemulsification) cataract extractions. (Phacoemulsification, the state-of-the-art cataract extraction method, uses ultrasonic vibration to shatter and break up a cataract, making it easier to remove.) This is the best way to tell if your doctor is both up to date and well trained. Dr. Walter Stark indicates that learning to do this operation properly requires between 50 and 100 procedures.

Experience

The doctor should do at least four to six cataract surgeries a week.

Results

SUCCESS RATE   Look for at least a 93% success rate in restoring vision to 20/40 or better.

Other Measures of Excellence

■ The doctor operates at a hospital specializing in eye care.

■ The surgeon plans to do follow-up her- or himself. The surgeon who removes the cataract should follow your care during the weeks and months following the operation. Top specialists frown on referring a patient to someone else for follow-up. You should ask about this beforehand.

EXPERT SOURCES

Although dozens of experts were interviewed for these chapters, Dr. Walter Stark, Director, Cornea Service, The Wilmer Ophthalmological Institute, Johns Hopkins Hospital, Baltimore, MD, is acknowledged for his significant contributions to this section.

REFERENCES AND SUGGESTED READING

Acheson, J., and others. Changing Patterns of Early Complications in Cataract Surgery with New Techniques: A Surgical Audit. *British Journal of Ophthalmology,* Vol. 72, No. 7 (July 1988), pp. 481–484.

Alpar, J. Preventive Cataract Surgery for the Prolongation of Life [letter]. *Ophthalmic Surgery,* Vol. 19, No. 4 (April 1988), p. 293.

Barrie, Jay. Cataract: Biochemistry, Epidemiology, and Pharmacology. *Lancet,* Vol. 338, No. 8770 (Sept. 28, 1991), p. 806.

Bensen, W. Increased Mortality Rates After Cataract Surgery. *Ophthalmology,* Vol. 95 (1988), pp. 1288–1292.

Bruce, David W., and Gray, Christopher S. Beyond the Cataract: Visual and Functional Disability in Elderly People. *Age and Ageing,* Vol 20, No. 6 (1991), pp. 389–391.

Chambless, W. Incidence of Anterior and Posterior Segment Complications in Over 3,000 Cases of Extracapsular Cataract Extractions: Intact and Open Capsules. *Journal of the American Intraocular Implant Society,* Vol. 11, No.2 (March 1985), pp. 146–148.

Dowling, J., and Bahr, R. A Survey of Current Cataract Surgical Techniques. *American Journal of Ophthalmology,* Vol. 99, No. 1 (1985), pp. 35–39.

Elam, J., and others. Functional Outcome One Year Following Cataract Surgery in Elderly Persons. *Journal of Gerontology,* Vol. 43, No. 5 (Sept. 1988), pp. M122–126.

Jaffe, Norman S., and others. *Cataract Surgery and Its Complications,* 5th ed. St. Louis: Mosby, 1990.

John, M., and Edsell, T. Advanced Versus Immature Cataracts—A Preliminary Report. *Annals of Ophthalmology,* Vol. 21, No. 6 (June 1989), pp. 222–224.

Krachmer, Jay H., and Palay, David A. Corneal Disease [editorial]. *New England Journal of Medicine,* Vol. 325, No. 25 (Dec. 19, 1991), pp. 1804–1806.

Massanari, R. M., and others. *Cataract Surgery: A Review of the Literature Regarding Efficacy and Risks.* University of Iowa Hospitals and Clinics and University of Iowa College of Medicine, 1990.

McCarthy, E., and others. National Trends in Lens Extraction: 1965–1984. *Journal of the American Optometric Association,* Vol. 59, No. 1 (1988), pp. 31–35.

Stark, W., and others. Changing Trends in Intraocular Lens Implantation. *Archives of Ophthalmology,* Vol. 107 (1989), pp. 1441–1444.

Steinberg, E. P., and others. Variations in Cataract Management: Patient and Economic Outcomes. In *Health Services Research,* Vol. 25 (Dec. 1990).

Burn Care

Risk of Inappropriate Care   HIGH

If you have a major burn and are not admitted to a specialized center, there is an excellent chance that you will not receive state-of-the-art care.

Potential Risk   VERY HIGH

After you suffer a major burn, you run a very high risk of developing a life-threatening infection—the larger the burn, the greater the chance. Of the 2 million people who suffer burns in the United States every year, 7,000 eventually die. (At least 50% of burns in adults and 90% of those in children could be prevented, according to the National Institute for Burn Medicine, a research organization.) Your chances of survival are much larger now than they were 20 years ago, as a result of advances in burn treatment. However, even with the best treatment, serious burns are often fatal. Here are the survival rates for patients whose burns cover over 50% of their body:

AGE (YEARS)	SURVIVAL RATE
0–14	62%
15–40	63%
40–65	38%
65+	25%

Step 1. Make Sure You Get the Best Care

The treatment of burns involves both short-term and long-term objectives. The immediate goals are to stabilize the victim and to prevent life-threatening complications; the overall goal is to return the patient to a useful and functional place in society.

If you or a member of your family is burned, there is only a short time within which to be transferred to a center of excellence, from as little as one hour to as much as 20 hours. You must make fast decisions. Survival may depend on it, and there's little margin for error. The American Burn Association and the American College of Surgeons have developed guidelines that can help determine if you need to be in a specialized burn center. They base them on the severity of the burn. Many local 911 emergency medical service staffs use these guidelines to make the initial decision about where to take victims.

Burn Categories

To begin making that determination you should be familiar with the following categories of burns:

First Degree   Damage is to the superficial layers of the epidermis (the first layer of skin), blood vessels are dilated, and the skin is red.

Second Degree   Varying layers of skin are damaged, and blisters are present. Some layers remain uninjured. Infection can increase the severity of the burn to third degree.

Third Degree   Destruction extends to all skin layers, with the surface appearing hard, dry, inelastic, and translucent and veins visible, with blood clots in them.

WHEN YOU NEED A TOP BURN CENTER   Anyone with a burn that is severe, has a questionable outcome, or may be disfiguring should be at a top burn center. This includes patients who have any of the following conditions:

■ Second- and third-degree burns on more than 10% of the body and under the age of 10 or over 50

■ Second- and third-degree burns on more than 20% of the body in any age group

■ Second- and third-degree burns that involve the face, hands, feet, genitalia, or skin overlying major joints

■ Third-degree burns on more than 5% of the body at any age group

■ Significant electrical burns, including lightning injury

■ Significant chemical burns

■ Inhalation injury

■ Preexisting illness that could complicate management, prolong recovery, or affect mortality

■ Other injuries that increase the risk of morbidity or mortality, such as gunshot wounds (The emergency team may stabilize such patients at a trauma center before transfer to a burn center.)

- Need for special social and emotional support or long-term rehabilitation and follow-up, including cases of suspected child abuse and neglect

- A child (Children should always be at a center of excellence.)

Step 2. Choose a Facility

Not all medical facilities provide equal care to burn victims. In general, however, the care at major burn centers is excellent. Alan Breslau, a burn survivor himself and the founder of the Phoenix Society, a support organization for burn victims, says: "In the United States the state of the art of burn care is terrific. It's a terrific specialty. It's fairly small so everyone knows everybody and everyone is pretty well up on the state of the art and pretty well practices it."

If you have a serious burn, you should look for a center with a multidisciplinary unit that includes social workers and physical therapists on its staff. The center should be in a separate location from the rest of the hospital. It should have programs for research in burn care and for training of medical personnel. Studies have found that survival is highest at burn centers staffed 24 hours a day and administered by a single clinical director. More than one administrator renders the care less effective.

Experience

It's generally true that you'll find the best care at centers that see the most patients. Experts dispute the exact minimum. The American Burn Association recommends that a center treat at least 75 patients a year. A better figure is 100 patients a year, according to Claudella Jones, R.N., Director of the National Institute for Burn Medicine in Ann Arbor, MI. Dr. Cleon Goodwin, Director of the Burn Center at New York Hospital, recommends that patients seek treatment at facilities that treat at least 200 burn victims a year. His center, the largest in the country, treats 1,200 patients annually.

Results

SURVIVAL RATES   The overall survival rate is a probably the most telling indication of a center's quality of care. As Claudella Jones points out, 80–90% of all hospital burn admissions have burns over less than 20% of the body. With good care these patients should survive. "If your center doesn't live up to these statistics, that's a red flag," Ms. Jones says. Mortality rates are difficult to judge, however, because hospitals estimate the size and severity of burns differently. Here are useful guidelines:

■ When few complications are present and the patient is between the ages of 2 and 50, the survival rate should be 100%.

■ For very severe burns the death rate should approach that of major centers. At New York Hospital in New York City, for instance, the rate is 7.8%.

■ The overall survival rate should not be below 95%.

Other Measures of Excellence

INITIAL CARE   The American Burn Association and the American College of Surgeons have developed standards for burn care. While these standards are excellent, you should be aware that enforcement is lax. According to these organizations you should look for the following:

■ Educational programs in emergency treatment and current concepts of patient care should be offered regularly.

■ Rehabilitation services should be present.

■ A single registered nurse should be responsible for administration of the burn unit. He or she should have two years' experience in intensive care or its equivalent and a minimum of twelve months of experience on a burn unit.

■ The burn center director should be a licensed, board-certified general or plastic surgeon with at least two years' experience in the management of burn patients in a specialized center. He or she should participate actively in the care of at least 50 acute burn patients a year.

■ There should be at least one full-time equivalent surgeon for every 200 patients admitted a year.

■ Prompt consultation should be available in these surgical and medical specialties:

cardiothoracic surgery	plastic surgery	nephrology
neurology	urology	pathology
obstetrics and gynecology	anesthesiology	pediatrics
ophthalmology	cardiology	psychiatry
oral surgery	gastroenterology	physiatry
orthopedics	hematology	pulmonology
otorhinolaryngology	infectious diseases	radiology

■ The following support personnel should be available:

social worker assigned to the unit permanently or for at least one year if rotated through units

dietitian available daily

respiratory therapist

psychologists and clergy, again permanently assigned or not rotated off the unit more than once a year

SKIN BANK   During your initial treatment you should be at a center that has a skin bank. That bank should conform to the standards of the American Association of Tissue Banks or have a protocol for the procurement and handling of skin from other sources.

DURING REHABILITATION   When rehabilitation therapy begins, you should check for the following:

■ The staff includes licensed or registered physical and occupational therapists assigned on a full-time basis. At least one full-time equivalent burn therapist should be present for every seven patients. If staff assignments are made on a rotational basis, rotations should be no more often than every three months.

■ Recreational and education services are available during hospitalization.

■ The needs and support capabilities of family and friends who are able to help after discharge are evaluated.

■ The availability and accessibility of community resources to assist in meeting physical, psychosocial, educational, and vocational needs after discharge are assessed.

■ Provision is made for periodic reevaluation of patient status after discharge from the hospital and for readmission, if necessary, for medical or surgical treatment or for rehabilitation.

Centers of Excellence for Burn Care

The following list of hospitals is provided only as a convenient starting place in your search for excellence. These hospitals are recommended on the basis of reputation, not experience and results. The list is not an endorsement. There may be hospitals just as excellent that have been omitted. You should apply the guidelines for experience, results, and other measures of excellence to any hospital you choose, whether or not it is on this list. Although hospitals from different sources have been combined into one list, the compilation in no way implies that one source has endorsed the hospital list of another source.

CALIFORNIA
University of Southern California   EX
Burn Unit
1200 No. State St
Los Angeles, CA 90033

FLORIDA
Jackson Memorial Hospital   EX
Burn Center
1611 NW 12th Ave
Miami, FL 33136

ILLINOIS
Sumner L. Koch Burn Center   EX
Cook County Hospital
1835 W Harrison St
Chicago, IL 60612

MASSACHUSETTS
Shriners Burn Institute   EX
51 Blossom St
Boston, MA 02114

Sumner Redstone Burn Center   EX
Massachusetts General Hospital
55 Fruit St
Boston, MA 02114

NEW YORK
New York Hospital–Cornell
    University Medical Center   EX
Burn Center
525 E 68th St
New York, NY 10021

OHIO
Shriner's Burn Institute   EX
202 Goodman St
Cincinnati, OH 45219

TENNESSEE
University Physicians Foundation   EX
(Affiliated with University
    of Tennessee)
951 Court Ave
Memphis, TN 38103

TEXAS
Parkland Memorial Hospital   EX
5201 Harry Hines Blvd
Dallas, TX 75235

U.S. Army Institute of
    Surgical Research   EX
Fort Sam Houston
San Antonio, TX 78234

WASHINGTON
Harborview Medical Center   EX
Burn Unit
325 Ninth Ave
Seattle, WA 98104

SOURCES
EX   indicates those hospitals recommended by experts interviewed.

Step 3. Select a Doctor

You should select a doctor who is board-certified in general or plastic surgery and has completed a one- to two-year fellowship. While shorter fellowships exist, you want a doctor who has more than the minimal training. In addition, the surgeon should have training in critical care and be on the staff of a burn center where he sees at least 50 hospitalized patients a year. Since most doctors will not have individual outcome figures, you will have to rely on the burn center's overall statistics. It is difficult to develop outcome figures for doctors because they are largely dependent on the nursing and clinical care offered.

Step 4. Become Your Own Expert

WHO TO CALL

American Burn Association This is primarily a professional education organization for doctors, nurses, and others in the field of burn care. To the public it offers the pamphlet "Burn Care Resources in North America," which contains telephone numbers, personnel resources, and the number of beds and specialties of burn centers in the United States and Canada. It also provides a listing of skin banks and burn fellowships, including duration and type of program, which can be very helpful.

716 Lee St
Des Plaines, IL 60016
708/824-5700

Phoenix Society This worldwide organization offers psychosocial support groups for burn survivors. Its services include: scholarships for children to 13 burn camps in the United States; a disaster response team, operated in conjunction with the American Red Cross, that will fly to any part of the United States to offer support to families and friends; pro bono reconstructive surgery for foreign children; and referrals to doctors and hospitals.

11 Rust Hill Rd
Levittown, PA 19056
215/946-BURN

National Institute for Burn Medicine Affiliated with the University of Michigan Medical Center, the NIBM has created a comprehensive program of research, prevention, treatment, and rehabilitation for burn care in the United States. It supports the National Burn Information Exchange, a voluntary physician's registry of over 100,000 case reports of patients admitted to specialized burn facilities. The NIBM can provide statistical information and guidance on organizing prevention programs and delivering burn care.

909 E Ann St
Ann Arbor, MI 48104
313/769-9000

International Society for Burn Injury   This organization provides a list of international burn centers.

2005 Franklin St
Denver, CO 20508
303/839-1694

National Burn Victim Foundation   This group provides counseling and legal and medical referrals. It evaluates pediatric patients in cases of suspected child abuse and has a volunteer disaster response team.

303 Main St
Orange, NJ 07050
201/676-7700

NIH CRISP System
301/496-7543

University-Affiliated Teaching Hospitals   See Appendix.

EXPERT SOURCES

Although we interviewed dozens of experts for these chapters, these specialists are acknowledged for their significant contributions to this section.

Dr. Cleon Goodwin, Director, Burn Center, New York Hospital–Cornell Medical Center, New York, NY

Dr. Jeffrey R. Saffle, Chairman, Committee on Organization and Delivery of Burn Care, University of Utah, Salt Lake City, UT

Claudella Jones, R.N., Director, National Institute for Burn Medicine, Ann Arbor, MI

REFERENCES AND SUGGESTED READING

American Burn Association. Hospital and Prehospital Resources for Optimal Care of Patients with Burn Injury: Guidelines for Development and Operation of Burn Centers. *Journal of Burn Care and Rehabilitation,* Vol. 11, No. 2 (Mar./Apr. 1990), pp. 97–104.

Cornell, R. G., and others. Evaluation of Burn Care Utilizing a National Burn Registry. *Emergency Medical Services,* Vol. 7, No. 6 (Nov./Dec. 1978), pp.107–112.

Feller, I., and Jones, C. A. Horizons in Burn Care. *Clinics in Plastic Surgery,* Vol. 13, No. 1 (Jan. 1988), pp. 151–159.

Feller, I., and Jones, C. A. The National Burn Information Exchange: The Use of a National Burn Registry to Evaluate and Address the Burn Problem. *Surgical Clinics of North America,* Vol. 67, No. 1 (Feb.1989), pp. 167–189.

Haab, M. E., and others. An Acute and Rehabilitation Burn Unit: Providing the Necessary Transition. *Journal of Burn Care and Rehabilitation,* Vol. 3, No. 4 (July/Aug. 1982), pp. 237–239.

National Institute for Burn Medicine. *Fire Safety, Burn Prevention, and Immediate Burn Care for Older Adults,* 1990.

Wolfe, R. A., and others. Mortality Differences and Speed of Wound Closure Among Specialized Burn Care Facilities. *Journal of the American Medical Association,* Vol. 250, No.6 (Aug. 12, 1983), pp. 763–766.

Chronic
Diseases

Acquired Immune Deficiency Syndrome (AIDS)

Risk for Inappropriate Care   VERY HIGH

Inappropriate care may cut an AIDS patient's life expectancy by a year or more. For those who are infected but not yet ill, even more years of useful life may be sacrificed. Finding the best care is fraught with error. The rules that apply so well to other diseases or operations don't apply here. Some major academic center may be poorly equipped to handle your day-to-day care. The best experts may be community AIDS doctors, not famous specialists. The best drug for you may not be FDA approved.

The American Foundation for AIDS Research (AMFAR) estimates that the virus infects 1.5 million people. By early 1992, the United States had reached 200,000 patients with full-blown AIDS. Over the last 10 years approximately 116,000 Americans have died of the virus.

AIDS activists have broken historic new ground in medical consumerism. Through aggressive lobbying they have generated billions of dollars in research funds, and pushed new drugs through the Food and Drug Administration in record time. Because of their efforts, new drugs have become widely available, improving the life expectancy and the quality of life for AIDS patients. But many patients, especially women, blacks, Hispanics, and those who live outside major metropolitan cities with their support networks, have a shortened life expectancy and reduced quality of life. Their risk for inappropriate care—inadequate or late medical treatment—is enormous. Many AIDS patients are unaware of the underground network of drug testing and manufacture. Many patients with AIDS have no health insurance and lack a support group that can point them to the right doctor, hospital, and treatment.

Last, you may be infected with the AIDS virus and not know it. That makes you a risk to others if you have unprotected sex, share intravenous (IV) drugs, or are a health care professional and don't rigorously follow established guidelines to protect your patients. You may also shorten your own life by not beginning treatment early enough. If you think you're at risk, get an AIDS test!

What It Is

Acquired Immune Deficiency Syndrome (AIDS) is a disease that damages the immune system with life-threatening consequences. When the body's immune system becomes weakened, the patient is vulnerable to a variety of infectious

diseases and cancers. Infection with the virus called HIV (human immune deficiency virus) causes the immune deficiency condition. Bodily fluids from HIV-
infected individuals transmit the infection. Blood and semen are the two most
dangerous bodily fluids, since they carry the greatest concentration of the AIDS
virus. Infection occurs most commonly through unprotected sex with infected
partners, intravenous drug use with contaminated needles or syringes, or contact
with contaminated blood as a result of transfusions or needle sticks. Receptive
anal sex is the most dangerous sex for both men and women. Though saliva does
carry the virus, it's considered unlikely that kissing can transmit the virus because
there is so little virus in saliva. Infected persons who are not yet ill are called sero-
positive or HIV-positive.

Many individuals experience no symptoms when first infected with HIV.
Some may suffer a brief viral-like illness characterized by fever, joint aches and
pains, itching, stomach cramps, and diarrhea. After you are infected, the average
length of time before you show symptoms of AIDS is ten years. If this chapter
encourages you to do nothing else, you should seek testing and counseling if you
practice any high-risk sexual behaviors, use intravenous drugs, or believe you
have been exposed to AIDS-infected blood. High-risk sexual behaviors are now
defined as having multiple sexual partners or having sex with IV-drug users. The
cornerstone of AIDS prevention and early treatment is voluntary testing of all
individuals who are at risk for carrying the virus.

Until recently, doctors assumed that AIDS proceeded in an inexorable progression from infection to death. With the introduction of early preventive measures
for sero-positive patients, this course may be delayed. According to the Centers
for Disease Control (CDC), on average, half of the people diagnosed with AIDS
will die within nine to 13 months. With excellent care, a quarter of them will live
two years, and another quarter will survive three years. Even if you are already ill
with AIDS, you may still be able to improve your chances of survival. This chapter
will tell you how.

Step 1. Make Sure You Get the Best Care

Reading this section on potential problems with your treatment carefully will aid
you in determining if there are discrepancies between your care and state-of-the-
art care. Use Step 2 to review shortcomings.

Diagnosis

Thousands of patients with early symptoms of AIDS-related infections are never
treated because their doctors don't pursue the diagnosis rigorously. Often they
don't suspect AIDS because the patients fail to fit the stereotypes of male homo-

sexual or IV-drug user. But the stereotypes are often wrong. Kimberly Bergalis alleged that she contracted AIDS from her dentist while a college student. She was not sexually active and had never used drugs. According to the American Foundation for AIDS Research (AMFAR), the disease is spreading more quickly among heterosexuals than among gays. The annual rate of increase is 26% for heterosexuals and 8% for homosexual men, estimates AMFAR. Sometimes even doctors who suspect the presence of AIDS don't look for the cause of opportunistic infections because they feel that nothing can be done.

This means that if you have AIDS, you must be prepared to be an activist on your own behalf. You have enormous battles ahead: You will have to fight to keep your insurance, to get into clinical trials, to find first-rate health care, to maintain your job, and to avoid discrimination on the basis of your disease. By being an activist you improve your chances of living longer. You will be prepared to prevent opportunistic infections and, if they do occur, to treat them as quickly and effectively as possible. The first step, if you are at risk for AIDS, is to get tested for the virus and to have counseling if the results are positive. This alone can add years to your life expectancy.

AIDS TESTS   The test commonly used to detect antibodies to the AIDS virus is known by the acronym ELISA (enzyme-linked immunosorbent assay). If the results are positive, a confirmation test, called the Western blot, is used. In the first six months of HIV infection, there may not be enough antibodies present for these tests to give positive results. As a result there is a danger that you may test negative even after you have been exposed to the AIDS virus. Although newer tests can disclose the presence of the virus in very small quantities, they are still research tools.

T-Cell Count   Doctors measure a specialized white blood cell, called the CD-4 cell or helper cell, to monitor the damage to the immune system. You should have CD-4 cell counts taken every six months if you are HIV-positive, even in the absence of symptoms, or according to the schedule in Table 3. The lower this count, the more likely you are to contract opportunistic infections such as Pneumocystis carinii pneumonia (PCP). As with much of AIDS, medications and guidelines are in constant flux. CD-4 counts serve as extremely useful guidelines. What you do at each of the levels shown in Table 3 is subject to change as doctors better learn when to use drugs that directly fight the AIDS virus and those that combat opportunistic infections. As this book goes to press, the Centers for Disease Control are expanding their definition of AIDS to include all patients who have CD-4 counts below 200. This makes CD-4 testing particularly important since a count below 200 qualifies you for a wide range of funding.

TABLE 3. Recommended Cell Count Schedule

CD-4 Cell Count	Recommended Schedule
1,000	Repeat every six months unless symptoms appear; if symptoms are present, test more regularly.
500–1,000	If no symptoms, repeat every three to four months.
250–500	Repeat count every three months. Some doctors would start Pneumocystis carinii pneumonia (PCP) prophylaxis and AZT (azidothymidine) at 250. At this count it is advisable to begin more frequent physical examinations, including a baseline chest x-ray, and to undergo a thorough education program about the early signs and symptoms of AIDS-related infections, such as fever and weight loss.
Under 200, with fever and weight loss	Have counts performed as often as necessary. The Public Health Service recommends starting PCP prophylaxis at this count.

Treatment Medications

Every doctor I consulted agreed that it's difficult to recommend specific medicines as state-of-the-art treatment because they change so frequently. During the writing of this book nearly a dozen new medications came into use. In the broadest terms there are two different kinds of medicines, those that fight the virus, and those that fight the opportunistic infections.

DRUGS TO FIGHT THE AIDS VIRUS   The first group of treatment drugs consists of medications that are active against the AIDS virus and improve your life expectancy. The first of these, and the best-known example, is azidothymidine (AZT).

While doctors differ on the appropriate time to begin the use of AZT, the U.S. Public Health Service has in the past recommended that physicians consider AZT treatment when the T-cell count reaches 500. Doctors who specialize in AIDS patients may wait even then. Dr. Joseph Sonnabend, Medical Director of the Community Research Initiative on AIDS in New York City, theorizes that AZT is effective for only two years in many cases, making it unwise to rush into using the drug. However, preliminary new research suggests that early AZT treatment may increase the chance of survival.

Other doctors argue that newer and better medicines inevitably will be developed, so AZT treatment might as well begin early on. Dr. Paul Volberding, Director of the AIDS program at San Francisco General Hospital, recommends that, since AZT can be highly toxic, especially in patients with advanced AIDS, doctors should not use it indiscriminately. If your doctor gives you AZT, be certain he or she has a good reason. This is particularly true if you are HIV-positive but have yet to develop symptoms of the disease.

There are dozens of other drugs in varying stages of clinical testing that also attack the virus. You need not consider them until you can no longer take AZT. That point comes when the drug becomes too toxic or stops working.

In the future, two or more of these drugs will probably be used together to treat the disease. That approach offers several advantages: Each drug can work on the AIDS virus in a different way, and doctors can use lower doses to avoid severe side effects. If this sounds like cancer chemotherapy, you're close. Researchers cured Hodgkin's lymphoma through a combination of several drugs, instead of one single magic bullet. Many experts believe that this multiple drug chemotherapy will be the future treatment of the disease. The FDA has approved the drug DDI and soon expects to approve DDC. Many physicians would consider these drugs only after AZT has failed or proved too toxic. Consideration should be given to their use along with AZT.

DRUGS TO FIGHT OPPORTUNISTIC INFECTIONS   The second group of drugs include those medications doctors use to treat opportunistic infections, the earliest and greatest threat to your life. Many of these medications are already available for other illnesses, although the FDA has not approved all for use against AIDS. Opportunistic infections are called just that because they take advantage of a weakened immune system to infect you and make you ill. Against a strong immune system, most would never cause illness. In fact, your life expectancy is determined by the number and types of opportunistic infections you contract.

In the treatment of AIDS the largest area of uncertainty is the prevention of infections. You should be familiar with the opportunistic infections that are most common in your area, for instance, histoplasmosis, a fungus that affects the lungs, in the mid-South. You and your doctor should undertake preventive measures if your T-cell counts have dropped and put you at risk. Trimethoprim/ sulfamethoxazole, for instance, has been proven effective in the prevention of PCP.

You should read the newsletters listed in Step 4 and discuss with your physician when to begin preventive treatment. Many academic centers won't even try preventive treatment (called prophylaxis). They may be wrong in that decision. Based on the experience of community doctors, prophylaxis has a reasonable chance of preventing the following diseases: cytomegalovirus, toxoplasmosis, tuberculosis and avian tuberculosis, and cryptococcus (an infectious fungal disease that begins in the lungs and may spread to other organs). Researchers have not worked out precise optimal dosages of these drugs (except in the treatment of PCP). Community AIDS physicians, including Dr. Sonnabend and Dr. Grossman, who practice in New York, feel that fewer patients are dying of infections because of the wider use of preventive measures. They feel some doctors undertreat all these conditions even when the infection becomes apparent.

Your doctor should respond quickly if you develop signs of infection. Right from the beginning he or she should be willing to use every tool of modern medicine to identify the source of all the infections that occur. Dr. Sonnabend says, "You can almost always find a diagnosis for fever and diarrhea." Your doctor must just be persistent. It is laziness to attribute it to HIV alone. Your doctor can often quickly and effectively treat opportunistic infections. "If your physician is really sharp and on the ball, he will pick up the diagnosis and you won't die," continues Dr. Sonnabend. You may develop a severe illness because preventive methods weren't taken. Doctors should aggressively track down fevers using blood cultures, marrow and liver biopsies, and gallium scans (which locate the site of infection with isotopes and special scopes to sample fluid or tissue from the lungs, stomach, or bowels). Here are some symptoms that should lead you to call your doctor immediately:

SYMPTOM	POSSIBLE OPPORTUNISTIC INFECTIONS
Shortness of breath during exercise	PCP (Pneumocystis carinii pneumonia)
Headache	Toxoplasmosis, cryptococcal meningitis, lymphoma
Visual blurring	Cytomegalovirus retinitis (infection caused by an agent in the herpes virus family)
Persistent fevers	Secondary infection, not the AIDS virus itself

In addition, your doctor also should be aggressive in the treatment of skin infections. Many doctors find these the least satisfying of AIDS-related infections to diagnose and treat. Many dermatologists are not helpful because they are unfamiliar with the conditions, according to AIDS specialists. You are entitled to a specific diagnosis and treatment for your condition.

The same is true if you are experiencing rapid weight loss. Your doctor should be able to identify the cause. Doctors can maintain your weight with intravenous feedings, although if you are very sick the cost can reach $100,000 a year.

You should be suspicious if your doctor is not willing to customize your treatment. I am critical of "cookbook" medicine in general, but it is a particular danger in the treatment of a disease that remains as unknown as AIDS. Community AIDS doctors say their colleagues at major medical centers want to "follow the book, when there is no book." Although AZT and pentamidine (to fight PCP) were the earliest preventive treatments, for instance, there are now a dozen or more other medications available through your doctor, clinical trials, and the

AIDS network. You should be familiar with all of them *before* you actually require them. If you can no longer use AZT, for example, you will want to look at drugs such as DDC and DDI.

Your doctor should be willing to explore the use of medicines that are still experimental when that seems justified. Medical schools teach doctors, first, to do no harm. Because of that caution some doctors, even at academic medical centers, are reluctant to prescribe drugs the Food and Drug Administration has not approved. Your doctor should have enough experience with experimental medicines to know the ones that might work in your case, and should be ready to experiment with different dosages of medicine to determine the therapeutic level. This is especially true of medications to prevent opportunistic infections. Since the FDA has not approved most of these medications, you won't find the correct dose in the conventional reference books. You can try cross-checking the amount prescribed with your pharmacist, with the AIDS network, and with the staff at centers such as the University of California at San Francisco. They may be willing to offer advice about experimental drugs.

Because AIDS has no known cure, many patients become discouraged and, mistrustful of the medical establishment, begin to pursue treatment on their own. This course can be fraught with disaster. One group of doctors currently offers a treatment to "bake" the AIDS virus out of the body. There is no evidence at all that this has ever succeeded. AIDS support groups have superb newsletters that can guide you to legitimate, if experimental, treatments under investigation in the United States or other countries (see Step 4).

Step 2. Look for Shortcomings

I hope you have gotten a good feeling about your treatment from reading Step 1, and that you understand much of it better. You'll learn even more by calling organizations listed in Step 4. But if you have an uncomfortable feeling that your treatment is not on track, you should study this section, which specifies some of the common and serious shortcomings that experts in the field recognize. If this section confirms your suspicions, you should go to Step 3. Some of these mistakes you can discover yourself; others only an expert can confirm.

MISTAKES IN DIAGNOSIS

You fail to get an AIDS test if you practice high-risk behaviors or are otherwise at risk.

You have an undiagnosed opportunistic infection.

Your health care provider doesn't pursue the diagnosis of AIDS-related skin diseases.

Your health care provider doesn't respond quickly and effectively to common symptoms of opportunistic infections.

Your health care provider doesn't diagnose the cause of AIDS-related weight loss.

MISTAKES IN TREATMENT

You're not an activist in your own behalf.

You are pursuing quackery.

You are given AZT before it is needed.

You are given the wrong doses of medications.

You aren't aware of clinical trials that could help you.

You are offered only a few approved treatments.

You are not treated for weight loss.

Your health care provider is not willing to customize your treatment or to consider empirical treatment.

Step 3. See a Specialist

If, from Step 2, you are concerned that your care is not state-of-the-art, this section will tell you how to choose an expert.

In New York City, the first doctors to see AIDS patients were physicians who specialized in venereal diseases. They diagnosed and treated AIDS patients before other physicians even recognized that it was a disease. They were unfamiliar with immunology and had little background that would help. These doctors, commonly referred to as community doctors, quickly acquired a wide variety of clinical experience and learned from their patients. Community doctors believe that treatment at the majority of medical centers is third-rate because their staff doctors don't have similar experience. Community doctors maintained then and maintain now that they can provide the best care for AIDS patients. Since there is no textbook for AIDS, they contend that academics have little to teach. In New York City and San Francisco, self-taught community doctors rate themselves ahead of the academic centers for outpatient medicine. Academic specialists we consulted sharply disagree, however.

In choosing the doctor who will monitor your care on a day-to-day basis you should consider the following.

EXPERIENCE   Your doctor should be managing several hundred AIDS patients at any given time. The longer your doctor has been treating AIDS the better. Some of the best community and academic physicians have been treating the disease since the beginning of the epidemic.

OUTCOME   Ask other patients about their experiences. While there are no formal measures of outcome in a private practice, you will find some doctors are pulling patients through one infection after another. They look for early symptoms, treat aggressively, and are willing to use whatever works.

PERSONALITY   You need to decide in advance what you're looking for. Your doctor may be an authoritarian who will tell you exactly what to do, or may become a health care partner who will make each decision with you.

WILLINGNESS TO TRY THE UNPROVEN   You face a variety of different opportunistic illnesses that threaten your life. You need to have a doctor who is willing to look at the best available evidence for each of a dozen or more *unproven* drugs. I emphasize *best available*—you certainly don't want a medicine cabinet full of quack remedies. However, many AIDS physicians have gained wide experience with experimental drugs and could save your life or prevent a serious illness with them.

FAMILIARITY WITH AIDS INFECTIONS   Your doctor needs to be very familiar with these infections. He or she should know the warning signs and treat you early.

OTHER SERVICES   Community doctors are willing to provide a wide range of services. These can include encouragement, willingness to listen, and education about early warning signs of infection. Some doctors also make appropriate referrals for financial counseling, support services, social services, and referral to AIDS advocacy groups.

Centers of Excellence for AIDS

These centers have significant numbers of patients with AIDS. They provide full clinical services in and out of the hospital and have a staff that can advise on all the social, legal, medical, psychiatric, and occupational problems that accompany the disease. To help you zero in on the most appropriate centers to choose from, the list of hospitals in this chapter is divided into several sublists: NIH AIDS Clinical Trials Group (ACTG) hospitals (which are further subdivided into general and pediatric hospitals); AMFAR Community-Based Clinical Trial (CBCT) Network hospitals; and NIH Community Programs for Clinical Research on AIDS (CPCRA) hospitals.

The lists of hospitals are provided only as a convenient starting place in your search for excellence. These hospitals are recommended on the basis of reputation, not experience and results. The lists are not an endorsement. There may be hospitals just as excellent that have been omitted. You should apply the guidelines for experience, results, and other measures of excellence to any hospital you choose, whether or not it is on these lists. Although hospitals from different sources have been combined into the lists, the compilation in no way implies that one source has endorsed the hospital list of another source.

CALIFORNIA

San Francisco General Hospital   US
Bldg 80, Ward 84
995 Potrero Ave
San Francisco, CA 94110

University of California, Los
   Angeles, Medical Center   US
Division of Hematology/Oncology
10833 Le Conte Ave, BH 412 CHS
Los Angeles, CA 90024

University of California, San
   Francisco, Medical Center   US
505 Parnassus Ave
San Francisco, CA 94143

MARYLAND

Johns Hopkins Hospital   US
600 N Wolfe St
Baltimore, MD 21205

MASSACHUSETTS

Massachusetts General Hospital   US
Infectious Disease Unit—Gray 5
55 Fruit St
Boston, MA 02114

NEW YORK

Memorial Sloan-Kettering
   Cancer Center   US
1275 York Ave
New York, NY 10021

SOURCES

US   indicates those hospitals recommended in *U.S. News & World Report.*

NIH National Institute of Allergy and Infectious Diseases, AIDS Clinical Trials Group (ACTG)

The following centers will test drugs to fight infections with HIV and related illnesses. At the end is a separate listing for children's hospitals.

ALABAMA

University of Alabama at Birmingham
1900 University Blvd
229 Tinsley Harris Tower
UAB Station
Birmingham, AL 35294

CALIFORNIA

LAC-USC Medical Center
1200 N State St, Rm 6442
Los Angeles, CA 90033

San Francisco General Hospital
Bldg 80, Ward 84
995 Potrero Ave
San Francisco, CA 94110

Stanford University School of Medicine
300 Pasteur Dr
Stanford, CA 94305

University of California, Los Angeles,
   Medical Center
Division of Hematology/Oncology
10833 Le Conte Ave, BH 412 CHS
Los Angeles, CA 90024

University of California, San Diego
Clinical Sciences Bldg, 4th Fl, Rm 430
Pediatrics/Infectious Diseases
9500 Gilman Dr, Mail Code #0672
La Jolla, CA 92093

COLORADO
University of Colorado Health Sciences
    Center
Infectious Disease Division
4200 E 9th Ave
Denver, CO 80262

CONNECTICUT
Yale University
155 Whitney Ave
New Haven, CT 06520

DISTRICT OF COLUMBIA
Georgetown University
Department of Medicine
3750 Reservoir Rd NW
Kober-Cogan, Rm 211
Washington, DC 20007

FLORIDA
University of Miami School of Medicine
Department of Medicine
First Fl, Elliot Bldg
1800 NW 10th Ave
Miami, FL 33136

ILLINOIS
NUMS, Comprehensive AIDS Center
Infectious Diseases, Ste 1106
680 N Lake Shore Dr
Chicago, IL 60611

INDIANA
Indiana University School of Medicine
Emerson Hall 435
545 Barnhill Dr
Indianapolis, IN 46202

MARYLAND
Johns Hopkins Hospital
600 N Wolfe St
Baltimore, MD 21205

MASSACHUSETTS
Massachusetts General Hospital
Infectious Disease Unit—Gray 5
55 Fruit St
Boston, MA 02114

MINNESOTA
University of Minnesota
Box 437 UMHC, 15-144 PWB
Harvard St at E River Rd
Minneapolis, MN 55455

MISSOURI
Washington University
Division of Hematology/Oncology
Box 8125
660 S Euclid Ave
St Louis, MO 63110

NEW YORK
Albert Einstein College of Medicine
Forchheimer 418
1300 Morris Park Ave
Bronx, NY 10461

Cornell University Medical Center
1300 York Ave, Rm A-421
New York, NY 10021

Mount Sinai Medical Center
Box 1042
One Gustave Levy Pl
New York, NY 10029

New York University Medical Center
Department of Medicine
550 First Ave
New York, NY 10016

SUNY Health Science Center
Box 56
450 Clarkson Ave
Brooklyn, NY 11203

University of Rochester Medical Center
Box 689
601 Elmwood Ave
Rochester, NY 14642

NORTH CAROLINA
University of North Carolina
School of Medicine
547 Burnett-Womack Bldg, CB7030
Chapel Hill, NC 27599

OHIO
Case Western Reserve University
School of Medicine, W-106
2109 Adelbert Rd
Cleveland, OH 44106

Ohio State University Hospitals
Rm N-1148, Doan Hall
Columbus, OH 43210

PENNSYLVANIA
University of Pennsylvania
Infectious Disease Section
536 Johnson Pavilion
Philadelphia, PA 19104

TEXAS
University of Texas Medical Branch
Department of Internal Medicine
Rm 218—Clay Hall, Rt H82
Galveston, TX 77550

WASHINGTON
Pacific Medical Center
Vaccine Unit, Rm 9307
1200 12th Ave S
Seattle, WA 98144

PEDIATRIC

CALIFORNIA
Moffitt Hospital
505 Parnassus Ave, Rm M-601B
San Francisco, CA 94143

University of California, Los Angeles,
 School of Medicine
22-404 MDCC
10833 Le Conte Ave
Los Angeles, CA 90024

UCSD Medical Center
Division of Infectious Diseases
Department of Pediatrics
225 Dickinson St, H-814-H
San Diego, CA 92103

COLORADO
University of Colorado Health Sciences
 Center
Pediatric Infectious Diseases
4200 E 9th Ave
Box C-227
Denver, CO 80262

DISTRICT OF COLUMBIA
Children's Hospital
111 Michigan Ave NW, Ste 2108
Washington, DC 20010

FLORIDA
University of Miami School of Medicine
Division of Pediatric Immunology and
 Infectious Diseases
PO Box 016960 (D4-4)
1550 NW 10th Ave, Rm 208
Miami, FL 33136

ILLINOIS
Northwestern University Medical
 School
2300 Children's Plaza
Chicago, IL 60614

LOUISIANA
Tulane University School of Medicine
Pediatric Infectious Diseases
1430 Tulane Ave
New Orleans, LA 70112

MARYLAND
Johns Hopkins Hospital
600 N Wolfe St, CMSC
Baltimore, MD 21205

MASSACHUSETTS
Children's Hospital
Division of Infectious Diseases
300 Longwood Ave
Boston, MA 02115

School of Medicine
Boston City Hospital
Children's Bldg 4
818 Harrison Ave
Boston, MA 02118

University of Massachusetts Medical
    School
Department of Pediatrics
55 Lake Ave N
Worcester, MA 01655

NEW JERSEY
Children's Hospital of New Jersey
AIDS Program
25 S 9th St
Newark, NJ 07107

NEW YORK
Albert Einstein College of Medicine
Rm 401—Forchheimer Bldg
1300 Morris Park Ave
Bronx, NY 10461

Bronx-Lebanon Hospital Center
Department of Pediatrics
1650 Grand Concourse
Bronx, NY 10457

Columbia University College of
    Physicians and Surgeons
Black Bldg
650 W 168th St, Rm 427
New York, NY 10032

Mount Sinai Medical Center
Box 1042
Rm 24-64, Annenburg Bldg
One Gustave Levy Pl
New York, NY 10029

New York University Medical Center
Division of Infectious Diseases and
    Immunology
550 First Ave
New York, NY 10016

NORTH CAROLINA
Duke University Medical Center
PO Box 2951
428 Jones Bldg, Research Dr
Durham, NC 27710

PENNSYLVANIA
The Joseph Stokes Jr Research Institute
Children's Hospital of Pennsylvania
34th St and Civic Center Blvd
Philadelphia, PA 19104

PUERTO RICO
University of Puerto Rico
University Children Hospital, AIDS
    Program
Fourth Fl, South Wing
Rm 4B-45, Gamma Project
GPO Box 365067
San Juan, PR 00936

TENNESSEE
St Jude Children's Research Hospital
332 N Lauderdale
Memphis, TN 38105

TEXAS
Texas Children's Hospital
6621 Fannin, Rm 0-321
Houston, TX 77030

WASHINGTON
Children's Hospital and Medical Center
4800 Sand Point Way NE
Seattle, WA 98105

AMFAR Community-Based Clinical Trial (CBCT) Network

*The Community-Based Clinical Trial Network provides an important complement to tradi-
tional academic research. Primary-care physicians conduct community-based clinical trials
in close cooperation with patients and AIDS advocates. The goals of the CBCT Network are
to produce data of the highest scientific quality, to accelerate the pace of AIDS research, and
to provide increased access to promising experimental therapies for people with AIDS and
HIV infection.*

ARIZONA
Phoenix Shanti Group Inc
1314 E McDowell Rd
Phoenix, AZ 85006

CALIFORNIA
AIDS Community Research
    Consortium
1048 El Camino, Ste A
Redwood City, CA 94063

Community Consortium
3180 18th St, Ste 201
San Francisco, CA 94110

East Bay AIDS Center
2640 Telegraph Ave
Berkeley, CA 94705

St Francis Memorial Hospital
900 Hyde St, 9th Fl
San Francisco, CA 94109

San Diego Community Research Group
3800 Ray St
San Diego, CA 92104

San Francisco Project Inform, Inc.
1965 Market St, Ste 220
San Francisco, CA 94103

Search Alliance
7461 Beverly Blvd, Ste 304
Los Angeles, CA 90036

Southwest Community Based AIDS
    Treatment Group
1800 N Highland, Ste 610
Los Angeles, CA 90028

COLORADO
Denver Community Program for
    Clinical Research on AIDS
Denver Public Health
605 Bannock St
Denver, CO 80204-4507

CONNECTICUT
Hill Health Center
400 Columbus Ave
New Haven, CT 06519

DELAWARE
Delaware Community Program for
    Clinical Research on AIDS
Medical Center of Delaware
501 W 14th St
Wilmington, DE 19801

DISTRICT OF COLUMBIA
Washington Community AIDS
    Program
VA Medical Center
Department of Infectious Disease
50 Irving St NW, Rm 4B102
Washington, DC 20422

Whitman Walker Clinic
1407 S St NW
Washington, DC 20009

FLORIDA
Bay Area AIDS Consortium
1222 S Dale Mabry Hwy, Ste 921
Tampa, FL 33629

Community Research Initiative of South
Florida
187 NE 36th St
Miami, FL 33137

GEORGIA
AIDS Research Consortium of Atlanta
131 Ponce de Leon, Ste 220
Atlanta, GA 30308

HAWAII
Hawaii AIDS Research Consortium
3675 Kilauea Ave, Young Bldg #16E
Honolulu, HI 96816

ILLINOIS
Chicago Community Program for
Clinical Research on AIDS
St Joseph Hospital
711 W North Ave
Chicago, IL 60610

KANSAS
University of Kansas School of Medicine
1010 N Kansas
Wichita, KS 67214

LOUISIANA
Louisiana Community AIDS Research
Program
Tulane University Medical Center
1430 Tulane Ave
New Orleans, LA 70112

MARYLAND
Baltimore Community Research
Consortium
Box 243
22 S Green St
Baltimore, MD 21201

MASSACHUSETTS
Community Research Initiative of New
England
338 Newbury St
Boston, MA 02115

MICHIGAN
Comprehensive AIDS Alliance of
Detroit
Wayne State University School of
Medicine
Division of Infectious Disease
Detroit Medical Center
4160 John R, Ste 202
Detroit, MI 48201

Henry Ford Hospital
Division of Infectious Disease and
Hospital Epidemiology
2799 W Grand Blvd
Detroit, MI 48202

MISSOURI
Kansas City AIDS Consortium
2411 Holmes
Kansas City, MO 64108

NEW JERSEY
North Jersey Community Research
Initiative
657 King Blvd
Newark, NJ 07102

NEW MEXICO
AIDS Wellness Clinic
811 St Michael's Dr
Santa Fe, NM 87501

NEW YORK
Addiction Research and Treatment
Corporation
22 Chapel St
Brooklyn, NY 11201

AIDS Treatment Center
Albany Medical Center Hospital
47 New Scotland Ave, Rm A-167
Albany, NY 12208

Bronx Lebanon Hospital—AIDS
Division
1276 Fulton Ave, Rm 223
Bronx, NY 10456

Clinical Directors Network of Region II,
Bronx, NY/Brooklyn, NY/
Newark, NJ
5601 Second Ave
Brooklyn, NY 11220

Community Health Network
758 South Ave
Rochester, NY 14620

Community Research Initiative on AIDS
(CRIA)
31 W 26th St
New York, NY 10010

Harlem AIDS Treatment Group
Harlem Hospital—Infectious Disease
Section
506 Lenox Ave, Rm 3107
New York, NY 10037

OREGON
Oregon AIDS Task Force
The Research & Education Group
2701 NW Vaughn St, Ste 770
Portland, OR 97210

PENNSYLVANIA
Philadelphia FIGHT
419 S 19th St, #201
Philadelphia, PA 19146

PUERTO RICO
Fundacion SIDA de Puerto Rico
Calle 16 SE
1200 Caparra Terrace
Rio Piedras, PR 00921

RHODE ISLAND
Brown University AIDS Consortium
Brown University
Box G-S204
Providence, RI 02912

TEXAS
AIDS Resource Center
Nelson-Tebedo Community Clinic
PO Box 190712
4012 Cedar Springs Rd
Dallas, TX 75219

HIV Study Group
Central Texas Medical Foundation
4614 North IH-35
Austin, TX 78751

Houston Clinical Research Network
4211 Graustark
Houston, TX 77006

VIRGINIA
Richmond AIDS Consortium
Box 49, MCV Station
Richmond, VA 23298

WISCONSIN
Wisconsin Community-Based Research
Consortium
c/o Milwaukee AIDS Project
315 W Court St
Milwaukee, WI 53212

CANADA
Community Research Initiative/Toronto
40 Gerrard St E, Ste 506
Toronto, Ontario
Canada M5B 2E8

NIH National Institute of Allergy and Infectious Diseases, Community Programs for Clinical Research on AIDS (CPCRA)

CPCRA involves community clinicians in the design and execution of AIDS clinical research protocols and the development of new research methodologies appropriate to community settings. It includes primary care physicians and nurses who care for large numbers of persons with HIV infection and who work in community health centers, hospitals, private clinics or practices, drug addiction treatment facilities, or a combination of locations. The CPCRA is particularly designed to reach out to all persons with HIV infection, including those in the population groups that have been underrepresented in AIDS studies: African-Americans, Hispanics, intravenous-drug users, and women. Through the program, HIV-infected people will gain increased access to experimental AIDS drugs.

CALIFORNIA
Community Consortium
San Francisco General Hospital
3180 18th St, Ste 201
San Francisco, CA 94110

COLORADO
Denver CPCRA
Denver Public Health
605 Bannock St
Denver, CO 80204-4507

CONNECTICUT
Hill Health Corporation
400 Columbus Ave
New Haven, CT 06519

DELAWARE
Delaware CPCRA
Medical Center of Delaware
Wilmington Hospital
14th and Washington Sts, Rm 453
Wilmington, DE 19801

DISTRICT OF COLUMBIA
Washington Regional AIDS Program
Veterans Administration Medical Center
50 Irving St NW
Washington, DC 20422

GEORGIA
AIDS Research Consortium of Atlanta, Inc
131 Ponce de Leon Ave, Ste 220
Atlanta, GA 30308

ILLINOIS
Chicago CPCRA
711 W North Ave
Chicago, IL 60610

LOUISIANA
Louisiana Community AIDS Research Program
Tulane University Medical Center
1501 Canal Blvd.
New Orleans, LA 70112

MICHIGAN
Comprehensive AIDS Alliance of Detroit
Harper Hospital Professional Bldg
4160 John R, Ste 202
Detroit, MI 48201

Henry Ford Hospital
Infectious Disease Division
2799 W Grand Blvd
Detroit, MI 48202

NEW JERSEY
North Jersey Community Research Initiative
657 King Blvd
Newark, NJ 07102

NEW YORK
Addiction Research and Treatment Corp
22 Chapel St
Brooklyn, NY 11201

Bronx-Lebanon Hospital Center
AIDS Division
1276 Fulton Ave
Bronx, NY 10456

Clinical Directors Network of Region II
5601 Second Ave, Ste 3
Brooklyn, NY 11220

Harlem AIDS Treatment Group
Harlem Hospital Center
Infectious Diseases Section
506 Lenox Ave, Rm 3107
New York, NY 10037

OREGON
The Research and Education Group
2701 NW Vaughn, Ste 770
Portland, OR 97210-5311

VIRGINIA
Richmond AIDS Consortium
Medical College of Virginia/Virginia
    Commonwealth University
Box 49, MCV Station
Richmond, VA 23298

Step 4. Become Your Own Expert

WHO TO CALL   AIDS has the most impressive support network of any disease in the United States. A well-reported series of newsletters provides in-depth coverage of the latest treatments. Your survival depends on being tapped into the network.

Gay Men's Health Crisis (GMHC)   This was the first group organized to help all people with AIDS, not just gays and lesbians. It operates several services in the New York metropolitan area:

Client assistance, including consumer advocacy and legal aid with creditors, insurance companies, hospitals, state and federal social service agencies. There is a buddy system that provides one-on-one assistance with shopping, housecleaning, laundry, drugs, and doctors.

Education, with monthly forums to discuss safe sex, treatment, nutrition, legal matters.

Support groups for AIDS patients, lovers, and parents run by social workers and psychotherapists. There are walk-in and regularly scheduled groups.

Public advocacy on the local, state, and federal levels to lobby for funding, social services, treatment, and research.

Referrals to about 30 local doctors through its hotline: 212/807-6655.

Gay Men's Health Crisis Treatment Issues, published every six weeks, updating developments in treatment.

129 W 20th St
New York, NY 10011
212/807-6664; 212/807-6655

People with AIDS Coalition   Staffed by people who are infected with the AIDS virus, this organization offers counseling and treatment information. The drop-in center provides informational brochures, support groups, meal programs, and a speakers' bureau. Two newsletters are published:

Newsline: One of the best resource newsletters, contains information on support groups, clinical trials, and hotlines. It is published monthly.

SIDA A'Hora: A Spanish-language quarterly for HIV-infected Hispanics.

31 W 26th St
New York, NY 10010
212/532-0290; 212/532-0568 in New York
800/828-3280

People with AIDS Health Group   This is a buyer's club that offers information on experimental medications not available in the United States. The newsletter, *Notes from the Underground,* describes the types and availability of experimental AIDS medications. It's considered by many to be the best AIDS drug treatment newsletter.

31 W 26th St
New York, NY 10010
212/532-0280

Body Positive   This organization provides educational information and peer support to HIV-positive individuals and their loved ones. Referrals are available to doctors in New York and New Jersey. The monthly newsletter, *Body Positive,* covers all aspects of the disease, including alternatives to conventional Western medical treatments.

2095 Broadway, Ste 306
New York, NY 10023
212/721-1346

American Foundation for AIDS Research   AMFAR is a major fund-raising organization and a sponsor of research on AIDS. It provides patient information and referrals to community medical centers. It publishes the *AIDS/HIV Treatment Directory,* a quarterly guide to new treatments for AIDS and opportunistic infections, considered the most comprehensive compendium of clinical trials in the United States.

1515 Broadway
New York, NY 10036
212/719-0033

San Francisco AIDS Foundation   This foundation can provide answers to all questions about AIDS treatment, safe sex, IV drug use, and other issues. In Northern California it makes referrals to doctors, lawyers, and dentists. For other areas it can provide contacts to local community organizations. It publishes the *Bulletin of Experimental Treatments for AIDS.*

PO Box 6182
San Francisco, CA 94101
415/863-AIDS

Project Inform   This group runs both an information clearinghouse on all stages of AIDS infection and an HIV treatment hotline. A newsletter, *PI Perspective*, and various fact sheets, are published three times a year and cover treatment issues.

1965 Market St, #220
San Francisco, CA 94103
415/332-6240, for administrative offices
415/558-9051, within San Francisco
800/334-7422, the rest of California
800/822-7422, outside California

HEAL   This group offers information about nontoxic, nonconventional treatments and spiritual healing. A support group meets weekly in New York City. The group's newsletter is *Heal Quarterly.*

PO Box 1103
Old Chelsea Station
New York, NY 10113
212/674-HOPE

National Institutes of Health   Their toll-free hotline can provide information about all federally sponsored clinical drug trials.

800/TRIALS-A

Centers for Disease Control   This hotline operated by the federal government is one of the best sources of information about support groups, medical treatment, and legal counsel.

800/342-AIDS
800/344-SIDA, Spanish language
800/AIDS-TYY, for the hearing impaired

National AIDS Information Clearinghouse   This group offers business and workplace information, educational resources, clinical trials information, and publications.

PO Box 6003
Rockville, MD 20850
800/458-5231

Community AIDS Treatment Information Exchange   This group's newsletter, *Treatment Update,* contains specialized information on experimental, conventional, and alternative treatments.

517 College St, Ste 324
Toronto, Ontario
Canada M6G 1A8
416/944-1916

Vancouver PWA Society Newsletter   This is a self-help, self-care group for HIV-positive individuals. It offers peer counseling, support groups, a resource library, and medical forums. The newsletter covers treatment information and updates.

1447 Hornby St
Vancouver, British Columbia
Canada V6Z 1W8
604/683-3381

Women and AIDS Resource Network   The network provides education, referrals, counseling, information, and support groups for women and their partners and children.

30 Third Ave, Ste 212
Brooklyn, NY 11217
718/596-6007

AIDS Project Los Angeles   This project offers over 20 programs for people diagnosed with AIDS. It may provide everything from food, temporary shelter, and dental care to support and mental health services as well as doctor referrals. It also maintains special counseling services regarding insurance and public and legal benefits.

6721 Romaine St
Los Angeles, CA 90038
213/962-1600

Chicago AIDS Foundation   This is the largest AIDS foundation in the Midwest. It provides extensive educational and outreach information and material as well as doctor referrals.

1332 N Halsted, Ste 303
Chicago, IL 60622
312/642-5454

AIDS Action Committee   This group provides counseling services, education, advocacy, and outreach services for people with AIDS in Massachusetts and their families. It publishes a monthly newsletter, *Wellspring.*

131 Clarendon St
Boston, MA 02116
617/437-6200
617/536-7733, information hotline
800/235-2331, for Massachusetts only

AID Atlanta   This organization can provide extensive information about AIDS. There is a speaker's bureau and a doctor referral system. It publishes a monthly newsletter, *Infolines.*

1132 W Peachtree St NW, Ste 112
Atlanta, GA 30309
404/876-9944 or 404/872-0600

Northwest AIDS Foundation   This group provides information and referrals for people throughout the United States and is an access point to special services for residents of Washington state with HIV or AIDS.

127 Broadway E, Ste A
Seattle, WA 98102-5711
206/329-6923

AIDS Treatment News   This is a twice-monthly newsletter that covers medical, social, and political issues.

P.O. Box 411256
San Francisco, CA 94141
415/255-0588
800/TREAT-12

ACT UP   This group, best known as a political action group, also offers extensive general information about the disease. It publishes a quarterly newsletter, the *ACT UP Report.*

135 W 29th St, 10th Fl
New York, NY 10001
212/564-AIDS

AIDS Forum   This group publishes a newsletter.

PO Box 1545
Canal St Station
New York, NY 10013

People with AIDS Health Group   This group provides help in obtaining medications unavailable in the United States.

150 W 26th St
New York, NY 10001
212/255-0520

NIH CRISP System
301/496-7543

University-Affiliated Teaching Hospitals   See Appendix.

EXPERT SOURCES

Although dozens of experts were interviewed for these chapters, these physicians are acknowledged for their significant contributions to this section.

Dr. Joseph Sonnabend, Director, Community Research Initiative on AIDS, New York, NY

Dr. Howard Grossman, New York, NY

David Barr, Gay Men's Health Crisis, New York, NY

Dr. Paul Volberding, Director, AIDS Program, San Francisco General Hospital, San Francisco, CA

REFERENCES AND SUGGESTED READING

American Foundation for AIDS Research. *AIDS/HIV Clinical Trial Handbook,* 1989.

American Foundation for AIDS Research. *AIDS/HIV Treatment Directory,* Fall 1991.

Barker, K. F., and Holliman, R. E. Laboratory Techniques in the Investigation of Toxoplasmosis. *Genitourinary Medicine,* Vol. 68, No. 1 (Feb. 1992), pp. 55–59.

Boucher, Charles A. B., and others. HIV-1 Sensitivity to Zidovudine and Clinical Outcome [letter]. *Lancet,* Vol. 339, No. 8793 (Mar. 7, 1992), pp. 626–627.

Centers for Disease Control. The HIV/AIDS Epidemic: The First 10 Years. *MMWR Morbidity and Mortality Weekly Report,* Vol. 40, No. 22 (June 7, 1991).

Coker, R. J., and others. Cavitating Pulmonary Cryptococcosis Developing in an HIV-Antibody Patient Despite Prior Treatment with Fluconazole. *Genitourinary Medicine,* Vol. 68, No. 1 (Feb. 1992), pp. 42–44.

Gay Men's Health Crisis. *Medical Answers About AIDS,* 1990 update.

Gazzard, B. G. When Should Asymptomatic Patients with HIV Infection Be Treated with Zidovudine? [editorial] *British Medical Journal,* Vol. 304, No. 6825 (Feb. 22, 1992), pp. 456–457.

Kyle, Walter S. Simian Retroviruses, Poliovaccine, and Origin of AIDS. *Lancet*, Vol. 339, No. 8793 (Mar. 7, 1992), pp. 600–601.

MacGregor, Rob Roy, and others. Efficacy and Tolerance of Intermittent Versus Daily Cotrimoxazole for PCP Prophylaxis in HIV-Positive Patients. *American Journal of Medicine*, Vol. 92, No. 2 (Feb. 1992), pp. 227–229.

Massachusetts Medical Society. HIV-Risk Behaviors of Sterilized and Nonsterilized Women in Drug-Treatment Programs—Philadelphia, 1989–1991. *Morbidity and Mortality Weekly Report (MMWR)*, Vol. 41, No. 9 (Mar. 6, 1992), pp. 149–152.

Massachusetts Medical Society. Street Outreach for STD/HIV Prevention—Colorado Springs, Colorado, 1987–1991. *Morbidity and Mortality Weekly Report (MMWR)*, Vol. 41, No. 6 (Feb. 14, 1992), pp. 94–95, 101.

McAllister, R. H., and others. Neurological and Neuropsychological Performance in HIV-Seropositive Men Without Symptoms. *Journal of Neurology, Neurosurgery and Psychiatry*, Vol. 55, No. 2 (Feb. 1992), pp. 143–148.

Miller, Riva, and Bor, Robert. Pre-HIV Antibody Testing—Too Much Fuss? *Genitourinary Medicine*, Vol. 68, No. 1 (Feb. 1992), pp. 9–10.

Paoli, Ivan, and others. Pharmacodynamics of Zidovudine in Patients with End-Stage Renal Disease [letter]. *New England Journal of Medicine*, Vol. 36, No. 12 (Mar. 19, 1992), pp. 839–840.

Persson, Elisabeth, and Jarlbro, Gunilla. Sexual Behaviour Among Youth Clinic Visitors in Sweden: Knowledge and Experiences in an HIV Perspective. *Genitourinary Medicine*, Vol. 68, No. 1 (Feb. 1992), pp. 26–31.

Powderly, William G., and others. A Controlled Trial of Fluconazole or Amphotericin B to Prevent Relapse of Cryptococcal Meningitis in Patients with the Acquired Immunodeficiency Syndrome. *New England Journal of Medicine*, Vol. 326, No. 12 (Mar. 19, 1992), pp. 793–798.

Schwarcz, Sandra K., and others. Crack Cocaine and the Exchange of Sex for Money or Drugs: Risk Factors for Gonorrhea Among Black Adolescents in San Francisco. *Sexually Transmitted Diseases*, Vol. 19, No. 1 (Jan.–Feb. 1992), pp. 7–13.

Sherr, L., and Strong, C. Safe Sex and Women. *Genitourinary Medicine*, Vol. 68, No. 1 (Feb. 1992), pp. 32–35.

Simonds, R. J., and others. Transmission of Human Immunodeficiency Virus Type1 from a Seronegative Organ and Tissue Donor. *New England Journal of Medicine*, Vol. 326, No. 11 (Mar. 12, 1992), pp. 726–732.

Smith, Peggy B., and others. Knowledge, Beliefs, and Behavioral Risk Factors for Human Immunodeficiency Virus Infection in Inner-City Adolescent Females. *Sexually Transmitted Diseases*, Vol. 19, No. 1 (Jan.–Feb. 1992), pp. 19–24.

Sperling, Rhoda S., and Stratton, Pamela. Treatment Options for Human Immunodeficiency Virus–Infected Pregnant Women [review]. *Obstetrics and Gynecology*, Vol. 79, No. 3 (Mar. 1992), pp. 443–448.

Stratton, Pamela, and others. Human Immunodeficiency Virus Infection in Pregnant Women Under Care at AIDS Clinical Trials Centers in the United States. *Obstetrics and Gynecology,* Vol. 79, No. 3 (Mar 1992), pp. 364–368.

U.S. Agency for International Development. *HIV Infection and AIDS: A Report to Congress on the U.S. AIDS Program for Prevention and Control.* Washington, D.C.: May 1991.

U.S. Department of Health and Human Services. *AIDS Clinical Trials: Talking It Over.* National Institutes of Health Publication No. 89–3025, Aug. 1989.

Wheat, L. Joseph, and others. Effect of Successful Treatment with Amphotericin B on Histoplasma Capsulatum Variety Capsulatum Polysaccharide Antigen Levels in Patients with AIDS and Histoplasmosis. *American Journal of Medicine,* Vol. 92, No. 2 (Feb. 1992), pp. 153–160.

Arthritis

Risk for Inappropriate Care   HIGH

"Attitude is the single biggest problem in the treatment of the disease," according to Dr. Joseph A. Markenson, an arthritis specialist at the Hospital for Special Surgery in New York City. Too many patients, and often their doctors, adopt an attitude that "everyone gets arthritis, there's nothing you can do about it, so why worry about it," Markenson says. Of the 37 million Americans who have arthritis, the Centers for Disease Control estimate that six million have never sought medical help. That attitude is not just wrong—it's dangerous. Arthritis can seriously impair your ability to perform simple tasks, erode your earning power, and destroy your ability to enjoy life. To take just one example: People with the disease lose a total of 45 million days of work, spend 156 million days in bed, and restrict their normal activities by 427 million days annually, according to the Arthritis Foundation. It's shocking that lives are being ruined by arthritis, because early, aggressive treatment can often prevent joint destruction.

What It Is

There are many forms of arthritis. The two most common forms are rheumatoid arthritis and osteoarthritis.

RHEUMATOID ARTHRITIS   This is the most serious form of arthritis, since it is a potentially crippling and debilitating illness. The Arthritis Foundation states that it affects 2.1 million Americans. The cause is not clear, but it is usually considered an autoimmune disease, meaning that the body's immune system, which normally destroys foreign microbes, turns on itself. It attacks joints and other body tissues. The normally delicate surface lining of the joints becomes inflamed, and the inflammation damages the joints, sometimes quickly, sometimes slowly. Rheumatoid arthritis involves more than just the joints. It is really a disease that affects the entire body, causing stiffness, chronic fatigue, and anemia among other symptoms.

OSTEOARTHRITIS   This, the most common form of arthritis, which afflicts 15.8 million Americans, is a degenerative disease of the joints. Again the cause is not clear, but it is generally thought of as wear-and-tear arthritis. The incidence of the disease increases with age and can be accelerated by joint injuries or fractures. Sports injuries are often the cause. Osteoarthritis may begin in one's twenties or thirties and occur without any symptoms at that early stage. By the age of 70 almost all individuals have some form of the disease. Osteoarthritis may be painful, but it is not the fast-moving, destructive disease that rheumatoid arthritis is. Therefore, much of this chapter is devoted to the management of rheumatoid arthritis.

Step 1. Make Sure You Get the Best Care

Read this section on potential problems with your treatment carefully to determine if there are discrepancies between your care and state-of-the-art care. Use Step 2 to review shortcomings.

Diagnosis

The treatment of rheumatoid arthritis is relatively straightforward. To the extent that it is possible, you want to control the inflammation and to preserve the function of afflicted joints. Medications decrease inflammation and slow the progression of the disease. Exercise and physical therapy maintain muscle strength and range of motion. Surgery can restore function in damaged joints. None of this is possible, however, unless you seek medical treatment.

COMPLETE EVALUATION   Without a complete diagnostic evaluation, an individual experiencing arthritis as joint pain can't know which form of the disease is present. Up to 50% of patients lack that basic knowledge, according to Dr. Markenson. It's also possible that you may attribute your aches and pains to arthritis when you have another disease entirely. Sometimes what one assumes is arthritis may be another illness. In one tragic case, a patient assumed that the swelling of his hands and wrists was caused by osteoarthritis. A year later doctors diagnosed an incurable lung tumor, which could have been treated successfully had it been found early on. For hot, inflamed, tender joints, "early on" means seeing a doctor within hours to a day or so after the condition begins. Women, in particular, should be quick to consult a doctor, for they are twice as likely as men to be afflicted.

IMPORTANCE OF EARLY DIAGNOSIS   There is no clear evidence that early treatment will help osteoarthritis; but if you have rheumatoid arthritis, your joints may be irreparably damaged by even a short delay in beginning treatment, says Dr. James McGuire of Stanford Medical School. Some rheumatologists claim that delay of prompt intervention can decrease life expectancy by a decade. A survey conducted for the Arthritis Foundation determined that 40% of patients with arthritis wait a year or more to seek help. This is far too long. In that time irreparable damage may be done to one or more of the joints. Dr. Markenson believes you may be injured permanently if you delay seeking help for even two weeks when you have acutely inflamed, tender joints. If you experience less severe aches and pains in your joints that, despite self-medication, increase in severity or last longer than two weeks, you need to see a doctor.

Again, if the joint feels red, hot, tender, and swollen, you need to see a doctor immediately. With an acutely hot, angry joint, you may not have arthritis at all, but rather an infection caused by bacteria. Take the case of the 23-year-old flight attendant who complained about a painful burning sensation in her wrist. She treated the pain for months with over-the-counter medications, totally unaware that these symptoms could be caused by serious infection. She sought help only after the joint became frozen and extremely difficult to use. By then it was too late. The pain's source was a gonococcal infection that had already caused irreversible damage to the joint.

RISK OF MISDIAGNOSIS   Unfortunately, even if you seek medical care promptly, there is a real danger that you may be misdiagnosed. Doctors may be as willing as their patients to dismiss arthritis as a trivial disease that does not require early, aggressive treatment. Because arthritis can affect many body systems, this attitude can be life-threatening. On the other hand, a doctor who rushes into a hasty diagnosis may do serious injury to patients.

There is no quick test to identify arthritis properly. In fact, you should be wary if your doctor relies heavily on high technology, such as CAT scans and MRIs, for a diagnosis. While these tests can be excellent tools for the diagnosis of disc problems in the back, for example, they are usually an unnecessary expense in the evaluation of arthritis symptoms. You should be suspicious, too, if your diagnosis is made from a blood test. Arthritis is not like high cholesterol, for instance, for which a doctor can order a fairly simple test and say, aha, you have high cholesterol. Although some physicians use the tests for that purpose, such tests can be misleading and should not be taken at face value. Based on tests alone, osteoarthritis can be mistaken for rheumatoid arthritis.

Far more than most diseases, arthritis—especially in its early stages—requires sophisticated clinical skills for an accurate diagnosis. Rheumatologists at the Hospital for Special Surgery are, first, internists who have specialized in the diagnosis and treatment of arthritis. You need a doctor who not only understands the disease but also spends enough time with you to make an old-fashioned diagnosis with a careful, detailed history and physical exam. Laboratory tests may lend support to that diagnosis, but they are not sufficient to identify your symptoms properly. Numerous diagnostic errors are made if a physician does not bother to examine the patient carefully. For instance, the classic description of rheumatoid arthritis holds that joints on both the right and left sides of the body are supposed to be inflamed, but early on, when diagnosis is most important, the joints may be affected on one side only. Your doctor should have the flexibility to cast aside textbook definitions if this will aid in the evaluation of your care.

Here are some of the dangers: An adult may have a painful back diagnosed as arthritis when it is caused by a severe infection. If the condition is left untreated, the patient may suffer long-term disability. A child with a particularly vicious form of juvenile rheumatoid arthritis may go blind if the disease is missed. That's because the physician will not know to refer her or him to an ophthalmologist for regular eye examinations, which would detect a well-known eye complication of juvenile rheumatoid arthritis. A careful clinician will look at a number of symptoms—persistently inflamed, swollen joints, fatigue, and anemia, for instance—before diagnosing the disease.

Perhaps because doctors tend to minimize the seriousness of arthritis, they also tend to undertreat the disease. This is the number-one error in the management of most forms of arthritis.

Treatment Medications

You deserve a doctor who will take the time to listen and help you to remain active and to cope with the inevitably high level of frustration that accompanies this disease, and to advise you on family and career problems that may arise. Individuals with rheumatoid arthritis are patients for life. Treatment should not be one-dimensional, although it often is. You should have a doctor who can take into account the physical, occupational, emotional, and lifestyle changes that result from the disease and who can devise a treatment regimen that will encompass all of them.

There is no single treatment for arthritis that is free of side effects and will accomplish all treatment objectives. However, the most effective treatment is to begin with an aggressive regimen of medications, starting with large doses, and then to try and obtain the same results with a lower dosage. This is the best way to ascertain if a particular drug will work. If a doctor starts conservatively and then attempts to treat the disease by escalating the amount of the drug, permanent damage may have occurred by the time the effective dosage has been discovered. Arthritis drugs will relieve pain before they cure the underlying inflammation. As a result, your symptoms could go away while your joints continue to get worse. Your doctor needs to give you a dose large enough to change the course of your illness, not just to eliminate the symptoms of the disease.

DRUGS THAT CONTROL INFLAMMATION AND PAIN

NSAIDs Nonsteroidal antiinflammatory drugs, known by the acronym NSAIDs, will probably be your very first therapy. NSAIDs treatment may go on for approximately several weeks to four months. The drugs should control pain and inflammation, although it may take time to discover the one that works best in your case. Many of these drugs are available as pain killers in over-the-counter medications such as Advil, Nuprin, and ibuprofen. Prescriptions are required for the larger-dose, longer-lasting antiinflammatory forms essential for the treatment of arthritis.

Although NSAIDs are very effective, they can have numerous gastric side effects, such as mild stomach pain, bloating, gas, heartburn, nausea, vomiting, indigestion, and ulcers. You are at higher risk for ulcers if you are over 60, smoke, have a prior history of ulcers, or suffer severe disability from other chronic illnesses. (See the chapter on Ulcers.) Other side effects include constipation, diarrhea, dizziness, mild headache, hearing problems, and fluid retention (such as unusual weight gain and swelling of the ankles, feet, or lower legs). Because NSAIDs interfere with blood clotting, you may bleed easily. You should be alert to such signs of internal bleeding as a burning feeling in or above the stomach, severe or constant pain at the bottom of the rib cage, occasional unexplained nausea or vomiting, and stomach pain that goes away after eating or taking antacids. If you vomit blood or find blood in your stool, you should contact your doctor immediately.

You can minimize the risk of the most severe side effects—ulcers and bleeding—by not smoking, by drinking alcohol only in moderation, by limiting your intake of the drugs to the amount prescribed, and by promptly reporting any side effects. A new drug called Cytotec (Misoprostol) can reduce the chances that your NSAIDs will produce an ulcer.

Allergic reactions to NSAIDs are also possible. You may be having such a reaction if you experience rapid breathing, wheezing, fainting, skin problems, rapid heartbeat, or puffiness in and around the eyes.

You can help your doctor to prescribe NSAIDs correctly if you keep him or her properly informed. Dr. Markenson suggests you make certain your doctor knows if any of the following are true.

LET YOUR DOCTOR KNOW IF:

■ You are allergic to any prescription or over-the-counter medicine. For example, if you've had an allergic reaction to aspirin—skin rash, wheezing, hives— you may have a similar response to NSAIDs.

■ You are pregnant or intend to become pregnant while you are taking the medication.

■ You are breast feeding.

■ You are taking other prescription or over-the-counter medicine, especially an anticoagulant such as a blood thinner or aspirin.

- You have certain other medical conditions: colitis, diabetes, ulcers, breast disease, asthma, bleeding, or other problems with your stomach, kidneys, or liver.

- You are taking medications for edema, hypertension, or heart disease.

While NSAIDs can be extremely beneficial, you won't benefit if you're not taking the drug correctly. Here is a checklist from the Arthritis Foundation that I have found very helpful.

TIPS FOR WISE DRUG USE

- Know why you are taking a drug and how it will help your arthritis.

- Always take the medicine with a full meal and plenty of liquids.

- If you are taking the medicine regularly and miss a dose, take it as soon as possible. However, if it is almost time for your next dose, skip the one you missed and go back to your regular schedule. Never take a double dose.

- Put your daily medicine doses in a pill organizer and place it where you will be when it is time to take your medication. Carry extra medicine with you if you are going to change your daily routine. Do not mix different medicines in the same container.

- Read the package insert that comes with the drug. If you have problems or questions, call your doctor.

- Never let another person use your medications, and never take medicine prescribed for someone else. Even though you both may have the same type of arthritis, a drug that works for another person may not help you.

- Never reduce your medication dose or stop taking it altogether without consulting your doctor. There may be times when you're feeling good and your arthritis isn't bothering you, but this doesn't mean the condition has gone away. You can still have inflammation without a lot of pain. Cutting down or stopping your medication on your own could have serious results and may even interfere with the progress of your treatment. Stop taking your medicine only if you have an allergic reaction or serious side effects. Call your doctor right away so you can resume treatment.

- Don't increase your medication if your pain becomes worse. Your dosage has been adjusted to meet your specific needs, and there is no advantage to taking more of it at difficult times. You will not make yourself feel better any faster by doing this, and you may even be doing yourself harm.

- Don't drive or operate machinery if your NSAID makes you drowsy or dizzy. Make sure you know how your medication affects you.

- Don't take NSAIDs with alcohol, coffee, or beverages such as tea, cocoa, and soft drinks that contain caffeine. These beverages may make your stomach problems worse.

- Don't take other medicines containing aspirin compounds (salicylate) or ibuprofen without checking with your doctor. This includes over-the-counter cold remedies and pain relievers and other prescription drugs. If you take these in addition to your prescribed medication, it may cause side effects from too much NSAID in your body or may increase stomach problems caused by NSAIDs. Always read the ingredients listed on the labels of these products. If ibuprofen, acetylsalicylic acid, or salicylate are listed, check with your doctor before taking the medicine.

These antiinflammatory drugs have a solid place in the treatment of arthritis, but they are also easily abused when large doses are taken without appropriate monitoring. Some physicians believe that the result is an unnecessarily large incidence of life-threatening stomach bleeding or kidney failure. Your doctor should order regular tests for anemia, kidney function, and gastrointestinal bleeding. If you self-medicate with large doses of drugs over an extended period of time, you put yourself at risk for a number of serious reactions. And, of course, you should not begin taking them until your doctor has made a solid diagnosis and determined that your condition is chronic.

Aspirin   Aspirin, the first NSAID, is still a very good drug. None of the newer NSAIDs has ever been shown to be more effective or safer. In addition, aspirin is also very inexpensive. The difficulty is this: The usual dose of aspirin for rheumatoid arthritis is 12 to 20 tablets a day. Since aspirin's effect wears off quickly, the tablets must be taken four or so times a day. Because many patients complain about the inconvenience, doctors tend to prescribe NSAIDs instead.

Steroids   Although NSAIDs are a standard treatment for arthritis, steroids may be prescribed if your case is unusually severe. They are *not* the same as anabolic steroids, which have deservedly received so much bad publicity. There is little question that steroids can be the single most effective of all the anti-inflammatory drugs. But they can also have disastrous side effects if taken at high dosages over an extended period. Certainly, no young or even middle-aged individual should take steroids for a long time. They are best used in small dosages, perhaps 5 milligrams of prednisone, to get older patients moving again or to help patients on standard therapy who are experiencing extreme tenderness, almost a smoldering, emberlike sensation, in their joints. In such cases steroids can be used as a short-term measure to bring the arthritis under control. They can be taken orally or through injections, which can bring excellent spot relief to painful joints. Steroid injections may also be given three times a year in severe cases of osteoarthritis when joints will eventually have to be replaced, and the effects last for weeks or months. One expert warned me these injections should not be given more than three times a year to any patient.

DRUGS THAT MODIFY THE COURSE OF YOUR ILLNESS   Such drugs actually modify the disease by slowing or even stopping the destruction of joints. The sicker you are, the faster you will need them. To assess that need for them, your doctor will look for the presence of one or more of the following conditions: stiffness that lasts more than one hour after awakening, persistent fatigue and anemia, the appearance of new rheumatoid nodules beneath the skin, and changes in your x-rays. Every rheumatologist I spoke to favored earlier use of these medications *before* signs of joint destruction appeared on x-ray. There are several drugs that fall into this category.

Gold Compounds   The time-honored treatment for advanced rheumatoid arthritis is the injection of gold compounds. Their safety has been well documented. There are two disadvantages, however: (1) You must visit your doctor every week for the shots. (2) You must also be patient. The injections can take up to 20 weeks to work. Sometimes gold compounds are given orally, which is more convenient for the patient but not quite as effective. As this book goes to press, a new study calls into question the effectiveness of gold. Dr. Markenson counters that the study is flawed and that gold is still an excellent choice.

Antimalarials   These are one of the safest of the second-line drugs. Originally used to treat malaria, they were found to reduce the symptoms of rheumatoid arthritis, especially when used over a long period of time. Most tolerate the drugs well, but side effects include damage to the retina and nausea. It is recommended that those patients taking an antimalarial drug have regular eye exams. Doctors consider these to be less effective than gold or penicillamine, but they have fewer side effects. Although antimalarials are weaker drugs, used in combination with other drugs, they are excellent.

Penicillamine   Like gold, this drug is used to treat people with rheumatoid arthritis who haven't responded well to other therapies. The purpose is to reduce inflammation and potentially retard the progression of the disease. There are serious and toxic side effects associated with long-term use, including nausea, rashes, hives, dryness, scaling, and the onset of other serious illnesses. Patients should be under close supervision of a physician when taking penicillamine. A trial period of several months is required to see if the drug takes effect. And it must be taken on an empty stomach, at least an hour before meals or after any other drug or food. Because of this toxicity, penicillamine is used a good deal less nowadays. The dosage may be increased at six-week intervals.

Cytotoxic Agents   These are gold's newer rivals. Some of them are only recently approved by the Food and Drug Administration. They work far more quickly, usually within four to eight weeks. The most widely used, methotrexate, has been proven very effective in long-term studies. Patient follow-up is available up to eight years. Cytotoxic agents usually are taken in pill form, so injections are not required. Imuran is another cytotoxic agent that is also prescribed.

DRUG INTERACTIONS   While you are taking any drugs for arthritis, you should be under the care of a single physician. Otherwise, you can end up with a dozen different drugs for a variety of illnesses, and these drugs can interact to cause severe side effects or to lower the effectiveness of the usual dose. One doctor needs to look at all your drugs. If you are taking beta blockers and diuretics for your high blood pressure, for example, they will be lowering the flow of blood through your kidneys. If you add NSAIDs and gold compounds for your arthritis, you are jeopardizing your kidneys further. This quadruple threat needs to be monitored carefully for decreases in kidney function.

DRUGS AND PREGNANCY   None of the drugs for arthritis are safe for pregnant women. Before you become pregnant, you should review your medication requirements with your doctor and the risk that pregnancy poses to your underlying disease. While you are on arthritis medication, you should practice effective birth control. If you become pregnant, you will need to consult an obstetrician who specializes in high-risk pregnancies.

TESTS THAT HELP YOUR DOCTOR MANAGE YOUR DRUG THERAPY   Since all of these drugs can have serious side effects, their use requires regular monitoring. Your doctor will order tests to aid in diagnosis and to check on the toxicity of medications. These tests include a complete blood count, uric acid, rheumatoid factor, ANA (antinuclear antibodies), ESR (erythrocyte sedimentation rate), chemical profile, and urine analysis. If you are on gold compounds, the urine analysis will be done weekly. During office visits, you should have a complete diagnostic workup that includes a detailed history and physical examination. As part of that workup, your doctor may order the following tests.

Bone Scan   This is a quick, effective method to evaluate numerous joints simultaneously and to distinguish between arthritis and other conditions that might be causing the symptoms, such as cancer and fractures. Based on this test, your doctor may order individual x-rays of suspicious joints. A decision will also be made about the use of more sophisticated tests, such as CAT scans and magnetic resonance imaging (MRIs). While these tests aren't appropriately used for the diagnosis of the disease, they may help in evaluating its progress and determining the best therapy. Some doctors believe that MRIs can reveal joint destruction two years before it can be picked up on x-ray and in time to initiate aggressive treatment. Moreover, a series of x-rays can be expensive. And while the amount of radiation in a single examination is not large, cumulatively it can be extensive over a lifetime.

Joint-Fluid Test   This test analyzes fluid withdrawn from an inflamed joint for the presence of crystals that can be a sign of gout or pseudogout. Cultures are taken to rule out infection. Removing fluid from an inflamed joint can also relieve pain and pressure, and restore normal range of motion. Sometimes steroids are injected into the joint at the same time.

Treatment Surgery

JOINT REPLACEMENT   Once pain limits your mobility and your ability to perform everyday tasks, you should consider joint replacement surgery. You will want a superspecialist. Total hip replacements have been the most successful operation in this category, followed closely by knee replacement. Other types, such as replacement of the shoulder, the elbow, and the knuckle joints of the hand have been performed less frequently but can be quite successful. When the joint damage is not extensive, partial replacement or resurfacing may be all that's necessary.

ARTHROSCOPY   Arthroscopic techniques are used to perform exploratory surgery inside certain joints, to remove joint debris, and to scrape off bone spurs. This operation is usually performed by a specialist in knee surgery or sports medicine. Arthroscopy avoids the long recovery time of major surgery, but may not be indicated if joint destruction is advanced. (See chapter on Arthroscopy for more information.)

ARTHRODESIS   Fusion of a joint (arthrodesis) is used for ankle, foot, and wrist joints when arthritic damage is severe. This procedure is used on the wrists, neck, and ankles of patients with rheumatoid arthritis. By fusing these joints, surgeons seek to relieve pain and to stabilize the joints. There will be some loss of motion and function. Pain relief is excellent. In rheumatoid arthritis, arthrodesis may be used to fuse an unstable area in the neck. Some motion is best. Patients who are prone to infection may do better with this technique than they would with a joint replacement operation, which carries the risk of infection. Since total joint replacement is not perfected for wrists and ankles, arthrodesis is performed. Sometimes physicians will try first to fuse the joint by splinting it.

KEY INDICATIONS FOR ARTHRODESIS

- Unresponsive to medications

- Joint completely destroyed

- Motion causing extreme pain

SYNOVECTOMY   This procedure removes the grossly inflamed diseased lining of the joint to bring relief of pain for patients with rheumatoid arthritis. Since the membrane sometimes grows back, a synovectomy is considered a temporary procedure that delays progression of the disease. After surgery, patients may often experience joint stiffness. When performed with an arthroscope, it is a relatively benign procedure. The patient is out of commission for only 24–48 hours. Synovectomy is performed in rheumatoid arthritis when the excessive synovial tissue is producing pain and joint stiffness despite medical treatment.

OSTEOTOMY   Cutting the bones near the joint corrects the misalignment that results from arthritis. Osteotomy is performed in younger patients to shift the load of weight-bearing away from the damaged segment of the joint. It may postpone the need for joint replacement for many years.

If you're young, you might prefer this operation over the replacement of joints, since artificial joints usually wear out in 10–20 years. An osteotomy buys time, usually 4–5 years, in order to postpone total joint replacement. It is used for this purpose in the under-45 population, and only for patients with osteoarthritis. The resulting fracture is immobilized in plaster for six weeks.

Physical Therapy

For the patient with rheumatoid arthritis, exercise and physical therapy play a crucial role in controlling pain due to muscle spasm and in maintaining strong functional joints. New research reveals that "weight-bearing exercise for incapacitating knee pain" shows significant benefit. Weight loss can dramatically lower the amount of pain you suffer. In both conditions it is crucial to seek out a physical therapist skilled in treating patients with arthritis.

Step 2. Look for Shortcomings

I hope you have gotten a good feeling about your treatment from reading Step 1, and that you understand much of it better. You'll learn even more by calling organizations listed in Step 4. But if you have an uncomfortable feeling that your treatment is not on track, you should study this section, which will specify some of the common and serious shortcomings that experts in the field recognize. If this section confirms your suspicions, you should go to Step 3. Some of these mistakes you can discover yourself; others only an expert can confirm.

MISTAKES IN DIAGNOSIS

Your swollen joint is misdiagnosed and leads to irreparable damage.

Your diagnosis is confirmed only by a blood test.

You don't know what kind of arthritis you have and may be mistreating yourself.

Your arthritis is passed off as trivial by your health care provider.

MISTAKES IN TREATMENT

You treat yourself without medical consultation.

You delay seeking treatment.

You pursue quackery.

Your health care provider is not trained to care for your arthritis.

You are undertreated with drugs too mild to slow your arthritis.

You take different drugs from different doctors without any coordination among your health care providers.

You are prescribed too many drugs by too many doctors.

You overuse steroids, which can have disastrous side effects if given at high doses over long periods.

The dose of your medication is too low to change the course of your illness.

You don't know how to take NSAIDs (nonsteroidal antiinflammatory drugs) correctly or you take them for long periods without medical supervision.

You take medications regularly for your arthritis but are not tested regularly for complications they may cause.

You are scheduled for joint surgery that is purely cosmetic.

Your health care provider delays recommending hand surgery until it is too late for it to be effective.

Your joints are manipulated when they are acutely hot, red, and tender.

You are not monitored during pregnancy by a high-risk expert.

Your treatment ignores physical and occupational therapy, emotional needs, and lifestyle changes.

You are disabled, and joint replacement surgery has not yet been offered.

Step 3. See a Specialist

If, from Step 2, you are concerned that your care is not state-of-the-art, this step will tell you how to choose an expert.

All patients with rheumatoid arthritis should have an expert review the management of their illness. If you have rheumatoid arthritis and don't consult a rheumatologist, you are making a major mistake, according to top experts. For most arthritis patients it is the biggest mistake they make. Even if you have a mild case that is responding well to treatment, you should see a specialist during the first year of treatment. If you have moderate-to-severe disease, that visit should be within the first few weeks. You should consult a rheumatologist if your diagnosis is unclear. Since most rheumatoid arthritis is not diagnosed by a specialist, your treatment may not be sufficiently aggressive. For the same reason you should see a rheumatologist if multiple joints are affected.

Many rheumatologists believe there is too much research being done on arthritis for any doctor who is not a specialist in the field to stay current on the newest developments. A specialist can provide your family doctor with a complete set of instructions for your care. If you had leukemia, for example, your doctor would send you immediately to a cancer specialist. But many doctors are afraid to say, "I don't know." In certain small rural areas doctors practice what has been called Good Samaritan medicine. Although they are doing their best, they may not have the knowledge, skills, or equipment to offer more than sympathy and support. However, any doctor should know when it is time to consult a specialist.

A board-certified rheumatologist is a doctor of internal medicine who has at least two years of advanced training in arthritis and rheumatic diseases. Both the American College of Rheumatology and the Arthritis Foundation can help you find a specialist in your area. You can also consult local centers of excellence in arthritis. All these addresses can be found at the end of this chapter.

You will want to see both a rheumatologist and an orthopedist who specializes in joint replacement if you are considering surgery. You shouldn't go directly to the orthopedist, who is likely to favor operating. You should undergo surgery if it will bring relief of pain or restore function. Rheumatologists warn against surgery for cosmetic purposes only. While you shouldn't rush into surgery, you shouldn't delay too long either. Patients who put off hand surgery, for instance, may have too much deviation in their tendons to make the operation technically possible. Arthritis should not be a totally disabling disease.

Your rheumatologist may recommend other specialists who can help you, too. Some top rheumatologists believe that chiropractors can offer excellent services to arthritis patients. They can increase joint mobility, strengthen muscles, and relax tendons and ligaments. If you decide to consult a chiropractor, remember that hot joints should never be exercised or manipulated. Physical therapists who specialize in arthritis patients can also substantially eliminate the pain that comes from sore ligaments, muscles, and tendons. Muscle atrophy and contractions create a large measure of the pain and disability of arthritis. This can happen with amazing speed. In five days you can lose a great deal of muscle power that will take months to regain. This is both treatable and preventable with physical therapy. Recently, doctors have also recognized that aerobic exercise can have a positive impact on arthritis. Physical therapy and aerobic exercise can increase your mobility and decrease your pain dramatically.

Remember, there should be a coordinating physician for a patient with arthritis. If you are on many drugs, these drugs can interact with each other to worsen side effects or to decrease the effectiveness of drug treatment. One doctor needs to look at *all* your drugs.

How to Choose a Surgeon

You want an orthopedic surgeon who works in an arthritis center. If your surgeon replaces only a few joints a year, you may have a higher likelihood of infection or poor fit. At least 60% of the surgeon's practice should consist of joint replacement operations. (Some experts even suggest 75% as a minimum.) It's not unreasonable to look for a medical center that replaces 1,200 joints a year, advises Dr. Markenson. At the Hospital for Special Surgery, 2,200 joint replacements are performed yearly. Smaller programs may lack staff sufficiently experienced or may not stock all sizes of joints.

FOR RHEUMATOID ARTHRITIS   A rheumatologist and a surgeon working together in a specialized center is your best bet. For rheumatoid arthritis, you want surgery performed where both the medical and the surgical teams are working together. You want comprehensive care. Make sure the majority of your doctor's patients are patients with rheumatoid arthritis.

FOR OSTEOARTHRITIS   If you're having total joint replacement, you want 60% of your surgeon's work to be total joints.

Centers of Excellence for Arthritis

The following lists of hospitals are provided only as a convenient starting place in your search for excellence. These hospitals are recommended on the basis of reputation, not experience and results. The lists are not an endorsement. There may be hospitals just as excellent that have been omitted. You should apply the guidelines for experience, results, and other measures of excellence to any hospital you choose, whether or not it is on these lists. Although hospitals from different sources have been combined into these lists, the compilation in no way implies that one source has endorsed the hospital list of another source.

RHEUMATOID ARTHRITIS

NORTH CAROLINA
Duke University School of Medicine   NIH
Box 3258
Durham, NC 27710

TENNESSEE
University of Tennessee   NIH
956 Court Ave, G326
Memphis, TN 38153

TEXAS
University of Texas Southwestern
    Medical Center at Dallas   NIH
5323 Harry Hines Blvd
Dallas, TX 75235

OSTEOARTHRITIS

ILLINOIS
Rush-Presbyterian-St. Luke's
    Medical Center   NIH
1653 W Congress Pkwy
Chicago, IL 60612-3864

INDIANA
Indiana University School
    of Medicine   NIH
541 Clinical Dr, Rm 492
Indianapolis, IN 46223

MINNESOTA
University of Minnesota   NIH
420 Delaware St SE
Box 189
Minneapolis, MN 55455

SOURCES

NIH indicates the specialized centers sponsored by the National Institutes of Health to do specialized research on rheumatoid arthritis and osteoarthritis.

Multipurpose Arthritis and Musculoskeletal and Skin Diseases Centers

The National Institute of Arthritis and Musculoskeletal and Skin Diseases has named the following centers to "develop and carry out programs in basic and/or clinical research; research related to professional, patient, and public education; and epidemiology and health services research." The goal is to explore innovative new directions for understanding the causes, treatment, and ultimate prevention of arthritis and musculoskeletal diseases. They are excellent centers to seek expert advice on the treatment of your arthritis.

GENERAL

ALABAMA
Department of Medicine — NIH
University of Alabama
University Station
Birmingham, AL 35294

CALIFORNIA
Stanford University Medical
   Center — NIH
701 Welch Rd, Ste 3301
Stanford, CA 94304

Stanford University School
   of Medicine — US
300 Pasteur Dr
Stanford, CA 94305

University of California,
   San Diego — NIH
Department of Medicine
P.O. Box 0945
La Jolla, CA 92093

University of California,
   San Francisco — NIH
P.O. Box 0868
San Francisco, CA 94143-0868

University of California
   School of Medicine — NIH/US
10833 Le Conte Ave
Los Angeles, CA 90024-1736

CONNECTICUT
University of Connecticut
   School of Medicine — NIH
263 Farmington Ave
Farmington, CT 06032

ILLINOIS
Northwestern University — NIH
McGraw Medical School
303 E Chicago Ave
Chicago, IL 60611

INDIANA
Division of Rheumatology — NIH
Indiana University School
   of Medicine
541 Clinical Dr
Indianapolis, IN 46223

MARYLAND
Johns Hopkins Hospital — US
600 N Wolfe St
Baltimore, MD 21205

MASSACHUSETTS
Boston University School
   of Medicine — NIH
818 Harrison St
Boston, MA 02118

Brigham and Women's
   Hospital — NIH/US
75 Frances St
Boston, MA 02120

Massachusetts General
   Hospital — US
55 Fruit St
Boston, MA 02114

MICHIGAN
University of Michigan
  Medical School   NIH
1500 E Medical Center Dr
Ann Arbor, MI 48109-0358

MINNESOTA
Mayo Clinic   US
200 First St SW
Rochester, MN 55905

NEW YORK
Hospital for Special Surgery   NIH/US
Cornell Medical College
514 E 71st St
New York, NY 10021

NORTH CAROLINA
University of North Carolina
  School of Medicine   NIH
932 Faculty Laboratory
  Office, Rm 231H
Chapel Hill, NC 27514

OHIO
Case Western Reserve University
  School of Medicine   NIH
2073 Abington Rd
Cleveland, OH 44106

SOURCES

NIH   indicates those centers funded by the National Institute of Health's National
Institute of Arthritis and Musculoskeletal and Skin Diseases.

US   indicates those hospitals recommended in *U.S. News & World Report.*

Step 3. Become Your Own Expert

WHO TO CALL

Arthritis Foundation   The foundation answers general questions, distrib-
utes literature, and provides contacts with local chapters. Your local chapter can
provide a list of board-certified rheumatologists or general practitioners whose
practice focuses on people with arthritis.

PO Box 19000
Atlanta, GA 30326
800/283-7800

**The National Institute of Arthritis and Musculoskeletal and Skin
Diseases**   The institute provides literature and brochures on arthritis.

9000 Rockville Pike
Bldg 31, Rm 4C05
Bethesda, MD 20892
301/496-3583

American College of Rheumatology   This medical society provides the names of fellows who are board-certified rheumatologists recommended for membership by two current fellows.

17 Executive Park Dr, #480
Atlanta, GA 30329
404/633-3777

NIH CRISP System

301/496-7543

University-Affiliated Teaching Hospitals   See Appendix.

EXPERT SOURCES

Although dozens of experts were interviewed for these chapters, these experts are acknowledged for their significant contributions.

Dr. Joseph A. Markenson, Hospital for Special Surgery, New York, NY

Dr. James McGuire, Associate Dean, Stanford University School of Medicine, Stanford, CA

Staff of the Arthritis Foundation

REFERENCES AND SUGGESTED READING

Allergic and Immunologic Disorders of the Eye. *Journal of Allergy and Clinical Immunology,* Vol. 89, No. 1 (Jan. 1992), pp. 1–15.

Amstutz, Harlan C. (ed). *Hip Arthroplasty.* New York: Churchill Livingstone, 1991.

Culling, Robert D., and others. Corticosteroid Injections for Chronic Low-Back Pain [letter]. *New England Journal of Medicine,* Vol. 326, No. 12 (Mar. 19, 1992), pp. 834–836.

Dalton, Thomas A., and Bennett, J. Claude. Autoimmune Disease and the Major Histocompatibility Complex: Therapeutic Implications [review]. *American Journal of Medicine,* Vol. 92, No. 2 (Feb. 1992), pp. 183–188.

Fries, James F. *Arthritis. A Comprehensive Guide to Understanding Your Arthritis,* 3rd ed. Reading, Mass.: Addison-Wesley, 1990.

Hirohata, Shunsei, and others. Regulation of B Cell Function by Lobenzarit, a Novel Disease-Modifying Antirheumatic Drug. *Arthritis and Rheumatism,* Vol. 35, No. 2 (Feb. 1992), pp. 168–175.

Kovar, Pamela A., and others. Supervised Fitness Walking in Patients with Osteoarthritis of the Knee. *Annals of Internal Medicine,* Vol. 116, No. 7 (April 1, 1992), p. 529.

Kremer, Joel M., and Phelps, Carlton T. Long-Term Prospective Study of the Use of Methotrexate in the Treatment of Rheumatoid Arthritis: Update After a Mean of 90 Months. *Arthritis and Rheumatism,* Vol. 35, No. 2 (Feb. 1992), pp. 138–145.

Rhodes, Valerie J. Physical Therapy Management of Patients with Juvenile Rheumatoid Arthritis. *Physical Therapy,* Vol. 71, No. 12 (Dec. 1991), pp. 910–919.

Taha, A. S., and others. Chemical Gastritis and Helicobacter Pylori–Related Gastritis in Patients Receiving Nonsteroidal Antiinflammatory Drugs: Comparison and Correlation with Peptic Ulceration. *Journal of Clinical Pathology,* Vol. 45, No. 2 (Feb. 1992), pp. 135–139.

Weinblatt, Michael E., and others. Long-Term Prospective Study of Methotrexate in the Treatment of Rheumatoid Arthritis: 84-Month Update. *Arthritis and Rheumatism,* Vol. 35, No. 2 (Feb. 1992), pp. 129–137.

Asthma

Risk for Inappropriate Care   **VERY HIGH**

"Asthma is underdiagnosed and undertreated. This is really the ultimate non-compliance disease. People don't know they have it and aren't treated for it. I've seen people who had a chronic cough and they weren't aware that it's asthma," says Dr. A. Sonia Buist, head of pulmonary and critical care medicine at Oregon Health Sciences University. If you are one of the 11 million Americans who suffer from asthma, there is a strong possibility you are not receiving state-of-the-art care.

This failure to treat asthma adequately has lead to a steady rise in death from asthma. While science and technology have been winning the war against heart disease, the fight against asthma is being lost. Between 1978 and 1987 the overall death rate for people ages 5 to 34 with asthma increased at an average *per year* of 6.2% and for children ages 5 to 14 the annual increase was 10.1%. The increase has been particularly striking in the inner city, where patients are denied access to medical treatment because of inability to pay for private health care, a limited number of public clinics, and a health system that is oriented toward emergency rather than routine care.

Asthma is—or should be—a very common, easy to treat disease. The great tragedy is that patients with asthma still die from a disease that can be so easily treated. There is rarely a legitimate reason why an asthma patient should die.

What It Is

In many respects asthma is a "good news" disease, because the damage is not permanent. It's unlike emphysema, for instance, where the destruction is irreversible if state-of-the-art treatment is delayed. Revolutionary new treatments are becoming available to treat the basic underlying inflammation rather than just the symptoms. Asthma patient Jackie Joyner Kersey triumphed over her disease and won an Olympic gold medal.

Asthma is very different from other chronic lung diseases. Although asthma obstructs the large and small airways that lead into the lungs, the obstruction is reversible. This obstruction may result from contraction of airway walls, inflammation of the lining of the air tubes, or increased mucus or phlegm production. Airways may be hyperactive and constrict easily when triggered to do so. Alternatively, an allergen triggers cells in the lining of the bronchi to release a variety of chemicals that constrict the airways. These cells almost explode, like terrorist bombs, when something in the environment triggers them to spew out these powerful chemicals. The result is wheezing, cough, sputum production, and shortness of breath.

SYMPTOMS   The most common symptoms of asthma are tightness in the chest, coughing, difficulty inhaling and exhaling, wheezing, and shortness of breath. If you have these symptoms, you may have asthma and should see a doctor to confirm the diagnosis. Asthma ranges from a mild form with infrequent short-lived attacks to a severe form in which attacks last for days and can require hospitalization. Virtually all asthma patients have a disease that is triggered by external factors.

CAUSES   According to the U.S. Department of Health and Human Services, allergy is the number one cause of asthma. About 90% of the people under age 10 who have asthma have allergies. If you are younger than 30 and have asthma, there is a 70% chance you are allergic. About half the people over 30 who have asthma have allergies. Attacks may be triggered by the stress of strong emotions, by vigorous exercise or pain, by allergies, or by reactions to yellow food coloring, metabisulfite (a preservative for fruit, vegetables, and wine), bacteria or chemicals in the workplace, viral respiratory infection, and environmental irritants such as cigarette smoke, perfume, air pollution, fumes and household chemicals. In a small group of patients with severe asthma, probably less than 1%, aspirin can be a trigger. If you are in this group and take aspirin or related compounds, such as ibuprofen, you will have a reaction.

Remember, asthma is not so much a *chronic* disease, as an *inflammatory* disease. If you and your doctor treat it that way, you will suffer far less from your illness. If you don't treat asthma early, chronic inflammation could cause permanent damage.

Step 1. Make Sure You Get the Best Care

Read this section on potential problems with your treatment carefully to determine if there are discrepencies between your care and state-of-the-art care. Use Step 2 to review shortcomings.

Before you can develop a treatment plan and start to bring the disease under control, doctors must diagnose you accurately. Since there is no easy diagnostic test, diagnosis can be elusive. It can also be difficult to judge accurately the disease's severity. This can't be done just by taking a medical history, performing a physical examination, and listening to the lungs through a stethoscope. Objective measures of pulmonary function are critical to making the diagnosis and judging the severity of your illness.

Diagnosis

SPIROMETER   This measures the volume of air that you can breathe in and out. It's a valuable tool for the initial assessment and periodic reevaluation of asthma patients. Here's how it works: You take the deepest breath you can, then you exhale, as fast and hard as you can, into a tube connected to the spirometer. Your doctor should take two readings. One, forced vital capacity (FVC), measures the amount of air you can forcibly expel from your lungs in a single breath. The other, FEV$_1$, measures the amount of air you can expel in one second. Both measures can help monitor the progress of the disease. As the airways become increasingly inflamed, the amount of air that can be expelled quickly decreases.

EXERCISE TEST   An exercise test employing a treadmill or stationary bicycle is sometimes used to provoke an attack of exercise-induced asthma. You'll be asked to walk, run, or bike at faster and faster speeds. Doctors will take spirometer readings before and after the exercise. If you move less air with each breath and can't get it out as fast after exercising, that clinches the diagnosis.

ALLERGY TESTING   Your doctor may test your skin's sensitivity to extracts of allergens known to cause asthma, such as pollen and cat dander. A positive reaction indicates that you may have an allergy to that particular substance. To confirm that allergic sensitivity, some doctors will order inhalation bronchial challenge testing. More often, a methacholine challenge is used, since allergen testing is considered dangerous by some top academic specialists.

PEAK-FLOW METER   This is a very inexpensive home testing device. It is a clear plastic tube that measures how fast you can forcibly expel air from your lungs. Since asthma narrows your airways, the worse your asthma, the slower you can expel air. In just a few seconds you can assess your own breathing capacity. If you have asthma, you should test yourself each morning. Here's how the test works: Take the deepest breath you can, then breathe out into the flow meter as fast and hard as you can. The meter will give you a reading. If your "peak" flow declines from one day to the next, you're headed for trouble and should let your doctor know. Any person with moderate or severe asthma that has daily or nightly symptoms should have and use a peak-flow meter.

Treatment

Although asthma should not be considered a fatal disease, it should be taken seriously. To control asthma, you must not neglect your care. That means you must understand the mechanisms of the disease, follow through on treatment, and take the medications your doctors prescribe. With education and understanding you will be less likely to panic if the disease becomes severe. You can guard against the psychological and social factors that may worsen asthma, and you will be more inclined to seek help when it is needed. I know from the members of my own family who have asthma that patients often fail to seek and especially to follow advice. Teenagers are often the worst offenders. As Dr. Buist points, out, "If people feel good, they don't treat themselves." Another asthma specialist, Dr. Lawrence J. Prograis of the National Institutes of Health, says "It's a perception problem. It's due to the fact that people still perceive it to be an episodic as opposed to a continuous disease. . . . Doctors have a real responsibility to their patients to distinguish between treatment and cure. It's a depressing thought: You have it for life. Doctors don't want to say it and people don't want to hear it. You are undergoing treatment for life. Public health officials have not marketed asthma like hypertension or diabetes as a chronic disease. You shouldn't forget that people do die from asthma."

FOR ACUTE SYMPTOMS　　If your symptoms become acute, you should seek emergency care. Some asthma patients have died in the emergency room because they delayed seeking medical attention until too late. Remember that if you don't take your disease seriously, your family and your doctor will be more likely to underestimate its gravity also. This can endanger your health. Since some asthma patients don't look ill in a conventional sense, even if you seek emergency medical care, there is a distinct possibility that health care workers may not initiate immediate therapy. Your airways may become so constricted that breathing is impossible. Unfortunately, this is not a rare occurrence.

INFECTIONS　　Infections can commonly trigger or worsen your asthma. You will want to take several preventive measures. Make certain you get the pneumococcal vaccine and a yearly flu shot. If you become infected, a virus is often the cause, so some asthma specialists will not start you on antibiotics.

However, if your sputum color changes, you have a fever, and you feel physically sick, then action must be taken. Your doctor will want to do an x-ray, take cultures of your blood, and examine your sputum for the source of infection. This is very important for patients with severe asthma. You should quickly begin taking a well-chosen antibiotic. New broad-spectrum antibiotics have few side effects and little resistance and can be used many times in a year. You shouldn't hesitate to take them early when indicated. If you have moderate-to-severe asthma, make certain you have a plan of action for infections.

Drug Therapy

In the last 15 years, as researchers have come to understand the basic mechanisms of asthma, state-of-the-art treatment has changed dramatically. We know now that patients will receive the maximum benefit if we treat the underlying problem, which is the inflamed airways. Doctors are switching from medications that merely relax the airways to drugs that soothe the agitated cells and reduce the inflammation. Only two years ago bronchodilators were the primary treatment for asthma. Now they are considered Band-Aids that can control symptoms but do little to alter the course of the disease. In fact, if you use bronchodilators (beta2-agonists—see later section) with increasing frequency in response to worsening symptoms, urgently needed help may be delayed. In addition, new studies point to dangers in overusing bronchodilators. After one canister has been used, each additional canister of beta2-agonists used during a month doubles the risk of death. Some doctors still don't prescribe antiinflammatory drugs, because they are unaware of this latest treatment or needlessly fear their side effects. Be sure your doctor uses these drugs to treat the disease and bronchodilators to control the symptoms. Here is what you need to know about the medications used to control asthma.

ANTIINFLAMMATORY AGENTS

Steroids Steroids are the most effective antiinflammatory drugs for the treatment of asthma. These are completely different from the anabolic steroids that are used to improve athletic performance. These steroids reduce inflammation and swelling in the airways and maximize the effect of other medications. They are very effective, but their potential for serious side effects limits their long-term use. However, you can avoid most long-term effects when you inhale the drug directly into your lungs rather than take it orally. If you take the drug in aerosol form, very little gets into the bloodstream. Make sure the following mistakes aren't being made:

- Failure to prescribe inhaled steroids early and aggressively enough
- Failure to monitor steroid medications after they've been prescribed

Never discontinue oral steroids abruptly, but rather wean yourself off of them very slowly, and under a doctor's supervision.

Oral Steroids A short course of oral corticosteroids can be useful when your disease is in the acute stages. If your doctor recommends oral steroids on a continuing basis, you should try inhaled steroids to determine whether oral corticosteroid treatment can be reduced or eliminated. Oral steroids should only be continued if your asthma cannot be controlled with inhaled steroids.

Long-term use of oral steroids on a daily basis is limited by the risk of significant adverse side effects: increased appetite, weight gain, fluid retention, growth of facial hair, acne, mood changes, high blood pressure, loss of bone mass, gastric ulcers, cataracts, blood coagulation disorders, and stunted growth in children. Because steroids can slow or halt normal growth in children and adolescents, younger sufferers should take them with particular caution. Drugs such as the antiinflammatory drug cromolyn should be tried as an alternative. Steroids may also activate hidden diabetes. Those symptoms frighten many doctors and patients who are considering long-term use.

Steroids should be reserved for patients with severe asthma, and the lowest possible dose should be used. You may want to try taking the drug in a single dose early in the morning every other day. By following this regimen carefully, many patients have used steroids for decades without serious consequences.

The steroid most commonly prescribed for asthma is prednisone. Methylprednisolone and prednisolone are also prescribed.

Inhaled Steroids   Inhaled corticosteroids are safe and effective and can reduce the need for the long-term use of oral steroids. Inhaled steroids are being used as the primary therapy for moderate and severe asthma. This is because they have far fewer side effects than oral steroids and because they treat the underlying cause of airway narrowing, inflammation. "For people with daily or nightly symptoms, the first-line therapy should be inhaled corticosteroids, second line is beta-agonists. We hardly ever use beta-agonists any more because the inhaled corticosteroids are so effective," says Dr. Buist.

Steroids can produce a sore mouth or throat. Hoarseness may be accompanied by a white lining in the throat. Inhalation through a "spacer" and regular gargling after each use sharply cut the risk of these side effects. (The spacer is simply a tube that lengthens the inhaler mouthpiece.)

Since inhaled steroids may not be effective for acute severe attacks of asthma, patients taking this medication should consult their physician immediately if their asthma worsens.

Inhaled steroids are available in higher dosage in Canada and England. Your doctor can write you a prescription that can be filled by mail. England often has new asthma medications on the market years before they appear in the United States. For these or other drugs, your doctor may write to any pharmacy in England. The practice is entirely legal. One source I've found reliable over the years is D. R. Harris & Co. Ltd., 29 St. James St., SW1, London, England. Right now some of these stronger medicines are being reviewed by the Food and Drug Administration and may be on the market here in a relatively short time. Check with your doctor first. This higher-potency inhaled steroid is called Becloforte and is strong enough that many patients who have been chronically dependent on oral steroids have been able to give them up entirely. There are few if any other drugs that I suggest you order from abroad. Since this drug is much safer than using oral steroids on a daily basis, I don't hesitate to recommend it.

Cromolyn Sodium   Cromolyn sodium is another inhaled drug that acts to prevent the narrowing of the bronchial airways by reducing their sensitivity to the factors that trigger asthma attacks. It can also decrease the acute narrowing that occurs after exposure to exercise, cold air, or sulphur dioxide. The drug can be very useful in preventing attacks, but it will not help once the symptoms have begun.

Since there is no way to predict who will respond, a trial may be required to determine its effectiveness. The side effects are relatively mild:

- Throat irritation and coughing (which can be controlled by bronchodilator drugs)

- Occasional skin rashes (which disappear when the medication is discontinued)

BRONCHODILATORS

Beta2-agonists These are the most widely used asthma drugs in the world. Manufacturers market them under the commercial names Proventil, Brethaire, Ventolin, and Alupent. Doctors once considered them the best drugs for the treatment of acute asthma. They are still excellent prevention for exercise-induced forms of the disease. Their long-term use is highly controversial, however. Some doctors believe their use on a daily basis to prevent asthma will actually worsen the disease.

You should adhere strictly to the prescribed amount. For every additional inhaler used each month over and above the recommended dosage of a single inhaler, the death rate rises. Much more than a canister a month is too much, according to the Food and Drug Administration.

The aerosol form of the drug is best, because this delivers it directly—and selectively—to the bronchial tubes. The pills cause more side effects and require higher doses to achieve similar results.

The chief advantage of beta2-agonists is that they have a powerful adrenalin-like effect on the airways, opening them without making the heart race, the way pure Adrenalin does.

Adrenalin (Epinephrine) Adrenalin can give temporary emergency relief when injected. Because it is quick acting, your doctor may recommend that you carry Adrenalin injectors for emergencies if you are prone to sudden severe attacks. Side effects include rapid heart rate, headache, jitteriness, irritated skin, nausea, and occasional vomiting.

Theophylline A recent study by the American Academy of Allergy and Immunology concluded that this is *not* the best drug for the majority of adults who require long-term therapy. It is rapidly becoming a back-up treatment instead of a first-line therapy. Inhaled steroids give better relief of symptoms and with fewer side effects. Theophylline can cause nausea, vomiting, loss of appetite, diarrhea, rapid heart beat, headaches, dizziness, insomnia, nervousness, and personality changes. However, if you find that theophylline is effective in your case, you may want to consider it. Because the drug is long-lasting, you don't have to remember to take it as often. Be sure your doctor monitors theophylline blood levels to guard against an excessive concentration of the medication. You can take theophylline by mouth or in an intravenous solution. Theophylline is most useful for those with nighttime symptoms not controllable with other medications.

Anticholinergics These drugs are most effective in patients who cough up a lot of mucus. They are not effective in all patients. The oldest of the drugs is atropine sulfate; a derivative of this drug which has fewer side effects is ipratropium (atrovent) which can be useful to break prolonged attacks. Both drugs are inhaled.

Safe Drug Use

Cromolyn, beta2-agonists, and steroids can all be delivered by inhaler. If your doctor prescribes them, he or she should provide instructions in their proper use so you can benefit more from the medications and suffer fewer and milder side effects. Your doctor should watch how you use them and critique your performance. A surprising number of people who have had asthma for years have little idea how to use inhalers properly. According to Dr. Buist, "Fifty percent of patients don't use inhalers correctly. Some people don't even take the cap off!" Often doctors and their office staffs don't actually know how to use this medication properly. You shouldn't be embarrassed to ask. Your doctor should instruct you properly and then monitor your subsequent use to make sure you have not fallen into any bad habits.

While a number of safe, effective asthma medications are on the market, you should be careful to try only one drug at a time. That is the only possible way to test for effectiveness and adverse reactions. The obvious exception is an acute attack that requires immediate medical intervention. Then doctors will probably clear your lungs with several medicines. Once you're back to normal, you'll still want to use each drug individually in order to gauge its degree of success in your case.

DISEASE SEVERITY AND DRUG TREATMENT You also should consider the severity of your disease when you decide which medication will work best for you. The following is adapted from National Heart, Lung and Blood Institute guidelines on asthma. It should provide some guidance about how well you should expect to fare with the severity of asthma you have.

Mild Asthma Attacks occur no more than twice a week and are characterized by wheezing, coughing, and shortness of breath. Each episode lasts less than one hour. Your peak-flow reading won't decline more than 20% from your best days. Your treatment should prevent any symptoms most of the time and return you to normal after an attack. You can judge "normal" by using your peak-flow meter.

Moderate Asthma   Like mild asthma, attacks occur no more than twice a week, but your normal activities and sleep are disturbed. Attacks may last several days, with wheezing, coughing, and shortness of breath. Occasional emergency care is needed. Your flow meter should decline no more than a 30% from normal. Treatment should reduce the frequency and severity of attacks.

Severe Asthma   Symptoms are continuous and will limit your level of activity. Attacks frequently get worse, particularly at night. Hospitalization and emergency treatment may be needed. At best, peak flow is only 40–60% of normal, and your peak-flow reading may decline 50% or more during attacks. Treatment should improve lung function, return you close to normal levels of activity, give you a good night's sleep, and reduce your need for bronchodilators and steroids.

Step 2. Look for Shortcomings

I hope that by reading Step 1 you have gotten a good feeling about your treatment and that you understand much of it better. You'll learn even more by calling organizations listed in Step 4. But if you have an uncomfortable feeling that your treatment is not on track, then study this section, which specifies some of the common and serious shortcomings that experts in the field recognize. If this section confirms your suspicions, you should go to Step 3. Some of these mistakes you can discover yourself; others only an expert can confirm.

MISTAKES IN DIAGNOSIS

You have coughing, wheezing, and shortness of breath and haven't been evaluated for asthma.

You aren't getting objective tests to assess the status of your disease.

You and your physician underestimate the seriousness of your symptoms.

MISTAKES IN TREATMENT

Your medications aren't being added one at a time or being chosen on the basis of the severity of your disease.

You aren't using nebulizers of inhalers properly.

Inhaled steroids aren't used early or aggressively enough in your care if you have moderate-to-severe asthma.

You overuse corticosteroids such as prednisone.

You overuse beta2-agonists.

Step 3. See a Specialist

If, from Step 2, you are concerned that your care is not state-of-the-art this section will tell you how to choose an expert.

The following are extremely important signs that your condition is not being properly managed:

- You cannot do what you want. (Asthma should not limit you.)

- You should not be waking up at night regularly. (The one exception may be that your asthma is so severe that no specialist can manage it.)

- You are using more than a canister (200 inhalations) of beta-agonists/bronchodilators per month.

You and your doctor should devise a long-term treatment plan that will accomplish four objectives: (1) minimize chronic symptoms, (2) decrease the frequency of acute attacks, (3) reduce the number of side effects to medication, and (4) produce objective improvement on pulmonary function tests and lessen the risk of death. Although I've seen it happen hundreds of times, you should not be given an inhaler after your first attack and just sent home. Although critics of our health care system complain, often justifiably, about overtesting and overtreating, asthma is a disease that is frequently undertreated. Your doctor should recommend follow-up diagnostic testing and continue to oversee your care. The expert you see may be a pulmonary physician (pulmonologist), who has broader training in pulmonary medicine, or an allergist, who is a single-disease specialist. The majority of the specialist's practice should be in the treatment of patients with asthma and other lung diseases. If you have poorly controlled exercise-induced asthma, consider seeing a doctor who specializes in exercise-induced asthma.

Dr. Buist says, "Knowledge is mushrooming so fast, many general practitioners or primary care specialists cannot keep up." The exception is the pediatrician who believes that *prevention* is the key.

Centers of Excellence for Asthma

The following list of hospitals is provided only as a convenient starting place in your search for excellence. These hospitals are recommended on the basis of reputation, not experience and results. The list is not an endorsement. There may be hospitals just as excellent that have been omitted. You should apply the guidelines for experience, results, and other measures of excellence to any hospital you choose, whether or not it is on this list. Although hospitals from different sources have been combined into one list, the compilation in no way implies that one source has endorsed the hospital list of another source.

CALIFORNIA

Children's Hospital of
   Los Angeles   BIM
4650 Sunset Blvd
Los Angeles, CA 90027

Scripps Clinic and Research
   Foundation   HC/BIM
10666 N. Torrey Pines Rd
La Jolla, CA 92037

University of California,
   Davis, Medical Center   BIM
2315 Stockton Blvd
Sacramento, CA 95817

University of California at
   Los Angeles   HC
Center for Health Sciences
   Building
Los Angeles, CA 90024

University of California,
   San Diego, Medical Center   HC
225 Dickinson St
San Diego, CA 92103

University of California at
   San Francisco   HC
Department of Medicine
400 Parnassus Ave
San Francisco, CA 94143

COLORADO

National Jewish Center for
   Immunology and
   Respiratory Diseases   BIM
1400 Jackson St
Denver, CO 80206

DISTRICT OF COLUMBIA

Georgetown University School
   of Medicine   HC
3900 Reservoir Rd, NW
Washington, DC 20007

ILLINOIS

Northwestern University
   Medical School   HC
303 E Chicago Ave
Chicago, IL 60611

Rush-Presbyterian-St Luke's
   Medical Center   BIM
1653 W Congress Pky
Chicago, IL 60612

IOWA

Division of Allergy and
   Immunology   HC
Dept of Internal Medicine
University of Iowa Hospitals
   and Clinics
650 Newton Road
Iowa City, IA 52242

MARYLAND

Johns Hopkins University
   School of Medicine   HC
Good Samaritan Hospital
5601 Lock Raven Blvd
Baltimore, Maryland 21239

NIAID, Building 10, Room
   11C205   HC
National Institutes of Health
Bethesda, MD 20892

MASSACHUSETTS

Brigham and Women's Hospital HC
75 Francis St
Boston, MA 02115

Children's Hospital
   Medical Center   HC/BIM
300 Longwood Ave
Boston, MA 02115

Tufts University   HC
School of Medicine
136 Harrison Ave
Boston, MA 02111

Massachusetts General Hospital   HC/BIM
55 Fruit St
Boston, MA 02114

MICHIGAN
University of Michigan Hospitals   BIM
1500 E Medical Center Dr
Ann Arbor, MI 48109

MINNESOTA
Mayo Clinic   HC/BIM
200 First St SW
Rochester, MN 55905

MISSOURI
Washington University School
   of Medicine   HC
660 S Euclid Ave
St Louis, MO 63110

NEW YORK
Columbia-Presbyterian
   Medical Center   BIM
622 W 168th St
New York, NY 10032

Cornell University   HC
1300 York Ave
New York, NY 10021

Health Sciences Center   HC
State University of New York
   at Stony Brook
Stony Brook, NY 11794

Mt. Sinai Hospital   BIM
One Gustave Levy Pl
New York, NY 10029

The Rockefeller University   HC
1230 York Ave
New York, NY 10021

NORTH CAROLINA
Duke University   HC/BIM
Box 2898
Durham, NC 27710

OHIO
Children's Hospital
   Medical Center   BIM
Elland and Bethesda Aves
Cincinnati, OH 45229

University of Ohio
   Children's Hospital Division   BIM
700 Children's Dr
Columbus, OH 43205

PENNSYLVANIA
Children's Hospital
   of Philadelphia   BIM
34th St at Civic Center Blvd
Philadelphia, PA 19104

Hospital of the University
   of Pennsylvania   BIM
3400 Spruce St
Philadelphia, PA 19104

TENNESSEE
LeBonheur Children's
   Medical Center   BIM
One Children's Plaza
Memphis, TN 38103

University of Tennessee
   Medical Center   BIM

956 Court Ave

Memphis, TN 38103

TEXAS

Baylor College of Medicine
   and Hospitals   BIM

One Baylor Plaza

Houston, TX 77030

WISCONSIN

Medical College of Wisconsin   HC

8700 W Wisconsin Ave

Box 122

Milwaukee, WI 53226

University of Wisconsin
   Medical School   HC

600 Highland Ave

Madison, WI 53792

SOURCES

HC   indicates those hospitals included on the *Health Care USA* list.

BIM   indicates those hospitals recommended by *The Best in Medicine.*

Step 4. Become Your Own Expert

WHO TO CALL

National Jewish Center for Immunology and Respiratory Medicine (Lung Line)   Lung Line nurses are prepared to answer questions about diagnosis, prevention, and treatment detection for diseases that include asthma, emphysema, chronic bronchitis, tuberculosis, occupational and environmental lung diseases, juvenile rheumatoid arthritis, and food allergies. They can provide answers to questions such as "Are there any new drugs for asthma?" or "What type of air filtering system should I use in my home?" They can provide names of local doctors who trained at the National Jewish Center or are recommended by its medical staff. Information about the center's patient care services and research studies are available.

1400 Jackson St
Denver, CO 80206
800/222-LUNG
800/355 LUNG (within Colorado)

American College of Allergy & Immunology   This medical society, which is responsible for certifying allergy specialists, will provide patient information and local doctor referrals.

800 E. Northwest Hwy, Ste 1080
Palatine, IL 60067
800/842-7777

Mothers of Asthmatics

10875 Main St, Ste 210
Fairfax, VA 22030
703/385-4403

American Academy of Allergy & Immunology   This information referral line offers patient information on a variety of topics and recommendations of local allergists who are members. Brochures and pamphlets are available.

611 E Wells St
Milwaukee, WI 53202
800/822-ASMA

American Lung Association   This association offers referrals to local lung associations, which can provide information about programs along with brochures and literature. They will know if your doctor is a member of the American Thoracic Society.

1740 Broadway
New York, NY 10019
212/315-8700

Asthma & Allergy Foundation of America   This is a patient education group that can supply information about asthma and a list of local doctors who are members of the American Academy of Allergy & Immunology.

1717 Massachusetts Ave NW, Ste 305
Washington, DC 20036
800/7-ASTHMA

National Heart, Lung and Blood Institute   This institute operates the National Asthma Education Program Clearinghouse, which provides patient information. No referrals are made.

9000 Rockville Pike
Bethesda, MD 20892
301/951-3260

National Institute of Allergy and Infectious Diseases

9000 Rockville Pike
Bethesda, MD 20892
301/496-5717

NIH CRISP System

301/496-7543

University-Affiliated Teaching Hospitals   See Appendix.

EXPERT SOURCES

Although dozens of experts were interviewed for these chapters, these physicians are acknowledged for their significant contributions.

Dr. A. Sonia Buist, Oregon Health Sciences University, Portland, OR

Dr. Lawrence J. Prograis, Chief, Asthma and Allergy Branch, National Institute of Allergy and Infectious Diseases, National Institutes of Health, Bethesda, MD

Dr. Kevin Weiss, George Washington University, Washington, DC

Dr. Ron Crystal, Chief, Pulmonary Branch, National Heart, Lung, and Blood Institute, National Institutes of Health, Bethesda, MD

Dr. Floyd Malveau, Chair, Microbiology, Howard University College of Medicine, Washington, DC

Staff at the National Jewish Center for Immunology and Respiratory Medicine, Denver, CO

REFERENCES AND SUGGESTED READING

Alexander, Andrew G., and others. Trial of Cyclosporin in Corticosteroid-Dependent Chronic Severe Asthma. *Lancet,* Vol. 339, No. 8789 (Feb. 8, 1992), pp. 324–328.

Bowie, Dennis M. The Asthma Self-Care Book: How to Take Control of Your Asthma [book review]. *Canadian Medical Association Journal,* Vol. 146, No. 4 (Feb. 15, 1992), p. 547.

Bruijnzeel, Koomen Carla, and others. Skin Eosinophilia in Patients with Allergic and Nonallergic Asthma and Atopic Dermatitis. *Journal of Allergy and Clinical Immunology,* Vol. 89, No. 1 (Jan. 1992), pp. 52–59.

Brunet, Chantal, and others. Allergic Rhinitis to Ragweed Pollen. I. Reassessment of the Effects of Immunotherapy on Cellular and Humoral Responses. *Journal of Allergy and Clinical Immunology,* Vol. 89, No. 1 (Jan. 1992), pp. 76–86.

Brunet, Chantal, and others. Allergic Rhinitis to Ragweed Pollen. II. Modulation of Histamine-Releasing Factor Production by Specific Immunotherapy. *Journal of Allergy and Clinical Immunology,* Vol. 89, No. 1 (Jan. 1992), pp. 87–94.

Buist, A. S. Reflections on the Rise in Asthma Morbidity and Mortality. *Journal of the American Medical Association,* Vol. 264, No. 13 (Oct. 3, 1990), pp. 1719–1720.

Carlson, Marie, and others. Degranulation of Eosinophils from Pollen-Atopic Patients with Asthma Is Increased During Pollen Season. *Journal of Allergy and Clinical Immunology,* Vol. 89, No. 1 (Jan. 1992), pp. 131–139.

Correlates of Asthma Morbidity in Primary Care. *British Medical Journal,* Vol. 304, No. 6823 (Feb. 8, 1992), pp. 361–364.

Cyclosporin in Chronic Severe Asthma [editorial]. *Lancet,* Vol. 339, No. 8789 (Feb. 8, 1992), pp. 338–339.

Hendeles, L. Asthma Therapy: State of the Art, 1988. *Journal of Respiratory Diseases,* Vol. 9, No. 3 (March 1988), pp. 82–108.

Herxheimer, Andrew, and others. Action Asthma: Privatising the Airways? [letter] *British Medical Journal,* Vol. 304, No. 6825 (Feb. 22, 1992), p. 505.

International Workshop on Etiology of Asthma. *Chest,* Vol. 91 (June 1987 Supplement), pp. 65S–198S.

Korenblat, P. E. An Integrated Approach to Asthma: Management Strategies. *Modern Medicine,* Vol. 57 (May 1989), pp. 84–89.

Larsson, Kjell, and others. Bronchodilator Treatment in Asthma: Continuous or on Demand? [letter] *British Medical Journal,* Vol. 304, No. 6825 (Feb. 22, 1992), p. 504

Lawton, Andy, and others. Bronchodilator Treatment in Asthma: Continuous or on Demand? [letter] *British Medical Journal,* Vol. 304, No. 6825 (Feb. 22, 1992), pp. 503–504.

Li, J. T. Five Steps Toward Better Asthma Management. *Practical Therapeutics,* Vol. 40, No. 5 (Nov. 1989), pp. 201–210.

Losada, Eloy, and others. Occupational Asthma Caused by Alpha-Amylase Inhalation: Clinical and Immunologic Findings and Bronchial Response Patterns. *Journal of Allergy and Clinical Immunology,* Vol. 89, No. 1 (Jan. 1992), pp. 118–125.

National Heart, Lung and Blood Institute. *Guidelines for the Diagnosis and Management of Asthma.* NIH Publication No. 91-3042, August 1991.

National Institute of Allergy and Infectious Diseases. What You Need to Know About Asthma. Bethesda, MD.

National Jewish Center for Immunology and Respiratory Medicine. *Allergy.* Denver, 1989.

National Jewish Center for Immunology and Respiratory Medicine. *Black Lung.* Denver, 1989.

National Jewish Center for Immunology and Respiratory Medicine. *Healthy Breathing.* Denver, 1989.

National Jewish Center for Immunology and Respiratory Medicine. *Immunology.* Denver, 1989.

National Jewish Center for Immunology and Respiratory Medicine. *Management of Chronic Respiratory Disease.* Denver, 1987.

National Jewish Center for Immunology and Respiratory Medicine. *Understanding Asthma.* Denver, 1989.

Page, C. P. One Explanation of the Asthma Paradox: Inhibition of Natural Anti-Inflammatory Mechanism by Beta2-Agonists. *Lancet,* Vol. 337 (1991), pp. 717–720.

Rosen, Mark J. Office Procedures: Treatment of Exacerbations of COPD. *American Family Physician,* Vol. 45, No. 2 (Feb. 1992), pp. 693–697.

Sterling, Graham. Respiratory Medicine in Clinical Practice [book review]. *Lancet,* Vol. 339, No. 8790 (Feb. 15, 1992), p. 416

Stewart, E. J., and others. Effect of a Heat- and Moisture-Retaining Mask on Exercise-Induced Asthma. *British Medical Journal,* Vol. 304, No. 6825 (Feb. 22, 1992), pp. 479–480.

Weiss, K. B., and Wagener, D. K. Changing Patterns of Asthma Mortality: Identifying Target Populations at High Risk. *Journal of the American Medical Association,* Vol. 264, No. 13 (Oct. 3, 1990), pp. 1683–1688.

Cancer

Risk for Inappropriate Care **VERY HIGH**

Every year 50,000 Americans die because they don't get early, aggressive, state-of-the-art cancer treatment. According to a government report, an even larger number fails to receive appropriate therapy. Here are the striking numbers of patients who did not receive state-of-the-art cancer treatment, according to a 10-year survey by the U. S. Congress' General Accounting Office.

PATIENTS NOT RECEIVING STATE-OF-THE-ART CARE	
Colon cancer	94%
Rectal cancer	60%
Breast cancer, Stage II	37%
Lung Cancer, Small-cell	25%
Lymphoma	21%
Hodgkin's Disease	20%

An estimated 30% of cancer patients never see a cancer specialist. Even those who do, may not get state-of-the-art care. Cancer care is a very fast-moving field. To keep up with new developments, health care providers must devote their entire clinical practice to cancer and work in a cancer center or at least at a hospital with a strong cancer program. While internists and general practitioners may be qualified to oversee your ongoing care, the initial treatment strategy is best devised by a cancer specialist, called an oncologist.

Surprisingly, your care is more likely to suffer if you have a choice of treatment centers. A major metropolitan area may have a dozen hospitals, all claiming to be cancer centers, although many may have old technology, outdated treatments, and a lack of trained cancer nurses. In many rural areas the choice is more clear-cut: You either travel to a major cancer center or stay in a small community hospital that lacks a cancer program. Rural doctors are more likely to refer patients to a major cancer center than their urban colleagues.

Dr. Robert F. Ozols, Chair of Medical Oncology at the Fox Chase Cancer Center in Philadelphia, points out the following: "The best chance to cure cancer is with the first treatment approach. Too often, patients go to cancer centers after they have failed treatments by local doctors. At that point, it is often too late."

What It Is

Cancer is the uncontrolled growth of abnormal cells. Normal cells in our bodies can become abnormal when they are exposed to carcinogens. Known carcinogens include radiation, tobacco, air pollution, certain medications, foods, and certain viruses. Normal cells may get a head start down the road towards cancer if they contain genetic changes or abnormalities that are inherited. Carcinogens transform the genetic material in normal cells so that these cells become abnormal. These abnormal cells grow faster than normal cells and can form large masses called tumors. Tumors can spread directly from one organ to another or spread to distant organs, such as bone, brain, lung, and liver.

Step 1. Make Sure You Get the Best Care

Read this section on potential problems with your treatment carefully to determine if there are discrepancies between your care and state-of-the-art care. Use Step 2 to review shortcomings.

Risk Factors

The sooner your cancer is found, the better. Certain high-risk individuals should receive regular cancer screening. Although a number of simple tests can detect cancer effectively, the majority of Americans simply ignore them. You should seek out and arrange with your doctor for the diagnostic tests that are appropriate to your age, sex, and specialized risk. For instance, if you have a history of panulcerative colitis, sporadic colon polyps, or colon cancer or a family history of colon cancer, genital cancer, or polyposis syndrome, you will want a customized cancer program. A big part of knowing you are at risk is knowing your family history. You should prepare a detailed history of who had what kinds of cancer for the last three generations.

The risk of developing cancer rises throughout life. By age 60, colon, lung, and prostate cancer are accelerating at an exponential rate. Cancer is a special problem in older Americans, for 50% of all cancers occur in this 11% of the population. But there is a dangerous tendency to let down your guard once you're over the age of 65. Though you may feel you've made it through the most dangerous period, nothing could be further from the truth.

Early Diagnosis

FOR WOMEN   If you are a woman, you should undergo special training to learn exactly how to examine your breasts once a month for lumps. And if you are a *young* woman, you should be especially vigilant about these self-examinations, because mammograms seem to be less accurate in this age group. Plan to win, plan to beat cancer before it has a chance to beat you. Sit down with your doctor and plan your cancer screening tests based on your age, sex, family history, and known risks.

WOMEN AND MEN   Here is the screening recommended by the National Cancer Institute and the American Cancer Society.

Cervical Cancer

- Pap smear and pelvic exam annually for women 18 years and older as well as for sexually active girls

Prostate Cancer

- Rectal examination annually for men 40 and older (Ultrasound and blood test are *not* recommended for general screening by the NCI. However, the blood test PSA (prostate-specific antigen) is showing tremendous promise in research studies. You should ask your doctor if it's appropriate for you.)

Breast Cancer

- Breast self-examination monthly for women age 20 and older

- Professional exam every 3 years for women 20–39, annually for women 40 and older

- Mammogram every 1 or 2 years for women 40–49, annually for women 50 and over (Many doctors recommend a baseline test be done at the age of 35. This schedule is accelerated for women at high risk.)

Ovarian Cancer

- Ultrasound and blood test (These promising new techniques are not recommended for general screening yet. Ask your doctor if you are at high risk.)

Colon Cancer

- Digital rectal examination annually for men and women 40 and older

- Stool blood test annually for men and women 50 and older

- Sigmoidoscopy every 3 to 5 years for men and women 50 and older

Lung Cancer

- X-ray not recommended for general screening

Early Warning Signs

Early screening and diagnosis can make all the difference in the world. Look at Ronald Reagan: He survived a massive cancer of the colon because of early screening. If he had waited for symptoms, he never would have lived to serve out a second term. Yet most Americans his age ignore cancer symptoms and avoid cancer screening. Cancer symptoms are often ignored because of a phenomenon called "cancer symptom confusion": New symptoms are written off because they are confused with the effects of aging. Here are some examples from the book *Principles of Geriatric Medicine and Gerontology:*

SYMPTOM	MISTAKEN DIAGNOSIS	CORRECT DIAGNOSIS
Increased skin pigmentation	Age spot	Melanoma
Rectal bleeding	Hemorrhoids	Colon cancer
Constipation	Old age	Rectal cancer
Shortness of breath	Getting old	Lung cancer
Decreased urinary stream	Enlarged prostate gland	Prostate cancer
Fatigue	Aging	Metastatic cancer
Bone Pain	Arthritis	Bone cancer

You can easily recall the early warning signs of cancer by remembering the word CAUTION. The following are the American Cancer Society's seven early warnings:

EARLY WARNING SIGNS OF CANCER

Change in bowel habits

A sore that does not heal

Unusual bleeding or discharge

Thickening or lump in the breast or elsewhere

Indigestion or difficulty in swallowing

Obvious change in a wart or a mole

Nagging cough or hoarseness

If you exhibit any of these early warning signs, don't be afraid—be aggressive!

Treatment

If you are among the nearly 1 million individuals who will be diagnosed with cancer this year, your goals are simple. You will want to aggressively find the center of excellence that has the best chances of curing your disease or achieving the longest, highest-quality survival with a minimum of risk and discomfort. But that is not easily done.

If you suspect you might have cancer, you need to boldly pursue state-of-the-art care from the beginning. Many patients, fearing their suspicions may be correct, delay seeing a doctor for three months to a year. Waiting can transform treatable cancer into a fatal cancer. Both the National Cancer Institute and the American Cancer Society believe that many more lives could be saved, even without further research advances, if patients sought help sooner. Patients often feel hopeless when they confront cancer and they assume a passive, pessimistic attitude toward their care. Even young, well-trained cancer doctors often inadvertently encourage this attitude by predicting their patients' life expectancy in a set number of weeks or months. By insisting on a so-called "realistic" approach, they undercut their patients' motivation to seek out new treatments or to improve their overall health. You want a doctor and a cancer treatment team that will give you a strong sense of optimism. If you leave your doctor's office with a death sentence, you need a new doctor.

While hundreds of potentially valuable, new treatments are being developed for cancer, you want to make sure you receive the maximum benefit from conventional therapies first. In some cases you may be cured; in other cases your disease may subside for a time. If your cancer is in remission, your doctor should establish an aggressive screening program, based on objective assessments, to check for recurrences. Some doctors fail to do this because of their ill-founded pessimism that a recurrence means a death sentence. But it is delay that can be fatal. For instance, a patient with brain cancer should have regular MRI brain scans. Otherwise, a recurrence will be discovered only after new symptoms appear, by which time a pea-sized cancer will have grown into a pear-sized tumor. Dr. Ozols says, "Again, I would emphasize the importance of the initial treatment plan. We often have only one chance for cure. Do not delay seeing an oncologist until your family doctor has failed."

Conventional cancer treatment consists of surgery, chemotherapy, and radiation. If a cancer cannot be removed through surgery alone, radiation and chemotherapy can be used to follow up.

SURGERY   The right surgeon can make an enormous difference to the successful outcome of your cancer operation. Experienced cancer surgeons often handle tissue differently than do general surgeons. Some experts believe that they can reduce the possibility that individual cancer cells will break off during surgery and spread through the body to invade other organs. Trained cancer surgeons may also be much more aggressive in operating, even after the cancer has spread. A senior surgeon at Memorial Sloan-Kettering Cancer Center in New York City has been known to perform as many as 17 procedures on a single patient, operating against all odds of success. Rather than abandoning a patient to fate, the surgeon is always willing to attack the most recent spread of cancer. Before an operation surgeons often approach the patient's bedside and say, "I know you feel terrible, but you're going to feel terrific as soon as I'm through." They are virtually always right, and the results are remarkable. Top-rated cancer surgeons are willing to operate again and again. Neurosurgeons may operate on a patient with brain cancer more than a dozen times for recurrences. A Boston surgeon, Dr. Henry

Sears, has enabled many patients who have colon cancer to survive far beyond their projected life expectancies through repeated operations.

A general surgeon should be willing to refer you to regional medical centers where experienced cancer surgeons operate. Cancer patient networks are another excellent source of referrals. As with any cancer treatment, the most important surgery is the first one. You will want the best surgeon you can get for this surgery.

You should be aware of regional biases in surgery that may influence your care. In New England, you are more likely than in the deep South to be offered the choice of a lumpectomy instead of a mastectomy for breast cancer. A survey of 42,000 women, released in 1991, shows a 40% chance of avoiding mastectomy in New England, as opposed to an 11% chance in the deep South. A 1992 study shows the risk by state. A lumpectomy is a harder operation to perform. This study felt surgeons were more likely to perform a lumpectomy if they were trained in the procedure during residency. Others feel it is a regional bias based on the surgeon's belief that one operation has a better long-term promise for cure than the other. If you have a lumpectomy for breast cancer, you will want a surgeon who is widely experienced with the technique. Some surgeons may not offer you the option because they fear cosmetic scarring. In 1991, the research firm MediQual reported that 30.98% of subtotal mastectomies they studied had none of the objective clinical findings documented in the hospital medical record they use to validate subtotal mastectomies at the time of surgery.

New research indicates that breast surgery during the correct phase of your menstrual cycle can make a big difference in survival. Make certain to discuss this when planning your surgery.

With breast cancer it is more appropriate to see a surgeon, radiotherapist, and medical oncologist *before* the surgery, to discuss the options. At the Fox Chase Cancer Center, a woman will see all three specialists on her first visit. A joint treatment plan is then constructed.

If you are told your cancer is inoperable, make certain you consult an experienced cancer surgeon to determine if there is any chance an operation might provide a cure. Numerous patients have not had surgery because their cancer was mistakenly diagnosed as inoperable. This can be a double-edged sword. Surgery is also abused in patients denied other treatments. A thorough review at a major cancer center can help you distinguish between abuse and potentially helpful treatment.

Surgeons may say, "We've got it all," when, in fact, they haven't removed all of the tumor. It's important that your cancer is classified properly at the time of the operation, with records of the extent of its spread and the involvement of other organs. The surgeon should see and feel this at the time, and the pathologist should identify the severity of the disease from tissue biopsies. If this is not done correctly, you may be undertreated and have a diminished chance of survival. After the operation you should be referred to a team of cancer specialists to coordinate your future care. This is best done at a comprehensive cancer center where follow-up chemotherapy and radiation are available.

CHEMOTHERAPY   If a cancer can't be removed surgically, doctors will seek an alternative means to kill the cells: drugs. Chemotherapy attempts to do that by poisoning cancer cells while minimizing damage to healthy cells. The treatment tries to take advantage of differences between the two kinds of cells. Since cancer cells multiply rapidly, some drugs strike at the cell's ability to reproduce quickly. Unfortunately, these chemicals almost always damage normal cells as well. Many patients undergoing chemotherapy lose their hair, because hair follicles, like the cancer cells, grow quickly.

For some the risk of chemotherapy's harmful side effects begins to exceed the benefits. Doctors can sometimes circumvent that limitation by combining drugs that work in various ways. A cure for Hodgkin's disease, for example, was found by using four different drugs on the same patient.

To plan your chemotherapy you will want to find an oncologist who has extensive experience with your type of cancer. You can learn whether a physician is a board-certified cancer specialist by consulting the *Directory of Medical Specialists,* your regional comprehensive cancer institute, or the National Cancer Institute (in Bethesda, Maryland). Doctors who work at a comprehensive clinical cancer center will have access to the latest combinations of drugs and ongoing research into their effectiveness. They are also apt to be much more aggressive about chemotherapy.

Some doctors, reluctant to push chemotherapy, undertreat the disease by adopting a "go easy" approach. Although you may feel better and have less severe side effects than you would under all-out chemotherapy, the National Cancer Institute believes that thousands of patients die each year because their doses of chemotherapy were inadequate. This is the single biggest mistake in chemotherapy. While low-dose chemotherapy appears to be kinder and gentler to the patient, this may be lowering the possibility of survival. You doctor should follow the side effects of chemotherapy closely. The drugs destroy many red and white blood cells and platelets. If they're not monitored, you could die. With too few platelets, you could bleed to death; with too few white cells, you may be vulnerable to a life-threatening infection. A well-trained cancer nursing staff is your best guarantee of surviving the complications of chemotherapy.

New medications in combination with chemotherapy can make the treatment much more successful. Among these is GM-CSF (granulocyte macrophage colony stimulating factor), which is available commercially. GM-CSF stimulates the bone marrow to grow additional white blood cells. As a result a patient can be given higher, perhaps even curative, doses of chemotherapy. If a bone marrow transplant is performed, GM-CSF helps to spur the new marrow into cell production much more quickly. That decreases the time during which a bone marrow recipient is most vulnerable to life-threatening infections. An even more powerful new therapy, called stem cell therapy, allows doctors to grow large quantities of fresh red and white blood cells from a simple blood sample instead of from the bone marrow.

Even if you are not taking GM-CSF, you will want to discuss with your physician the kind of chemotherapy you will receive. You may be surprised at the number of different chemotherapy programs for your kind of cancer. Although doctors may have personal favorites, not all are equally effective. You may find you are being given "standard" chemotherapy because that's all your insurance will cover. Get the opinion of several senior oncologists before you commit to a series of chemotherapy treatments.

EPO is another drug that stimulates bone marrow production. EPO makes more red blood cells. Doctors use this with or after chemotherapy to get your blood back up toward normal levels.

Expert Chemotherapy Staff   If you and your physician decide on chemotherapy, you will want to be sure the hospital has a properly trained medical staff. You are taking significant risks if you undergo major chemotherapy at a small community hospital, for they are simply not prepared to deal with a wide range of complications, which may include severe bleeding and infection (for example, cisplatin, a common and extremely powerful chemotherapeutic agent, can be severely dehydrating and destructive to the kidneys). The hospital should have a ward set aside for chemotherapy and staffed by trained oncology nurses. Your local hospital, however, may be fully equipped to handle milder forms of chemotherapy.

Adjuvant Chemotherapy   Adjuvant therapy is used to kill stray cancer cells after surgery. If you are not offered this treatment, you should ask your doctor about it. While many early trials of adjuvant chemotherapy failed to show significant results, more recent research, especially in cases of colon and breast cancer, have shown promise. Sometimes adjuvant therapy is not offered even in cases where its effectiveness has been proven. Adjuvant chemotherapy in stage II breast cancer is mandatory.

A final cautionary note: Chemotherapy regimens are rapidly changing, and both insurance companies and the FDA are slow to recognize the benefits of new treatments.

RADIATION   Doctors use radiation, one of the oldest cancer treatments, to target specific tumors and destroy as many cells as possible. Its usefulness is limited by the sensitivity of nearby normal tissue to radiation exposure: The more sensitive that tissue is, the less radiation that can be used. In addition, the skin's ability to tolerate radiation is also limited.

While new forms of radiation may offer greater effectiveness with less risk of injury or side effect, they are extremely costly, sometimes requiring the use of multimillion-dollar cyclotrons. This therapy is available only at specialized centers. Your health care plan may try to limit your access to them because of the extra expense. You can learn about the different radiation treatments by contacting the regional cancer centers and the National Cancer Institute.

Not all radiation centers are created equal. You should look for an on-site physicist, computer modeling of the tumor that limits the amount of radiation reaching surrounding tissues, and the use of a radiation shield, called a custom block, that is designed for individual patients. The best centers employ multiple radiation fields on a daily basis and a linear accelerator. This equipment is needed to treat tumors that require a razor-sharp margin between normal and cancerous cells. In Hodgkin's disease, for instance, many lymph nodes need to be irradiated in the chest while the surrounding tissue must remain unharmed. Older cobalt-radiation machines can be used successfully to treat some forms of cancer, such as breast and lung, but they won't give the highly defined margins necessary to treat small tumors.

Clinical Trials

For decades, desperate cancer patients have fled to the Bahamas, Germany, Mexico, and elsewhere seeking last-ditch but ultimately futile "cures" for their disease. With stunning new discoveries in cancer research, patients can find the best experimental therapies at America's most prestigious cancer institutes, including the National Cancer Institute, Dana-Farber, Memorial Sloan-Kettering, Fox Chase, and the Mayo Clinic. They offer treatment to cancer patients through clinical trials; yet only 25,000 people a year enroll. In fact, as few as 1% of those eligible enter them. Although these treatments have not yet been proven effective, patients participate in the research. In some cases you will be helping to advance science; in other instances you may be one of the first to benefit from a powerful new treatment. You should be prepared to travel long distances if necessary. Often, doctors are conducting only a few trials of a particular treatment for the entire country.

All clinical trials have been approved by institutional review boards, which ensures that all patients in a clinical trial receive first the best-known treatment to date. The National Cancer Institute and the FDA monitor and approve the use of experimental drugs.

After you have assembled information about the various clinical trials, you should call or write the sponsors. You want to learn what their results are and how they compared to other programs. Your physician may be able to help you with these contacts. Some physicians running trials are very tight-lipped; others will be genuinely helpful. Don't be afraid to be pushy. This may be the most important information you'll ever get. Various support groups can provide useful information about their experience with various centers and treatments.

After considering all the options, you need to learn if you are eligible. If so, you will need a physician to apply for you.

As research progresses on a new drug, doctors acquire more knowledge about a treatment's effectiveness. There are three key phases in clinical trials:

Phase I   Doctors test a potential drug for its toxicity, searching for dangerous side effects. If you participate at this stage, it's unlikely (but possible) that you will benefit; however, you may help others by volunteering.

Phase II   If enough people can tolerate the drug, research begins on its effectiveness in patients who have had a recurrence following standard therapy. When a drug has progressed to this point, you are more likely to be helped, but no long-term success is guaranteed.

Phase III   When the drug shows some measure of effectiveness, the trials are expanded to include a much broader patient population, with whom it is compared to standard therapy. If a drug shows effectiveness on this group, it is likely to become an accepted treatment. If the drug is being tested at numerous centers under the same treatment protocol, doctors undoubtedly have reason to believe the treatment is promising.

You can obtain details for all three stages, at no charge, through the Physician's Desk Query (PDQ) system. (See Step 3 for how to use PDQ.) This is a system I use almost every day in my own office to find the latest information on treatment. Your doctor can use it to search for:

- the latest information about the treatment of most types of cancers

- descriptions of clinical trials that are accepting patients and the criteria for participation

- physicians and medical centers conducting clinical trials, including the stage of research and specifics about the therapies being used

Your doctor then can call the physicians who are running the individual trials to ask about their successes and your chance of acceptance. Here are the questions you need to have answered:

What is the purpose of the study?

How is it being done?

What is likely to happen in my case?

How long will I be hospitalized?

What are the results up to now?

These results may be very hard to determine, since the data is analyzed infrequently in Phase II and Phase III trials. Once efficacy is determined, the trial is closed.

TYPES OF CLINICAL TRIALS TREATMENTS

Advanced Conventional Therapy Many experimental therapies are variations on the standard combination of chemotherapy, radiation, and surgery. But don't be fooled. Cancer cures have emerged from fairly conventional treatment, as they did for Hodgkin's disease by using four different drugs at the same time. In many cancers doctors are still searching for the ideal combination of existing chemotherapies. In fact, most chemotherapy is considered experimental.

Biologics In the past 25 years, despite a government-declared war on cancer, little progress has been made in curing the biggest killers: breast cancer, colon cancer, pancreas cancer, kidney cancer, stomach cancer, and lung cancer that is inoperable. Many scientists believe the next major advances for these incurable cancers will come from the so-called biological response modifiers, or *biologics,* so called because they are cancer-fighting drugs produced by the human body. Interferon may be the most famous of the biologics; IL-2 (interleukin-2) also shows great promise. IL-2 performs no anticancer activity by itself, but works by stimulating immune cells to attack the cancer.

Doctors hope that the biologics, as naturally occurring substances, will have less severe side effects than other cancer drugs. IL-2 appears to be very toxic, however. TNF (tumor necrosis factor) also shows promise but can be quite toxic. Doctors hope to customize it, by changing the way it attaches to cells, so that it triggers only good responses, not bad ones.

Scientists hope to use a number of biologics together to coordinate an attack on cancer cells, not unlike mounting a combined air, sea, and land attack on an enemy military target. Hairy-cell leukemia, which can be cured with alpha interferon, is the first big success story. So far few biologics have been approved for general use, but hundreds of trials for cancers, now considered incurable, are under way.

Gene Therapy   In the end, a cure for cancer may be found in the genes. There are two different kinds of cancer genes, oncogenes and antioncogenes. Antioncogenes act as brakes on cancer cell growth, whereas oncogenes act as accelerators for cancer cell growth. Cancer can result from too much accelerator or not enough brake. Researchers can now insert the correct gene into the body using what are called stem cells. Doctors hope these will provide effective long-term treatment for currently incurable cancers. Oncogenes direct healthy cells to become cancerous when they are activated by environmental factors such as ultraviolet rays, cigarette smoke, automobile exhaust, and dietary toxins. Antioncogenes normally repair damage to the chromosomes. But when these antioncogenes also become injured, the cell's natural protection from cancer-causing agents is lost.

Although no gene therapy is now approved, scientists are looking for ways to prevent the activity of the cancer-promoting genes. Since proteins often carry the cancer-causing instructions, scientists are experimenting with counteracting agents. Dr. Steve Rosenberg at the National Cancer Institute is experimenting with another form of gene therapy. He "stitches" cancer-fighting genes into special white blood cells, producing a new kind of superkiller cell, beginning a new era in cancer treatment.

A Note about Pain Medication

If your cancer is not in remission and you are in pain, your doctor should be willing to search for the right type and amount of pain medication. Millions of cancer patients suffer needlessly because the health care community is too conservative in administering pain medications to patients with incurable cancers. Time and again it has been shown that restricting pain medicines is much more likely to induce dependence than giving sufficient quantities to work effectively. This management error accounts for enormous suffering by both cancer patients and their families.

Special Impact of Cost Cutting on Cancer Care

Cost cutting affects a wide range of medical services, but the severity and length of cancer as an illness makes it particularly prone to malicious cost-cutting measures. If you are in a managed health care program, you will find that it's difficult to go beyond the most conventional of therapies.

Many patients in certain prepaid health plans face long delays before they can arrange diagnostic tests. Many such group programs are reluctant to provide the full range of screening tests. Mammograms and Pap smears are the two most widely overlooked. One member of a health maintenance organization waited nearly a year before learning he had colon cancer. The HMO took months to schedule the diagnostic tests that had been ordered. As a result of this bottom-line orientation in medicine, you may be refused referral to appropriate specialists, comprehensive cancer centers, or treatment deemed experimental though considered state-of-the-art by specialists.

That's not to say that all HMOs are bad. One—U.S. Healthcare—aggressively sought out patients for breast cancer screening. The result? A review of their breast cancer patients showed a much higher number in early rather than late stages.

The case of Bob, a young and energetic father of two small children, illustrates the problems created by bottom-line cancer medicine and the difficulty of finding excellent care. He worked for an electronics firm in southern California that offered health coverage at a large HMO. During a routine visit his physician found a mass in his right kidney; diagnostic tests confirmed that it was a cancerous tumor. After surgeons removed the kidney, Bob was assured that "we got it all." Several weeks later Bob felt a deep gnawing pain in his left leg that seemed to get worse as the days passed. He called his surgeon, who did not return the phone calls. During the next two and a half weeks he left dozens of messages with the surgeon's secretary. Finally his surgeon agreed to see him. Bob pleaded for further diagnostic tests. Those requests were refused. At this HMO, as at many, access to specialists and diagnostic tests is limited, to hold down costs and to increase profits. Eventually his surgeon relented and ordered an x-ray, which revealed a large mass in his leg. Scans of the bones, lungs, and liver showed that the cancer had spread widely.

Bob was referred to one of the HMO's oncologists, a physician who specializes in treating inoperable cancers. Bob described the oncologist as a 9-to-5 clock watcher who displayed little interest in his case. The physician glanced at the scans in an x-ray reading box on the office wall. He returned to his desk, dashed off a prescription, and handed it to Bob. "Pain medication," he explained. "But what about my treatment?" Bob asked. "There is no treatment," the physician answered. "If you have more pain, I'll have the pharmacy get you a refill." Bob asked about experimental treatments. The oncologist said none existed, at least to his knowledge. Although the physician volunteered to find out, Bob never heard from him again.

Convinced there had to be some treatment, Bob followed the usual route of desperate, terminally ill cancer patients. He called clinics in Mexico and the Bahamas, sent for information on a cancer nutrition clinic in West Germany. Finally a friend, spotting a news story in the *Los Angeles Times,* alerted Bob to a treatment program in California that used the body's immune system to fight cancer. Hoag Memorial Presbyterian Hospital, less than 30 minutes away in Newport Beach, offered the treatment. He arranged an appointment for later that week. Physicians there explained the treatment: As Bob's blood was run through a machine similar to the ones used in kidney dialysis, white blood cells were withdrawn from the body through a process called plasmaphoresis. The white blood cells were washed in the new drug, IL-2, which converted them into "superkillers" that destroyed cancer cells on contact. Afterward, the "superkiller" cells were returned to the body just as if it were a standard blood transfusion.

During the treatment Bob suffered some shortness of breath and gained 25 pounds through fluid retention. Both were temporary side effects. Several weeks later he returned to Hoag for bone, liver, and lung scans, which revealed no cancer. The treatment had succeeded, at least temporarily. Bob sent the $20,000 bill to his HMO for reimbursement. It was returned unpaid. He protested, but after a meeting of the HMO board to reconsider his case, the decision stood. "We can't make an exception. We will not pay for experimental treatment," he was told.

Bob and patients like him can represent a substantial drain on HMO profits. This HMO could point to a policy that disallowed coverage for experimental treatment. Other HMO's refuse to use even conventional treatments for cancer patients, to avoid the high cost of chronic care. An Illinois HMO simply told patients that due to a backlog, they would have to wait six months to begin radiation. One woman with breast cancer was told she could not have a second round of chemotherapy. Although Bob was refused diagnostic tests and further treatment by his health care program, the most distressing aspect of his case may be that his doctors eliminated all hope. There was no counseling, no referral, no compassion for a young man facing death.

Step 2. Look for Shortcomings

By reading Step 1, I hope you got a good feeling about your treatment and that you understand much of it better. You'll learn even more by calling organizations listed in Step 4. But if you have an uncomfortable feeling that your treatment is not on track, then study this next section, which specifies some common and serious shortcomings that experts in the field recognize. If this section confirms your suspicions, you should go on to Step 3. Some of these mistakes you can discover yourself; others only an expert can confirm.

MISTAKES IN DIAGNOSIS

You're in a high-risk group and don't get regular, early screening or practice cancer prevention.

You don't self-monitor for cancer.

Your health care provider doesn't screen for cancer.

You don't seek medical attention fast enough after warning signs develop.

You have a more serious stage of cancer than doctors diagnose, which leads to undertreatment.

Your health care provider is not monitoring your cancer for recurrence.

MISTAKES IN TREATMENT

You have cancer and haven't seen a cancer specialist.

Your treatment is based on a regional bias.

Your health care provider is not prescribing biologics, such as GM-CSF, for maximum benefit, when indicated.

You fail to receive adjuvant therapy.

Your health care provider does not refer you to the specialists you need.

You are undertreated.

Your primary care provider doesn't provide state-of-the-art care.

You receive inadequate chemotherapy, radiation, or surgical removal.

You have an incurable cancer and haven't been informed of the appropriate experimental medicine.

Your surgeons won't operate again to remove recurrent cancer, when surgery could help.

You receive major chemotherapy in a hospital that is ill-equipped and ill-staffed to deal with complications.

You wait until "standard" therapy has failed before going to a cancer center. Remember, your first chance is your best chance.

You are not well informed about the kind, location, and stage of cancer you have.

You "accept" your fate without determining what the chances are for curative treatment or for treatment that can significantly improve your life expectancy or quality of life.

You inadvertently lock yourself out of promising new treatments by starting the first treatment recommended without researching others and your eligibility for them.

Your health care provider fails to use adequate amounts of pain medication.

You don't undertake lifestyle changes in the areas of nutrition, exercise, and stress.

Step 3. See a Specialist

If, from Step 2, you are concerned that your care is not state-of-the-art, this section will tell you how to find an expert.

Choosing a Doctor

Most physicians are delighted to have patients who are interested in their disease and eager to learn about it. This is the kind of doctor who should be enlisted in your battle against cancer. Ideally, this is your family practitioner or internist. The doctor who follows your care need not be a cancer specialist. He or she should recognize the desirability of consulting with different experts, however. Many physicians are reluctant to refer patients to regional cancer centers. Although many community hospitals are conveniently located and have the expertise to care for some cancers, the staff doctors may be unaware of the latest and most promising therapies. Chemotherapies, for instance, are constantly undergoing change as doctors refine their use. Your doctor should know about the leading cancer centers and oncologists in your area. He shouldn't feel threatened if you seek treatment at a large cancer center, although he may reasonably expect that your treatment will continue at the local community hospital. Your doctor should open doors, make referrals, find information, call experts on your behalf. Remember, this is a fight for your life. Cancer patients have died because they were unwilling to go behind their physicians' backs to locate medical care, out of fear that their doctors would feel slighted. You won't make friends if you're confrontational, but you will win a powerful ally if you ask for your physician's help in your search for a cure. If your physician's attitude is "take me or leave me," look for another doctor. Chances are, however, that will not be the case.

MEDICAL ONCOLOGIST   A medical oncologist is board-certified in internal medicine and the subspecialty of oncology. An oncologist must go through a minimum two-year fellowship program. Dr. Robert J. Mayer, Clinical Director of the Department of Medicine at Dana Farber Cancer Institute in Boston and a board member of the American Society of Clinical Oncology, offers the following advice:

■ The bulk of your oncologist's practice should be cancer patients. There are some oncologists who, for some reason, maintain a great deal of their work in the broad field of internal medicine.

■ Your oncologist should have been trained at a major cancer center or university with a cancer center, as opposed to a community cancer center.

- Your oncologist should be affiliated with a National Cancer Institute (NCI) comprehensive cancer center or NCI cooperative group where he or she will be attending meetings and have access to new treatments and protocols.

SURGICAL ONCOLOGIST   There is no board certification in surgical oncology. Try to find out whether or not your surgeon is recognized regionally as a cancer specialist, that is, is an expert in a given area. You want a surgeon who performs the type of surgical procedure you will be going through, and does so once a month (at an absolute minimum), not once a year.

TEAM ONCOLOGY   If you are having a major procedure, you want a team. Your surgical oncologist should work closely with a medical oncologist. Ask your doctor whether or not he or she is attending hospital-based tumor boards. These are weekly conferences where problems and management issues are discussed.

Step 4. Choosing a Hospital

If your doctor and local hospital can't provide state-of-the-art care, you should go to a major cancer institute where the staff has acquired extensive knowledge and expertise in the treatment of a wide variety of cancers. Especially for a second opinion, you want advice from skilled doctors at a center that is nationally recognized for cancer treatment. You should be acquainted with the following types of centers. Doctors credentialed at such centers will have the most comprehensive cancer training and will be up to date on the most current treatments.

NATIONAL CANCER INSTITUTE   With an annual budget in excess of $1 billion, the National Cancer Institute (NCI), which is part of the National Institutes of Health, sponsors thousands of clinical trials of new drugs around the country as well as research on promising treatments for incurable cancers at its own hospital on the Bethesda, Maryland, campus. You can find out if you're eligible to participate in clinical trials by asking your doctor to contact the institute, or call 800/4-CANCER yourself for preliminary information. If you are accepted, the NCI will pay for the entire treatment. The NCI has a reputation of treating patients extraordinarily well and of offering the last, best hope for a cure for many. The National Cancer Institute does not provide routine care for cancers for which there are already well-established treatments.

COMPREHENSIVE CANCER CENTERS   These institutions, which include some of the best-known hospitals in the country, are designated by the National Cancer

Institute as comprehensive cancer centers. You are best advised to be evaluated and to begin your treatment at one of these centers, which offer the latest high-technology diagnostic tests and therapies. You will receive the benefit of a team approach in which research and clinical staff work closely together to share knowledge. If you have breast cancer, for instance, you will be seen by a radiologist, a surgeon, a chemotherapist, a pathologist, and a social worker, all of whom have expertise in your disease. You may be able to continue your treatment closer to home, with periodic return visits. Your cancer center physician will refer you to a local hospital and medical team and coordinate your care with them. Marion Morra, a staff member at the Yale University Comprehensive Cancer Center, says: "Small hospitals just don't make it. You have all these horror stories of people who go to small local hospitals and are told that they're going to die. They should prepare their will. Then they go to a comprehensive cancer center and learn that their cancer is being treated with fairly good results."

To be designated a comprehensive cancer center, the hospital must conform to rigid standards to get the initial NCI grant and then be inspected by a panel of experts. Each such center must meet these requirements:

- Strong core of basic lab research

- Technology-transfer programs that tie together basic and clinical research and link them to outside organizations

- Proven record of innovative clinical research studies

- Active program of high-priority clinical trials

- Significant amount of cancer prevention and research control

- Effective research training and continuing education system

- Wide range of cancer information services for patients, doctors, health professionals, and the surrounding community

- Substantial commitment to community service and outreach programs

Centers of Excellence for Cancer

The following list of hospitals is provided only as a convenient starting place in your search for excellence. The list is not an endorsement. There may be hospitals just as excellent that have been omitted.

COMPREHENSIVE CARE CENTERS FOR CANCER These are the comprehensive cancer centers designated by the NCI.

ALABAMA
University of Alabama Comprehensive
 Cancer Center
1918 University Blvd
Basic Health Sciences Bldg., Rm 108
Birmingham, AL 35294

ARIZONA
Arizona Cancer Center
University of Arizona Cancer Center
1501 No. Campbell Ave
Tucson, AZ 85724

CALIFORNIA
Jonsson Comprehensive Cancer Center
 (University of California at Los
 Angeles)
10-247 Factor Bldg
10833 Le Conte Ave
Los Angeles, CA 90024-1781

The Kenneth Norris Jr. Cancer Center
University of Southern California
1441 Eastlake Ave
Los Angeles, CA 90033-0804

CONNECTICUT
Yale University Comprehensive Cancer
 Center
333 Cedar St
New Haven, CT 06510-8028

DISTRICT OF COLUMBIA
Vincent T. Lombardi Cancer Research
 Center
Georgetown University Medical Center
3800 Reservoir Rd, NW
Washington, DC 20007

FLORIDA
Sylvester Comprehensive Cancer Center
University of Miami Medical School
1475 NW 12th Ave
Miami, FL 33136

MARYLAND
Johns Hopkins Hospital
600 No. Wolfe St
Baltimore, MD 21205

MASSACHUSETTS
Dana Farber Cancer Institute
44 Binney St
Boston, MA 02115

MICHIGAN
Meyer L. Prentis Comprehensive Cancer
 Center
110 E Warren Ave
Detroit, MI 48201

University of Michigan Cancer Center
101 Simpson Dr
Ann Arbor, MI 48109-0752

MINNESOTA
Mayo Comprehensive Cancer Center
200 First St SW
Rochester, MN 55905

NEW HAMPSHIRE
Norris Cotton Cancer Center
Dartmouth-Hitchcock Medical Center
2 Maynard St
Hanover, NH 03756

NEW YORK
Columbia University Cancer Center
College of Physicians and Surgeons
630 W 168th St
New York, NY 10032

Kaplan Cancer Center
New York University Medical Center
550 First Ave
New York, NY 10016

Memorial Sloan-Kettering Cancer
 Center
1275 York Ave
New York, NY 10021

Roswell Park Memorial Institute
Elm and Carlton Sts.
Buffalo, NY 14263

NORTH CAROLINA
Cancer Center of Wake Forest University
Bowman Gray School of Medicine
300 So. Hawthorne Rd
Winston-Salem, NC 27103

Duke University Comprehensive Cancer
Center
P.O. Box 3843
Durham, NC 27710

Lineberger Cancer Research Center
University of North Carolina School of
Medicine
Chapel Hill, NC 27599

OHIO
Ohio State University Comprehensive
Cancer Center
410 West 12th Ave
Columbus, OH 43210

PENNSYLVANIA
Fox Chase Cancer Center
7701 Burholme Ave
Philadelphia, PA 19111

Pittsburgh Cancer Institute
200 Meyran Ave
Pittsburgh, PA 15213

University of Pennsylvania Cancer
Center
3400 Spruce St
Philadelphia, PA 19104

TEXAS
University of Texas M.D. Anderson
Cancer Center
1515 Holcombe Blvd
Houston, TX 77030

VERMONT
Vermont Cancer Center
University of Vermont
1 South Prospect St
Burlington, VT 05401

WASHINGTON
Fred Hutchinson Cancer Research
Center
1124 Columbia St
Seattle, WA 98104

WISCONSIN
Wisconsin Clinical Cancer Center
University of Wisconsin
600 Highland Ave
Madison, WI 53792

CLINICAL CANCER CENTERS These centers, known for their excellence in cancer treatment, are also designated by the NCI. They focus on both basic and clinical research within the same institution.

CALIFORNIA
City of Hope National Medical Center
Beckman Research Institute
1500 E Duarte Rd
Duarte, CA 91010

University of California at San Diego
225 Dickinson St
San Diego, CA 92103

COLORADO
University of Colorado Cancer Center
4200 E 9th Ave
Box B190
Denver, CO 80262

ILLINOIS
University of Chicago Cancer Research
   Center
5841 So. Maryland Ave
Box 444
Chicago, IL 60637

NEW YORK
Albert Einstein College of Medicine
1300 Morris Park Ave
Bronx, NY 10461

University of Rochester Cancer Center
601 Elmwood Ave
Box 704
Rochester, NY 14642

OHIO
Case Western Reserve University
University Hospitals of Cleveland
Ireland Cancer Center
2074 Abington Rd
Cleveland, OH 44106

RHODE ISLAND
Roger Williams General Hospital
825 Chalkstone Ave
Providence, RI 02908

TENNESSEE
St Jude Children's Research Hospital
332 No. Lauderdale St
Memphis, TN 38101

TEXAS
Institute for Cancer Research and Care
8122 Datapoint Dr
San Antonio, TX 78229

UTAH
Utah Regional Cancer Center
University of Utah Medical Center
50 No. Medical Dr, Rm 2C10
Salt Lake City, UT 84132

VIRGINIA
Massey Cancer Center
Medical College of Virginia
Virginia Commonwealth University
1200 E Broad St
Richmond, VA 23298

CONSORTIUMS FOR CANCER CARE   These centers represent several medical institutions that have combined their services to form a major cancer program and
are designated by the NCI.

CALIFORNIA
Drew-Meharry-Morehouse Consortium
   Cancer Center
Charles R. Drew University
12714 So. Avalon Blvd, Ste 301
Los Angeles, CA 90061

ILLINOIS
Illinois Cancer Center
200 So. Michigan Ave, Rm 1700
Chicago, IL 60604-2404

BASIC CENTERS FOR CANCER CARE   These NCI-designated centers are almost
entirely devoted to basic research.

CALIFORNIA
Cancer Research Center
La Jolla Cancer Research Foundation
10901 N Torrey Pines Rd
La Jolla, CA 92037

Armand Hammer Center for Cancer
   Biology
Salk Institute
P.O. Box 85800
San Diego, CA 92186-5800

INDIANA
Purdue Cancer Center
Purdue University
S University St
West Lafayette, IN 47907

MAINE
The Jackson Laboratory
600 Main St
Bar Harbor, ME 04609-1500

MASSACHUSETTS
Worcester Foundation for Experimental
   Biology
222 Maple Ave
Shrewsbury, MA 01545

Center for Cancer Research
Massachusetts Institute of Technology
40 Ames St
Cambridge, MA 02139

NEBRASKA
Eppley Institute
University of Nebraska Medical Center
600 S 42nd St
Omaha, NE 68198-6805

NEW YORK
Cold Spring Harbor Laboratory
P.O. Box 100
Cold Spring Harbor, NY 11724

Institute of Environmental Medicine
New York University Medical Center
550 First Ave
New York, NY 10016

American Health Foundation
320 E 43rd St
New York, NY 10017

PENNSYLVANIA
Fels Research Institute
Temple University School of Medicine
3420 N Broad St
Philadelphia, PA 19140

Wistar Institute
3601 Spruce St
Philadelphia, PA 19104

VIRGINIA
Cancer Center
University of Virginia Medical Center
Box 234 Health Science Center
Charlottesville, VA 22908

WISCONSIN
McArdle Laboratory for Cancer
   Research
University of Wisconsin
1400 University Ave
Madison, WI 53706

COMMUNITY HOSPITALS FOR CANCER CARE   The convenience of staying close to home when you have prolonged cancer therapy is a key issue in your care. Still, you are best advised to be evaluated at a leading cancer center immediately. You may be able to continue treatment and evaluation at your community hospital. That decision is one you should make with your oncologist. One way to do that is to look for a Community Clinical Oncology Program (CCOP). Through such a program, community physicians work with scientists conducting NCI-supported clinical trials designed to answer specific questions about the effectiveness of new ways to prevent, detect, diagnose, and treat cancer. Facilities participating in a CCOP are required to affiliate with at least one research base (such as a public health department or an NCI-supported clinical cooperative group or cancer center).

ARIZONA
Greater Phoenix CCOP
925 E McDowell
Phoenix, AZ 85006

CALIFORNIA
Bay Area Tumor Institute CCOP, Ste 204
2844 Summit St
Oakland, CA 94609

California Healthcare System CCOP
P.O. Box 1333
Ross, CA 94957

Central Los Angeles CCOP
2131 W Third St
Los Angeles, CA 90057

Sacramento CCOP
Sutter Cancer Center
5275 F St
Sacramento, CA 95819

San Diego Kaiser Permanente CCOP
Kaiser Permanente Medical Center
Department of Oncology
4647 Zion Ave
San Diego, CA 92120

San Joaquin Valley CCOP
P.O. Box 1232
Fresno Community Hospital and
    Medical Center
Fresno, CA 93715

DELAWARE
Medical Center of Delaware CCOP
P.O. Box 1668
Wilmington, DE

FLORIDA
Community Clinical Oncology Program
Department of Surgery
Mt. Sinai Medical Center
4300 Alton Rd
Miami Beach, FL 33140

Florida Pediatric CCOP
Florida Association of Pediatric Tumor
    Programs
P.O. Box 13372
Gainesville, FL 32604-1372

GEORGIA
Atlanta Regional COOP
St Joseph's Hospital
5665 Peachtree Dunwoody Rd NE
Atlanta, GA 30342-1701

ILLINOIS
Carle Cancer Center CCOP
Carle Clinic Association
602 W University Ave
Urbana, IL 61801

Community Clinical Oncology Program
Kellogg Cancer Center
Evanston Hospital
2650 Ridge Ave
Evanston, IL 60201

Illinois Oncology Research Association
    CCOP
Ste 780
900 Main St
Peoria, IL 61603

INDIANA
Indiana Regional Cancer Center CCOP
Community Hospitals of Indianapolis
1500 No. Ritter Ave
Indianapolis, IN 46219

Methodist Hospital of Indiana CCOP
Methodist Hospital Cancer Center
Box 1367
1701 No. Senate Blvd.
Indianapolis, IN 46206

IOWA
Community Clinical Oncology Program
Cedar Rapids Oncology Project
788 8th Ave SE
Cedar Rapids, IA 52401

Iowa Oncology Research Association
  CCOP
1044 Seventh St
Des Moines, IA 50314

KANSAS
Wichita CCOP
P.O. Box 1358
Wichita, KS 67201

LOUISIANA
Ochsner CCOP
Ochsner Cancer Institute
1514 Jefferson Hwy
New Orleans, LA 70121

MICHIGAN
Grand Rapids Clinical Oncology
  Program
100 Michigan St NE
Grand Rapids, MI 49503

Kalamazoo Clinical Oncology Program
1521 Gull Rd
Kalamazoo, MI 49001

MINNESOTA
Duluth CCOP
The Duluth Clinic, Ltd.
400 E Third St
Duluth, MN 55805

W. Metro-Minneapolis CCOP
5000 West 39th St
St Louis Park, MN 55416

MISSOURI
Kansas City Clinical Oncology Program
Baptist Medical Center
6601 Rockhill Rd
Kansas City, MO 64131

Ozarks Regional CCOP
1000 E Primrose St, Ste 450
Springfield, MO 65807

St Louis–Cape Girardeau CCOP
Tower B, Ste 3018
Mercy Doctor's Building
621 So. New Ballas Rd
St Louis, MO 63141

NEVADA
Southern Nevada Cancer Research
  Foundation CCOP
501 So. Rancho Dr, Ste C-14
Las Vegas, NV 89106

NEW JERSEY
Bergen-Passaic CCOP
Hackensack Medical Center
30 Prospect Ave
Hackensack, NJ 07601

NEW YORK
Brooklyn CCOP
Cancer Institute of Brooklyn
927 49th St
Brooklyn, NY 11219

North Shore University Hospital CCOP
Don Monti Division of Oncology
300 Community Dr
Manhasset, NY 11030

Syracuse Hematology-Oncology CCOP
Hematology-Oncology Associates of
  Central New York
North Medical Center
7209 Buckley Rd, Ste 1P
Liverpool, NY 13088

NORTH CAROLINA
Southeast Cancer Control Consortium
  CCOP
2062 Beach St
Winston-Salem, NC 27103-2614

NORTH DAKOTA
St Luke's Hospitals CCOP
Roger Maris Cancer Center
820 4th St N
Fargo, ND 58122

OHIO
Columbus CCOP
1151 So. High St
Columbus, OH 43206

Dayton Clinical Oncology Program
Cox Heart Institute
3525 Southern Blvd
Kettering, OH 45429

Toledo Community Hospital Oncology
    Program
3314 Collingwood Blvd.
Toledo, OH 43610

OKLAHOMA
Saint Francis Hospital/Natalie Warren
    Bryant CCOP
6161 So. Yale Ave
Tulsa, OK 74136

OREGON
Columbia River Oncology Program
4805 NE Glisan Rd, Rm BG 10
Portland, OR 97213

PENNSYLVANIA
Allegheny CCOP
Allegheny-Singer Research Institute
320 E North Ave
Pittsburgh, PA 15212-9986

Geisinger Clinical Oncology Program
Geisinger Medical Center, 20-01
No. Academy Ave
Danville, PA 17822

Mercy Hospital CCOP
General Services Bldg, Ste 205
746 Jefferson Ave
Scranton, PA 18501

Twin Tiers CCOP
Robert Parker Hospital
Guthrie Healthcare System
Guthrie Square
Sayre, PA 13840

SOUTH CAROLINA
Spartanburg CCOP
P.O. Box 2768
1776 Skyline Dr
Spartanburg, SC 29304

SOUTH DAKOTA
Rapid City Regional CCOP
P.O. Box 4097
Rapid City, SD 57709

Sioux Community Cancer Consortium
    CCOP
Central Plains Clinic, Ltd.
1000 E 21st St, Ste 2000
Sioux Falls, SD 57105

VERMONT
Green Mountain Oncology Group
Rutland Regional Medical Center
160 Allen St
Rutland, VT 05701

WASHINGTON
Community Clinical Oncology Program
The Virginia Mason Clinic
1100 9th Ave
P.O. Box 900
Seattle, WA 98111

Northwest CCOP
Tacoma General Hospital
314 So. K St, Ste 204
Tacoma, WA 98405-0986

WISCONSIN
Marshfield Medical Research Founda-
    tion CCOP
Marshfield Clinic
1000 No. Oak Ave
Marshfield, WI 54449

Milwaukee CCOP
2901 W Kinnickinnic River Pky, Ste 516
Milwaukee, WI 53215-3690

CLINICAL TRIALS COOPERATIVE GROUP PROGRAM FOR SPECIFIC CANCER
TYPES   Composed of academic institutions and cancer treatment centers throughout the United States and Canada, cooperative groups share with the NCI the responsibility of identifying important questions in cancer treatment research and designing carefully controlled clinical trials to answer these questions. The groups are heterogeneous in their structures and research focuses. Some groups concentrate on treatment of a single type of cancer, some study a specific type of cancer therapy, and others focus on a group of related cancers. Some cooperative groups have a range of research emphases. Together, the groups share a common purpose: to develop and conduct large-scale trials in multiinstitutional settings.

ARIZONA
Brain Tumor Cooperative Group
  (BTCG)
Barrow Neurological Institute
St Joseph Hospital and Medical Center
350 W Thomas Rd
Phoenix, AZ 85013

CALIFORNIA
Children's Cancer Study Group (CCSG)
440 E Huntington Dr, Ste 300
P.O. Box 60012
Arcadia, CA 91006-6012

MINNESOTA
North Central Cancer Treatment Group
  (NCCTG)
Mayo Clinic
200 First St SW
Rochester, MN 55905

NEW HAMPSHIRE
Cancer and Leukemia Group B
  (CALGB)
444 Mount Support Rd, Ste 2
Rural Route 3, Box 750
Lebanon, NH 03766

NEW YORK
National Wilms' Tumor Study Group
  (NWTSG)
Roswell Park Cancer Institute
Elm and Carlton Sts.
Buffalo, NY 14263

PENNSYLVANIA
Gynecologic Oncology Group (GOG)
1234 Market St, Ste 1945
Philadelphia, PA 19107

National Surgical Adjuvant Project for
  Breast and Bowel Cancers (NSABP)
University of Pittsburgh
914 Scaife Hall
3550 Terrace St
Pittsburgh, PA 15261

TEXAS
Pediatric Oncology Group (POG)
4949 West Pine Blvd.
Houston, TX 77030

Southwest Oncology Group (SWOG)
5430 Fredericksburg Rd, Ste 618
San Antonio, TX 78229-6197

VIRGINIA
Intergroup Rhabdomyosarcoma Study
  (IRS)
Medical College of Virgina
MCV Box 646
Richmond, VA 23298

WISCONSIN
Eastern Cooperative Oncology Group
   (ECOG)
Wisconsin Clinical Cancer Center
University of Wisconsin
600 Highland Ave
Madison, WI 53792

BELGIUM
European Organization for Research on
   Treatment for Cancer (EORTC)
Institute Jules Bordet
Rue Heger, Bordet 1
1000 Brussels, Belgium

MAKING A FINAL CHOICE   With most illnesses there are objective measurements that can be used to judge institutions. In cancer the most helpful rates to remember measure survival, response, and partial and complete remission. Radiation therapy departments generally keep reliable records that will enable you to compare hospitals. These rates are difficult to obtain for standard chemotherapy and surgery at an individual institution. In general, you are looking for the greatest amount of expertise in the kind of cancer that you have and the type of treatment you will receive.

Step 5. Become Your Own Expert

To ensure that you will receive excellent care, you need to become your own consumer advocate. It's tremendously important to educate yourself about your illness. Within a few hours you can acquire an enormous amount of knowledge about the treatment options being used. While a wide range of people is available to help, you don't want just any second opinion. You want advice from skilled doctors at a center that is nationally recognized for cancer treatment. And remember that the health care system doesn't speak with one authoritative voice.

You should write down your questions beforehand and take notes of your conversations. Have with you the following information: your diagnosis, including the type, location, and classification of your cancer; the results of diagnostic tests, such as x-rays and scans of your liver, brain, lungs, and bones; records of blood tests and biopsies; discharge summaries; and a description of treatments to date. When you talk to experts in person, bring along a tape recorder. And bring another person with you—people hear different things in conversations. If you have a friend or relative who is good at negotiations with large bureaucracies, you should ask him or her to accompany you. The health care system is a large bureaucracy. And as with all such organizations, the people who lack power are apt to get lost. While you will want to develop your own list of questions, first and foremost you should know what is conventional and what is experimental *before* you begin *any* treatment. Here are some additional suggested questions to ask.

What do I need to know to understand my kind of cancer?

Is my cancer curable?

What treatment is considered the "cure"?

If my cancer is not curable, are there promising new treatments?

What treatment do you recommend, and why?

Where is treatment available?

Has one institution been more successful than others at treating this type and stage of cancer?

How do experimental treatments compare with the standard treatment?

What results can be expected?

Who will pay for these treatments?

How much research has been done so far on the experimental treatments and what are the results?

How safe is the procedure?

What are the side effects?

How and when will I know if the treatment is working?

Exactly what will the surgeon do?

What are the relative benefits and risks of not having a particular treatment?

You will want to learn of the centers that specialize in your cancer, the available treatments, including both the conventional and experimental therapies, and the research programs that may be available. In many experimental treatment programs you need to be a relatively "virgin" patient. You must not have received treatments that may confuse research results. It is very important to review all options before beginning a new course of treatment, or you may be disqualified from therapy that could prove beneficial. Here are the institutions we have found most helpful.

WHO TO CALL

National Cancer Institute   This is a phone center service of the National Cancer Institute. A trained staff member answers the telephone. All calls are confidential. Staff members have access to a large computerized database and can send you written materials. This is a good first step that can provide valuable leads to ongoing clinical trials with the names of physicians to contact and state-of-the-art care. Their most important service is the multidisciplinary second-opinion center, where a cancer specialist will review your medical records and your doctor's treatment plan. If you do nothing else from reading this chapter, you should take this step. You also can receive detailed research reports summarizing the cause, incidence, symptoms, diagnosis, and treatment of your type of cancer.

800/4-CANCER

American Cancer Society   The telephones at the ACS are staffed by volunteers, including many physicians, who can provide general information or more specifics from an extensive database. They can arrange for a second opinion or put callers in touch with health care professionals who can help. They will individualize information. If you have pancreatic cancer, they'll send information on new and experimental treatments.

You can also call the ACS to discuss their position on unproven treatment methods, to ensure that you are not pursuing futile or even harmful therapies.

The American Cancer Society also sponsors numerous local support groups:

■ *Road to Recovery* provides transportation to and from treatments.

■ *Reach to Recovery* brings together breast cancer patients and people who have already learned to cope with the disease. Patients are visited by volunteers who share a similar medical history.

■ *I Can Cope* program offers psychological and emotional support groups. Families are welcome.

■ *Look Good, Feel Better* helps women who are suffering ill effects of cancer treatment, especially hair loss from chemotherapy. Trained cosmetologists provide wigs and makeup.

1599 Clifton Rd
Atlanta, GA 30329
800/ACS-2345 or 404/329-7629

American Red Cross   The ARC provides a range of services for emergency situations.

431 18th St, NW
Washington, DC 20006
202/737-8300

Cancer Research Institute   This group has an excellent cancer information network. It has a toll-free hot line and offers an excellent booklet containing information on second opinions, financial aid, and how to take charge.

National Headquarters
133 E 58th St
New York, NY 10022
800/99-CANCER

Corporate Angel Network   This group locates empty seats on corporate planes and makes them available to cancer patients. If you can't afford to fly to a distant cancer center, this network may be able to get you there.

Westchester County Airport, Bldg 1
White Plains, NY 10604
914/328-1313

International Bone Marrow Transplant Registry   Most bone marrow teams throughout the world participate in this registry, which was created to improve efficiency and effectiveness in the search for unrelated donors.

Medical College of Wisconsin
8701 Watertown Plank Rd
414/257-8325

Leukemia Society of America   The 57 local chapters of this group can provide public and professional educational materials, limited financial aid—up to $750 per year for qualified patients—and information on leukemia, lymphoma, and Hodgkin's disease.

733 Third Ave
New York, NY 10017
212/573-8484

National Marrow Donor Program   This organization maintains a registry of people who want to be donors. It's used to treat over 30 fatal blood diseases, including leukemia. Information on bone marrow transplants is also available.

3433 Broadway St, NE, Ste 400
Minneapolis, MN 55413
800/654-1247

Cancer Consulting Group   This group provides expert information, through oncologists, on state-of-the-art treatment and knowledge. The consulting doctors, about 50 nationwide, can work with you alone or together with your doctor. The oncologists are research-oriented doctors in various cancer fields. The basic fee is $250 per hour.

990 Grove
Evanston, IL 60201
708/866-7711
800/383-4636

CANHELP, Inc.   This organization offers cancer treatment information, including a worldwide search for conventional as well as alternative therapies. Working from copies of your medical reports, such as scans, x-rays, and lab work, the staff will provide you with a 5- to 15-page report on treatment and management options, including doctor referrals. The fee is $400.

3111 Paradise Bay Rd
Port Ludlow, WA 98365
206/437-2291

The Health Resource   This group's fee ranges from $150 to $225 for a computer search of medical journals and books on different diseases, including cancer.

209 Katherine Dr
Conway, AZ 72032
501/329-5272

National Coalition for Cancer Survivorship   This group serves as an information clearinghouse, particularly on insurance and employment discrimination issues, and offers referrals to support groups throughout the United States.

1010 Wayne Ave
Silver Spring, MD 20910
301/585-2616

DES (Diethylstilbestrol)   This consumer organization works with daughters of women who took the synthetic estrogen DES during pregnancy. It produces a quarterly newsletter and makes referrals to doctors.

1615 Broadway
Oakland, CA 94612
415/465-4011

American Self-Help Clearinghouse   This group makes referrals to over 30 state or local self-help clearinghouses that can put callers in contact with support groups.

St Clare's–Riverside Medical Center
Pocono Rd
Denville, NJ 07834
201/625-7101

Candlelighters   This is a Pediatric Cancer Support Group where parents can get information on treatment, clinical trials, referrals, psychological support, and reimbursement. They'll also help you communicate with your physician, and coach you on how to use the medical system, how to cope with cancer in the workplace, and how to deal with children.

1312 18th St NW, Ste 200
Washington, DC 20036
800/366-2223
202/659-5136

NIH CRISP System

301/496-7543

University-Affiliated Teaching Hospitals   See Appendix.

PHYSICIAN'S DATA QUERY (PDQ)   The most helpful and current cancer information is found in the National Cancer Institute's very powerful computerized database called PDQ (physician's data query), which can be accessed 24 hours a day through any personal computer with a modem and a communications software program. You can ask one of the health care professionals familiar with the program to assist you. If you want to enter these databases on your own, you can sign up with one of the computer databases listed below. Many hospitals, libraries, and doctor's offices also have these databases available.

PDQ can help you discover the medical centers offering the most up-to-date treatment for your cancer and to locate experimental clinical trials if there is no known cure.

Cancer Information File   According to the National Cancer Institute, the Cancer Information file (PDQC) contains prognostic and treatment information on over 80 different major types of cancers. Each summary provides a prognostic statement, including information on the relevant staging and cellular classification systems and options, by stage of disease and/or cell type. Each summary also cites key references from the literature and references to ongoing research whenever appropriate. The information in this file was reviewed by over 400 cancer specialists. An editorial board composed of 72 prominent oncologists reviews each summary on a monthly basis to maintain the currency and accuracy of the file, and modifies the content of the summaries based on new data. This is the database you want to start with.

For an actual search, you will need the following information:

- Cancer type

- Cell type (determined by a pathologist, based on a biopsy)

- Cancer stage

- Prior treatment

- Medical complications

PDQ Protocols   The Protocols file (PDQP), updated on a monthly basis, contains summaries of active treatment protocols that are open for patient entry. Either the protocols are those supported by the National Cancer Institute (NCI) or the descriptions have been submitted to NCI by investigators at institutions throughout the country. The title, the unique protocol identification number, the protocol chairperson, study objectives, the patient entry criteria, the details of the treatment regimen, and information about where the study is being conducted are provided. Protocols are investigational and are intended for use by trained oncologists.

PDQ Directory File   The PDQ Directory file contains the names, addresses, telephone numbers, and affiliations of physicians who spend a major portion of their clinical practice treating cancer patients, and health care organizations that have organized programs of cancer care. Each physician in the PDQ Directory is either a member of one or more of the 14 professional societies established for physicians who treat cancer patients that list their membership directories in PDQ or a principal investigator for one or more active protocols. Each society determines its own criteria for membership in the society. The Directory does not necessarily encompass all cancer specialists located in a particular geographic area, and does not constitute an endorsement of professional competence. All records in the Directory are updated annually.

WHAT TO READ   The Office of Cancer Communications will send you a wide variety of materials on cancer. You may receive them by writing to the following address.

Office of Cancer Communications
National Cancer Institute
Bldg 31, Rm 10A30
Bethesda, MD 20894

Computer Databases

Medlars Management Section
National Library of Medicine
Bldg 38, Rm 4N421
8600 Rockville Pike
Bethesda, MD 20894
301/496-4000

Data Star
485 Devon Park Dr, Ste 10
Wayne, PA 19087
800/221-7754

BRS Information Systems
Maxwell Online Limited
8000 Westpark Dr
McLean, VA 22102
800/468-0908

DIALOG Information Services, Inc.
3460 Hillview Ave
Palo Alto, CA 94304
800/3-DIALOG

EXPERT SOURCES

Although dozens of experts were interviewed for these chapters, these physicians are acknowledged for their significant contributions to this section.

Dr. Robert F. Ozols, Chair, Medical Oncology, Fox Chase Cancer Center, Philadelphia, PA

The staff of the National Cancer Institute

REFERENCES AND SUGGESTED READING

Bentley, Christopher R., and others. Tamoxifen Retinopathy: a Rare but Serious Complication. *British Medical Journal,* Vol. 304, No. 6825 (Feb. 22, 1992), pp. 495–496.

Boice, John D., Jr., and others. Cancer in the Contralateral Breast After Radiotherapy for Breast Cancer. *New England Journal of Medicine,* Vol. 326, No. 12 (Mar. 19, 1992), pp. 781–785.

Brennan, Michael J., and Weitz, Jody. Lymphedema 30 Years After Radical Mastectomy. *American Journal of Physical Medicine and Rehabilitation,* Vol. 71, No. 1 (Feb. 1992), pp. 12–14.

Buter, J., and others. Infection After Subcutaneous Interleukin-2 [letter]. *Lancet,* Vol. 339, No. 8792 (Feb. 29, 1992), p. 552.

Cohen, Harvey. *Principles of Geriatric Medicine and Gerontology.* New York: McGraw-Hill, 1990, p. 78.

Curtin, J. J., and Sampson, M. A. Need for Open-Access Non-Screening Mammography in a Hospital with a Specialist Breast Clinic Service. *British Medical Journal,* Vol. 304, No. 6826 (Feb. 29, 1992), pp. 549–551.

Farrow, D. C., and others. Geographic Variation in the Treatment of Localized Breast Cancer. *New England Journal of Medicine,* Vol. 326, No. 17 (April 23, 1992), pp. 1097–1101.

Freimuth, V. S., and others. *Searching for Health Information: The Cancer Information Service Model.* National Cancer Institute, Cancer Information Service, 1989.

Greenfield, Marjorie. Reduced Spinal Bone Mass in Patients with Uterine Cervical Cancer [letter]. *Obstetrics and Gynecology,* Vol. 79, No. 3 (Mar. 1992), pp. 479–480.

Haskell, Charles, M. *Cancer Treatment,* 3rd ed. Orlando, Fla.: Saunders, 1990.

Inoue, Masaki, and others. CA 19-9, CA 125, Carcinoembryonic Antigen, and Tissue Polypeptide Antigen in Differentiating Ovarian Cancer from Benign Tumors. *Obstetrics and Gynecology,* Vol. 79, No. 3 (Mar. 1992), pp. 434–440.

Morra, Marion, and Potts, Eve. *Choices: Realistic Alternatives in Cancer Treatment.* New York: Avon Books, 1987.

National Cancer Institute. *Questions to Ask Your Doctor About Breast Cancer.*

National Coalition for Cancer Survivorship. *Charting the Journey: An Almanac of Practical Resources for Cancer Survivors.* Consumer Reports Books, 1990.

Nattinger, A. B., and others. Geographic Variation in the Use of Breast-Conserving Treatment for Breast Cancer. *New England Journal of Medicine,* Vol. 326, No. 17 (April 23, 1992), pp. 1102–1107.

O'Brien, M. E. R., and others. Blindness Associated with High-Dose Carboplatin. [letters to the editor] *Lancet,* Vol. 339, No. 8792 (Feb. 29, 1992), p. 558.

Oka, Kuniyuki, and others. Adenocarcinoma of the Cervix Treated with Radiation Alone: Prognostic Significance of S-100 Protein and Vimentin Immunostaining. *Obstetrics and Gynecology,* Vol. 79, No. 3 (Mar. 1992), pp. 347–350.

Reiter, Robert C., and others. Ovarian Cancer in Women with Prior Hysterectomy: A 14-Year Experience at the University of Miami [letter]. *Obstetrics and Gynecology,* Vol. 79, No. 2 (Feb. 1992), pp. 317–319.

Sidransky, David, and others. Clonal Origin of Bladder Cancer. *New England Journal of Medicine,* Vol. 326, No. 11 (Mar. 12, 1992), pp. 737–740.

U.S. Department of Health and Human Services. *What You Need to Know About Cancer.* NIH Publication No. 90-1566, Nov. 1989.

Coronary Artery Disease

Risk for Inappropriate Care VERY HIGH

Many patients with coronary artery disease do not get the medication, surgery, or procedures that could improve their quality of life, slow the course of their illness, or increase their life expectancy. Heart disease kills hundreds of thousands of Americans every year before they ever reach a hospital. If many had sought early accurate diagnosis through the appropriate testing, their doctors could have saved thousands of lives. Two acquaintances of mine died this past year, one at age 37, the other at 41. In both cases, testing would have found large heart blockages that through surgery could have been bypassed, thus possibly saving their lives.

Cardiac procedures may also be inappropriately used. Many academic cardiologists say pacemakers are used like water. In 1991, the research firm MediQual reported that 67.81% of pacemaker insertions they studied had none of the objective clinical findings documented in the hospital medical record they use to validate pacemaker insertions at the time of surgery.

Risk for Inappropriate Care If You Are a Woman

If you are a woman, recent scientific research shows that some doctors may take your symptoms a great deal less seriously than a man's. A recent study showed that even when doctors admitted to a hospital women with more advanced disease than men, the men were still 28% more likely to receive state-of-the-art diagnostic testing and 45% more likely to have surgery or other procedures to reroute blood to coronary arteries. Some new studies disagree, but one prominent cardiologist told me: "If a man's having chest pain, he's having a heart attack; if a woman's having chest pain, she's having an anxiety attack." If you're a woman, doctors may take you less seriously at every stage of the disease. You're less likely to get early, sophisticated testing, less likely to undergo angioplasty, and less likely to have bypass surgery. When you do have those procedures, the statistics say you will be older, sicker, and at higher risk than a man. The director of the National Institutes of Health, Dr. Bernadine Healy, says, "We have to start seeing heart disease as a woman's disease and not as a man's disease in disguise."

If you have chest pain or substantial risk factors, you will want to have a full cardiac evaluation so you can undertake aggressive, early measures. Dr. Jeffrey Borer, a cardiologist at the New York Hospital–Cornell Medical Center, points out that coronary artery disease is a different disease in women. "It's peak incidence is 15–20 years later in life than in men. Events are much less likely to be heralded by chest pain in women than men. Sudden death as a first event is much more common in women than men. The conclusion is that women in the high-risk age group, 65–80, should be screened even if they are asymptomatic!"

What It Is

Coronary Artery Disease is the progressive narrowing of coronary arteries, which deprives heart muscle of the blood flow it needs to pump effectively during exercise and when at rest. This lack of blood flow can lead to angina, a condition in which chest pain occurs because of lack of oxygen to working heart muscle. Clots may also form in these narrowed arteries, causing a heart attack or sudden death. There is considerable controversy about what really causes the fatty deposits to form in coronary arteries, although researchers know the contributing factors well: high blood pressure, elevated cholesterol, a family history of heart disease, obesity, and diabetes.

The exact causes of this disease that afflicts 37 million Americans are unknown. The effect, however, is apparent. The arteries that supply blood to your heart are narrowed by cholesterol deposits, calcium, and other materials. The longer you have the disease, the harder and more extensive the deposits become. Most heart attacks are thought to occur when a blood clot finally blocks the already-restricted flow of blood through these narrowed arteries.

Step 1. Make Sure You Get the Best Care

Read this section on potential problems with your treatment carefully to determine if there are discrepancies between your care and state-of-the-art care. Use Step 2 to review shortcomings.

Risk Factors

If your risk of heart attack is high, the earlier you identify risk factors the better. You and your health care providers can sharply lower them. (That's not true for a variety of other equally serious diseases. A woman with a high risk of breast cancer, for example, has few risk factors she can change that will cut her chances of cancer.) Some key risk factors are:

- High blood fats (for example, high cholesterol)
- Personal history of arteriosclerosis (already affecting your brain or legs)
- More than 30% overweight
- High blood pressure

- Smoking (more than 10 cigarettes day)

- Low HDL cholesterol (the "good" cholesterol)

- Diabetes

- Living alone (after a first heart attack)

- Family history of premature heart attack (before age 55)

Of these, only the last risk, a family history of heart disease, can't be modified. If you have one or more of these risk factors and have, as yet, not been evaluated, make an appointment with your doctor to be screened for coronary artery disease.

Diagnosis

A large and powerful armamentarium of drugs, devices, and procedures, up to and including surgery, can now make a big difference in quality of life and cut your risk of an early, premature death. This makes early diagnosis of paramount importance. The earlier you find out, the more you can do. Many patients who have early warning signs of heart disease delay seeking medical attention for months to years. Jim Fixx, author of *The Complete Book of Running*, was said to have symptoms characteristic of heart disease only days before he died while running. He may have believed that rigorous physical exercise alone would prevent a heart attack. It does not. Although there are simple screening tests for heart disease, the majority of Americans simply ignore them. Remember that the longer you wait for testing and treatment, the greater your chance of suffering a heart attack or dying.

You should not adopt the passive or pessimistic attitude that nothing can be done for the disease. Nothing could be further from the truth. If you have an abnormal sensation in your chest area that occurs consistently during exertion, you need to see a doctor who will take those symptoms seriously. If your doctor isn't worried, you should be. Just because this sensation is not in the middle of your chest does not mean it should be disregarded. You may still have heart disease.

Patients often describe the sensations associated with coronary artery disease as a choking, squeezing, suffocating, heavy, or pressurelike quality. The sensation may appear to travel to the left shoulder, arms, back, neck, stomach, or even teeth. Now, many of us are concerned any time we have a new sensation in our chest, but it is quite clear that such may not be related to heart disease. As an example, a pain that feels like a stitch in your side and gets worse with breathing is not due to a lack of blood flow to your heart. Cardiologists often are excellent sleuths and can tell by asking. But even the best diagnostician can be wrong, which is why they adopt a rather-safe-than-sorry stance on testing and hospitalization. You should too. Never take a chance with abnormal sensations in your chest. I can't count the number of times I've had to console someone at the emergency room door over the death of a spouse because a fatal heart attack was mistaken for indigestion. Don't be confused by a lack of what you call "pain." If you have an abnormal sensation in your chest, call your doctor!

Tests

State-of-the-art diagnosis begins with a complete medical history and physical exam by a physician who sees and treats a wide range of patients with coronary artery disease. Dr. Thomas B. Graboys, Director of the Lown Cardiovascular Center and Professor at Harvard Medical School, says, "The most important aspect of any evaluation for coronary disease is a thorough history and a physical examination. Only then should further testing be contemplated."

Your doctor will be able to establish a preliminary diagnosis by taking a detailed history and carefully examining you. If the doctor recommends a major diagnostic test after this exam, always ask him or her two questions:

- How will my therapy change if the test is positive?

- Does that therapy have a strong likelihood of helping me?

For example, if your doctor recommends an angiogram but is considering neither surgery nor angioplasty, you are wise to resist the procedure. An angiogram, an invasive test in which the doctor threads a long, narrow tube into your heart, carries a small risk of disability or death. For this level of risk, you deserve to derive some benefit. (See the chapter on Angiogram.)

GENERAL SCREENING   Some very simple laboratory tests can tell your doctor a great deal. For instance, a urine analysis may uncover diabetes or kidney disease, both of which can worsen heart disease. A resting EKG may show evidence of a past heart attack or abnormal heart rhythm. Here are the general screening tests:

Blood   Cholesterol, HDL cholesterol, glucose (diabetes), creatinine (kidney function), hematocrit (for anemia), thyroid function (an overactive thyroid caused President George Bush's irregular heart rate).

Chest X-Ray   May show calcium in coronary arteries. (Some experts do not consider this a very good screening test.)

Resting EKG   A technician, nurse, or doctor performs this test while you lie quietly on a table. It's not the same as a stress test, for which you must exercise.

SPECIFIC TESTS FOR CORONARY ARTERY DISEASE   The tests just listed can suggest heart disease and its risk factors but have no degree of precision in determining how well your heart is working and what the possibilities are for making it work better. More sophisticated tests are the only objective assessment of the severity of the disease. Symptoms are a notoriously poor way to evaluate heart disease. Recent studies show that patients often have a more advanced stage of the disease than initially suspected by their doctors. As a result, they are undertreated. Our health care system is not reaching a lot of people. If you're at risk of heart disease, you should have the best testing available to make certain you are safe.

The following section is a little more technical than most in this book, so lets first look at the basics. The stress test is often your doctor's first test of choice. It won't tell you what part of your heart is affected or what your heart function is like. It's really a yes-or-no test. Yes, you have heart disease, or no, you don't. The difficulty is that too often it ends up being a maybe test: Maybe you have heart disease, but then maybe you don't. Newer technology seeks to improve this.

This leads doctors to order heart scans. These can be much more specific. Most use radioactive tracers. Different tracers let doctors look at different kinds of heart function. Some specifically label areas of heart muscle that are badly damaged or destroyed. Others look at how well your heart works as a pump. These tests let your doctor know how bad things are. But the most specific tests show which areas of your heart are not getting the amount of blood flow they should. These tests have the greatest value for future planning. The most valuable of them find areas of the heart that would perform better if only blood flow could be improved.

You needn't understand or remember all of this, but you should be able to ask *why* the test is being done. There are several basic reasons:

- To make a positive diagnosis of coronary artery disease

- To grade how severely your heart's function has deteriorated

- To find areas of the heart that are already damaged

- To find areas of the heart that can be improved by angioplasty or surgery

You can improve the level of your care by finding out why your doctor wants to do a certain test and what he or she plans to do with the result, for instance, refer you for surgery or angioplasty, or change a program of medical therapy. If surgery or angioplasty is the aim, all that a scan can tell you is that an area of heart muscle supplied by a specific blood vessel is not getting the blood flow it should. It doesn't tell you precisely what the problem is. Is the artery severely narrowed throughout its length? And if so, is that blockage able to be bypassed? Or is it too long, too hard, and too difficult to operate on? If so, you'll need an angiogram. In a sense, all tests lead you further toward an angiogram. They're a prelude, unless you end up with a clean bill of health or heart disease too severe to benefit from an operation.

Here are more detailed descriptions of the tests your doctor may order.

EKG Stress Test   This is the granddaddy of cardiac tests. It is a crude measure of coronary artery disease that is best used with patients who already have characteristic symptoms. You will be asked either to progressively walk faster on a treadmill or to progressively pedal on a stationary bicycle. A doctor will monitor changes on an EKG that show that some areas of heart muscle are not getting enough oxygen as you go faster. If you begin to have cardiac symptoms, the doctor will stop the test. Again, at best, stress testing tells you have heart disease and what your exercise tolerance is (see the chapter on Stress Tests). A positive stress test is most likely to be associated with underlying coronary artery disease in a patient who has symptoms. The key issue is the next step. In a patient without symptoms, a negative test confers a relatively high degree of confidence that important coronary artery disease is not present. However, a positive stress test in a patient who has no symptoms provides far less information and would lead to another test of some sort. If the patient has risk factors or a high-risk lifestyle (such as a 60-year-old who plays basketball every evening), then the exercise EKG is a poor choice. This patient is better off choosing a more expensive, more definitive heart scan test from the start.

Echocardiogram   When President Bush developed heart arrhythmia in the spring of 1991, his doctors relied on an echocardiogram to see if his heart was OK. This is a completely safe first step. It provides images made by ultrasonic waves. The echocardiogram helps confirm the presence of an enlarged heart or poor heart function after a heart attack. It may also uncover other reasons you suffer chest pain, such as a narrowed heart valve. The test is good for marked changes, such as an entire section of heart muscle that is diseased and therefore moving poorly when the heart pumps blood. Combined with a doppler device (to assess blood flow) and special imaging techniques, the heart's output (cardiac output) can be measured. This was once possible only with a much more invasive, and potentially risky, test called an angiogram (see the chapter on Angiogram). Cardiac output is an excellent indirect measure of poor heart function when it is low. When your cardiac output is low, your heart's function is poor. All that said, the resting echocardiogram really provides very little useful information for the patient with suspected coronary artery disease. It is not a good prognostic tool for the evaluation of angina. While an exercise or drug-stress echo can be done, it is less useful than the nuclear scans described next. The echo should be used in the evaluation of the patient with known or suspected coronary artery disease if there is a specific question that can be answered with the test. However, there are few such questions. Some cardiologists believe the resting echo is taken as a knee-jerk reaction when a specific question is not being asked, and simply adds to the high cost of health care. The bottom line for you? Make sure you know why the test is ordered.

Cardiac Scans   Heart scans are increasingly impressive as tools to show the location and severity of coronary artery disease. You should exhaust the information that scans can give you before undergoing an angiogram, unless you are in a potentially life-threatening situation or your symptoms cannot be adequately controlled with drugs. Each major medical center has its favorite scans for which they have a large amount of experience. Each scan type is named after the radioactive label employed in that particular scan. Special cameras can see the radioactive material as it flows through the body. In overview, these tests can show three important facets of heart function: the amount of blood your heart can eject with each heartbeat (the less it ejects, the poorer your heart function), areas of heart muscle that have been damaged by a heart attack, and areas of the heart muscle that aren't getting enough blood flow because of blocked or narrowed coronary arteries (so doctors can see what areas can be improved with surgery or angioplasty). As science and technology improve, newer tests will allow your doctor to actually watch a drug work as it's given to determine its effectiveness in you. As newer, cutting-edge scans continue to improve, they may replace much of the need for the angiogram.

Here's specifically what different scans can show.

Radionuclide Ventriculogram (Technetium 99^m)   Should the main pumping chamber of the heart, called the left ventricle, be badly damaged by a heart attack or receive too little blood flow through blocked and narrowed coronary arteries, it will be a much less effective pump. Doctors can tell that because only a small fraction of the blood in the left ventricle is pumped out, technically referred to as a low ejection fraction. Technetium 99^m is attached to red blood cells. In this test, cameras photograph these radioactively labeled red blood cells as they flow through the heart and out into the great vessels. While this test is highly effective in the diagnosis of coronary disease, it is particularly useful for its predictive value: If the result is markedly abnormal, even in the absence of symptoms, then the risk of events is relatively high. In this situation, aggressive treatment, even surgery, may be appropriate. If it's completely normal after exercise, statistically there is a very low chance that you will die from a heart attack in the near future. If it's strongly positive, your heart function is poor, but you probably won't know why or what to do about it until you have further tests.

Acute Infarct Scan (Technetium 99^m)   An infarct scan lights up areas of the heart—"hot spots"—that have been irreversibly damaged by a heart attack. The test is best done 2–3 days after a suspected heart attack to confirm the diagnosis of heart attack. It is little used in cardiology today, having been supplanted by other tests.

Blood Flow Perfusion Imaging Scan (Thallium 201 or Technetium 99^m Isonitrile)   Thallium is actively taken up by working heart muscle cells. If areas of heart muscle are badly damaged or get very little blood, they aren't able to pick up thallium, and so show up as a "cold spot." When combined with gradually increasing exercise, these cold spots begin to appear in areas of the heart that don't get enough blood. That tells doctors that the arteries supplying those areas of muscle are probably narrowed or blocked. Like radionuclide ventriculography, the technique is versatile enough to demonstrate the effectiveness of grafted vessels after coronary artery bypass surgery or the effectiveness of drug or balloon angioplasty. The results can tell your doctor if your heart muscle is not getting enough oxygen, if you have had a heart attack, or if a bypass graft has closed or narrowed after surgery. Since the test can be difficult to interpret in young to middle-age females, it may be a poor choice for them. In recent years, thallium has been replaced in some forms of this test with a new technetium-based agent. The basic concepts involved in this newer form of test are similar to those with thallium.

Positron Emission Tomography (PET) Scan   This test provides beautiful color of the heart. Like the thallium scan, it can find and localize areas of the heart that are getting an inadequate flow of blood. Advocates say there are far fewer false positives than with the thallium scan. Detractors say the technology has not been proven superior to thallium. Here's PET's biggest advantage: One kind of PET scan allows doctors to identify heart muscle that could improve with more blood flow. In other words, this muscle could be salvaged with bypass surgery or balloon angioplasty. (Of note, however, is that critics say thallium performs just as well.) It can also predict if clot-dissolving drugs can save heart muscle damaged during a heart attack. PET scans have limited availability and can be expensive, up to $2,000 for a study.

Magnetic Resonance Imaging (MRI)   This test does not require the injection of radioactive material. That's a real advantage if you are allergic to such substances or want to avoid the radiation. This technique has a great future. For the present, a version called cine MR can determine the amount of blood the heart pumps out with each beat. That gives your doctor a good indication of overall heart function. However, for evaluation of the patient with coronary artery disease, this does not add to the information available from other tests, though there are high expectations for future development.

Angiogram   The most precise method of locating blockages in the arteries and measuring the degree of obstruction is an angiogram, performed at cardiac catheterization, also called an A-gram or a heart cath. In addition to providing information about the coronary arteries, the cath also permits blood flow to be clearly visualized to assess if the heart is functioning normally or if there is a faulty valve or a hole in the heart wall. It also carries the greatest risk, which is why you will want to have an angiogram only if absolutely necessary.

RECOMMENDED ORDER OF TESTS   The rules are not hard and fast for determining the order in which tests are performed. Theoretically, you want to begin with the least dangerous, least costly tests. Dr. Thomas Graboys recommends the following order:

1. Stress test

2. Echocardiogram

3. Scans

4. Angiogram

If an angiogram has been suggested, read the complete chapter on Angiogram in this book. Unless surgery or angioplasty is being seriously considered, you should try to learn as much as you can from other, safer tests first. Dr. Jeffrey Borer, a cardiologist at the New York Hospital–Cornell Medical Center, seriously questions the use of the resting echocardiogram. It may be both irrelevant and unnecessary for most patients with coronary artery disease.

FREQUENCY OF TESTS   Since coronary artery disease is progressive, testing must be repeated. In the absence of a change of symptoms, objective testing should be repeated each year for moderate-to-severe disease. Once a year is a reasonable schedule for stable disease, since the rate of progression is relatively slow and patients seldom change appreciably on objective testing in less than a year. This presupposes that there are no changes in the patient's symptoms and the patient doesn't deny or misinterpret symptoms. A visit to the doctor every six months would be prudent. If you don't repeat the tests, says Dr. Borer, "It's sticking your head in the sand." If, for instance, you suffer from congestive heart failure, a condition in which the heart pump begins to fail and fluid accumulates in the lungs, objective testing is critical to be certain that a heart valve isn't leaking. Stress tests and heart scans are the most logical tests to repeat. An angiogram is too dangerous a test to be done on a routine basis to follow the progress of disease. Last year, a friend of mine's brother died suddenly of a heart attack in his late 30s. He'd had an extremely strong family history and very high cholesterol levels, and he'd skipped his periodic testing. A regular testing schedule would most likely have found a severe narrowing early enough to do something about it.

While symptoms are not good predictors of the seriousness of your disease, you should seek immediate help if they change. This could save your life. In general, if you know you have heart disease, then even if you feel well, a visit to the doctor at six-month intervals is wise, to be certain that potentially important, though subtle, symptoms and signs have not developed.

Treatment

There is no single state-of-the-art treatment for coronary artery disease. You will probably be managed with a variety of medications and procedures over the years you have the disease. The basic tradeoff is risk. Medications carry little risk of causing death or disability. If you opt for surgery or angioplasty, you may feel dramatically better in a very short time, but you risk complications or even death. Therefore, these procedures are often reserved for intolerably severe symptoms or for situations in which objective testing indicates a risk to life which can be significantly reduced. By reading the chapters on Coronary Artery Bypass Surgery and Angioplasty, you will learn how to reduce the risk of these procedures significantly. Hundreds of new devices are being constructed and tested to reduce that risk even further and to increase your doctor's ability to restore blood flow even to completely blocked vessels. (One new laser can stop a heart attack in progress!)

For the day-to-day management of coronary artery disease, there are no new, breakthrough medications. You will probably end up on several drugs. But how judiciously these drugs are combined is a very real art. Since medications carry the lowest risk, if objective testing doesn't reveal important life-threatening disease, you may want to undergo a trial of drug therapy first. If the side effects are intolerable or you cannot return to the activity level you wish, then you will want to explore angioplasty or surgery with your physician. In some cases there is no choice. Acute changes in your condition brought on by large blockages in arteries that threaten your life will force you to consider surgery or angioplasty. This chapter concentrates on the use of medications to treat coronary artery disease.

You may well ask that if medications aren't great and surgery is dangerous, what choice is left? The most stunning new developments in cardiology are preventive. Reversal of coronary artery disease was something scientists once dreamed of. Now it is a reality, with drastic changes being possible with lifestyle alterations or drug therapy. If the disease is caught early enough and before it poses any immediate threat to your health, these preventive measures are the future.

PREVENTIVE TREATMENT   Actual reversal of the narrowing found in coronary arteries is the most important new breakthrough in the treatment of coronary artery disease. A decade ago no one thought it possible. It's not accomplished with high-tech lasers or angioplasty balloons but with decidedly low-tech preventive medicine. Dr. Dean Ornish, a San Francisco physician, has shown that a very low-fat diet, stress reduction, and regular exercise can open narrowed arteries for those who have the motivation to drastically change their lives. He has an excellent book on his program. For others, drug therapy can have the same dramatic effect. Recent studies show that several cholesterol-lowering drugs can open narrowed arteries. A look into the future shows vigorous changes in lifestyle, with diets extremely low in fat (5% and below).

Many of the biggest gains in the battle against coronary artery disease have come through simple measures: diet, exercise, stress management, and control of high blood pressure and cholesterol. The most important change you can make is to quit smoking. Smoking will rapidly accelerate the progress of the disease. It will also reduce your ability to exercise. The most important positive measure you can take is to begin a well-supervised exercise program. If you have diabetes, excellent control of that disease will lower your risk of having a heart attack (see the chapter on Diabetes).

If you are not fighting heart disease with a wide frontal assault, you are taking unnecessary risks. Medication and surgery have their place in the treatment of coronary artery disease, but each carries with it certain risks. Behavioral changes are risk free.

MEDICATIONS BEFORE YOU'VE HAD A HEART ATTACK, TO DECREASE CHEST PAIN Nitrates, beta blockers, and calcium channel blockers all work to reduce chest pain. Your doctor will probably begin with nitrates. By skillfully combining these three medications, your doctor has very powerful tools with which to make you more comfortable. Drugs are best added one at a time, to observe their effect and side effects. The use of all three together is extremely potent and requires great care.

There is no current evidence that these drugs affect the basic underlying process of coronary artery disease. In other words, they are excellent medications for pain relief but won't slow the progress of your disease. Only with a low-fat diet, exercise, stress reduction, cholesterol-lowering drugs, and other disease-modifying measures can you do that.

Nitrates For chest pain relief, nitrates are usually the drugs of first choice. The most effective is nitroglycerin, because it enters your system so quickly and at such high levels. A common form is the small nitroglycerin tablet that is placed under your tongue. There are other, longer-acting forms of nitrates available as skin patches, gum, or pills. Nitrates work by decreasing the workload of your heart. If nitrates alone do not ease or remove your chest pain, your doctor may add a beta blocker or calcium channel blocker.

A note of caution: If there is any dramatic worsening in the intensity or duration of your chest pain, the faster you are in the hands of emergency medical personnel, the better. If the pain does not improve after 10–15 minutes on nitroglycerin, you may be suffering a heart attack and should make arrangements to be seen in an emergency room. Side effects include headache and dizziness.

Beta Blockers   Beta blockers work to reduce chest pain by sharply dropping the force of the heart's contractions, the heart rate, blood pressure, and the heart's output during exercise. The decreased work the heart has to do reduces the chest pain. These drugs are not well tolerated by some patients, because they can cause fatigue, depression, cold extremities, and impotence. Beta blockers may worsen asthma and diabetes. These drugs not only prevent angina but also reduce the risk of another heart attack among patients who have suffered a heart attack recently. Many experienced cardiologists believe they can prevent a heart attack even if you haven't already had one, although research doesn't yet bear that out. They use beta blockers both for risk reduction and to decrease chest pain. Beta blockers still don't affect the basic underlying disease.

Calcium Channel Blockers   Calcium channel blockers work very effectively to reduce chest pain, by reducing blood pressure and the force of the heart's contractions in order to decrease the heart's workload. These are the newest pain-reduction drugs. They are excellent for reducing high blood pressure. However, if you are taking these drugs to slow the steady progression of coronary artery disease, the evidence is not there yet. They may be used alone or in combination with beta blockers and/or nitrates. The three together are a formidable triple threat, but carry high potential for adverse effect if improperly managed. Two additional notes: You may also be given certain calcium channel blockers for arrhythmias such as paroxysmal atrial tachycardia and atrial fibrillation. A November 1991 American Heart Association Abstract showed that patients taking calcium channel blockers when they had a heart attack had higher death rates than comparable patients on no drugs or on beta blockers. However, animal studies suggest calcium channel blockers may slow down the progress of coronary artery disease. There is no clear evidence in humans to date. Side effects include flushing, skin rash, and constipation.

MEDICATIONS THAT CAN PREVENT OR STOP HEART ATTACKS

Aspirin   Aspirin may be the most effective medicine available to reduce your risk of heart attack. It does not accomplish that by changing your underlying disease or slowing the narrowing of your coronary arteries, as cholesterol-lowering medications might. It prevents the onset of a heart attack by preventing clot formation in narrowed coronary arteries. In other words, aspirin is a great safety belt, but isn't going to slow the progression of your illness and isn't a substitute for preventive measures.

Precisely how much should be used and under what circumstances is not fully known. Most cardiologists recommend limiting aspirin use to one tablet a day (325 mg is a full adult-sized aspirin). As little as 30 mg of aspirin may be enough to provide protection against a heart attack without increasing the risk of internal bleeding, ulcers, or stroke. Many cardiologists compromise by prescribing baby aspirin, which are 80 mg each. While aspirin may benefit any patient with coronary artery disease, those who have unstable chest pain or who have had a previous heart attack are most likely to benefit.

Clot-Dissolving Drugs (Thrombolytics)   These drugs have been the most miraculous breakthrough cardiology drugs of the last several decades. They can literally stop a heart attack in its tracks. They work to dissolve the blood clot that has completely closed a narrowed coronary artery and caused the heart attack. Even though these drugs are given once a heart attack has begun, I mention them in this section for a good reason: They can quite literally save your life. In the best of cases they stop a heart attack in progress and prevent much of the damage to heart muscle that would occur without it. If you have coronary artery disease, you should discuss these drugs with your doctor in advance, to determine if they are right for you by looking at risk factors you may have for their use, including bleeding tendencies, uncontrolled high blood pressure, and older age. In that way, should you have a heart attack, you can be given one of these drugs as soon as possible for the greatest possible advantage. The two most widely used thrombolytics are TPA and streptokinase. Future thombolytics will probably work with even less risk or complication.

MEDICATIONS FOR AFTER A HEART ATTACK

Aspirin   If you've already had a heart attack, aspirin can prevent a second attack and sudden death. You should consider an aspirin a day if you have had a heart attack. If you have had a stroke or near stroke, called a transient ischemic attack (TIA), then take note that research has demonstrated that aspirin therapy can prevent both strokes and heart attacks.

Beta Blockers   The patients most likely to benefit from beta blockers have had a recent heart attack. The drugs are most effective in the first six months following that attack, but current research shows that the beneficial effect may last for two or more years. If you've recently had a heart attack, ask your doctor about taking beta blockers.

Vasodilators   These drugs may help the heart repair itself in a healthier way after a very large heart attack, called an anterior myocardial infarction. If you've had a major heart attack, you should ask if vasodilators might help you. It is quite clear that they can also improve life expectancy if you have congestive heart failure. One drug in this category, enalapril, has been shown to reduce the chance of death by 16%. In combination, the vasodilators of hydralazine and isosorbide dinitrate improve your survival and your ability to exercise, if you have congestive heart failure.

Anticoagulants   If you've had a major heart attack, these drugs can prevent the formation of blood clots that may dislodge from your heart and cause a stroke. They may also prevent a second heart attack.

Angiotensin-Converting Enzyme (ACE) Inhibitors   Newly published research shows that ACE inhibitors can cut your long-term risk of death after suffering a heart attack. These are not yet in widespread use, but be certain to ask your doctor whether they may be right for you.

MEDICATIONS TO TREAT ATRIAL ARRHYTHMIAS   A majority of Americans suffer irregular heartbeats on occasion. You've probably felt your heart skip a beat from time to time. Physicians classify heart rhythms by the part of the heart they occur in. Those that occur in the heart's booster pump, or atrium, are called atrial arrhythmias. President George Bush had one of those called atrial fibrillation. The key danger with atrial arrhythmias is that they will drive your heart too fast, causing you to feel short of breath or to suffer chest pain. In Bush's case, there was the additional risk of blood clots forming in his atrium. Otherwise, however, physicians worry a great deal less about atrial arrhythmias because they are generally not life-threatening. They may be treated with a variety of medications to slow the rhythm to an acceptable level or even to try to convert it to a normal rhythm. Because you may lose the normal "booster" effect of the atrium, doctors would like you to have a normal heart rhythm.

This is sometimes achieved by using an electrical current in a procedure called cardioversion. The newest technique involves surgery in which doctors sever flawed electrical circuits in the heart, a technique currently being performed on patients with atrial fibrillation. When there is only a single bad circuit, or "pathway," doctors can now cut that pathway using a long catheter that they thread into the heart. The catheter may deliver a laser pulse, a special radio frequency, or other power source as a means of precision destruction of the flawed pathway. A condition called Wolf-Parkinson-White syndrome is widely and successfully treated with this technique. In fact, a friend and patient of mine—Sam Osborne, the great cross-country ski racer—used to become weak and wobbly-kneed when he raced. His coaches thought he had a head problem. I stress-tested him in my laboratory and found his heart racing at over 240 beats a minute. He had Wolf-Parkinson-White syndrome. For 10 years, he couldn't compete or work out hard without the threat of a very fast heart rhythm. Then last year he had a catheter threaded into his heart, enabling doctors to destroy the flawed pathway. Within a few months, he was able to complete the New York Marathon, and now no longer has any signs or symptoms of his former illness.

MEDICATIONS TO TREAT VENTRICULAR ARRHYTHMIAS   While medications can be enormously helpful in the prevention and treatment of heart disease and for the treatment of atrial arrhythmias, you should be alert to the inappropriate use of antiarrhythmia drugs for what are called ventricular arrhythmias. These occur in the heart's main pumping chamber, called the ventricle. If you have no other symptoms, it's doubtful you belong on medication. "Only a fraction of patients with extra beats will ever require therapy," states Dr. Thomas Graboys.

In the past, medications were prescribed widely for this condition. Doctors whose patients were known to have ventricular arrhythmias and later had fainting episodes or even died were justifiably anxious about "doing nothing." However, research does not support the use of medications most of the time. There are, of course, dangerous heart rhythm disturbances. They are dangerous because they can keep your heart from pumping blood effectively enough to keep you alive. Given this danger, there is a real temptation for physicians to "do something" for a disturbance of heart rhythm that might be a precursor to these fatal rhythms. You should resist this effort until special tests are performed to determine if this problem poses any risk to you. In most cases it doesn't.

In those cases where the rhythm is potentially dangerous, it isn't clear that treatment is any better than doing nothing at all. You want to be very conservative about the use of drugs, because they can be dangerous in and of themselves. Several studies among people recovering from heart attacks have shown that more patients died by taking certain medications for ventricular arrhythmias than by not taking them. Many cardiologists no longer prescribe antiarrhythmia drugs for ventricular arrhythmias except in clearly life-threatening circumstances. You can check with a cardiologist, the American Heart Association, the Food and Drug Administration, or the National Heart, Lung and Blood Institute for the latest list of dangerous antiarrhythmia drugs. In many cases where something *must* be done, cardiologists will appropriately insert a type of pacemaker, called an implantable defibrillator, which can restore your heart rhythm to normal once it senses a dangerous arrhythmia.

The best way to find out if you need medication and to see if that medication actually works for you is to undergo state-of-the-art diagnostic testing, in a special electrophysiology unit where doctors can probe and test your heart's electrical system. They will try to provoke the most dangerous electrical disturbance in your heart they can to see if you are vulnerable to life-threatening arrhythmias. If you are, they will place you on your drug of choice and then retest to make certain it is working properly. Without that proof, treatment is a gamble.

Treatment is a huge dilemma because patients complain about multiple irregular heartbeats that worry them and their doctors. Many patients force their doctors to "do something" even though it is not in their best interest. This is one clear-cut case where a trip to a cardiologist who specializes in arrhythmias at a major center with an electrophysiology lab is time and money well spent.

WISE USE OF MEDICATION   If you become light-headed or short of breath on medication or if you suffer other intolerable side effects, let your doctor know immediately.

To minimize side effects, start using drugs one at a time to determine which works best, with the fewest side effects. Many health care providers pile on heart medications one after another. They fail to monitor the side effects closely enough. You could easily end up on eight different medications, ranging from anticholesterol and antihypertensive agents to drugs that alleviate chest pain and prevent heart attacks. Be suspicious if you are given a handful of prescriptions after your first trip to the doctor for chest pain. Often there is little rationale for so many drugs. Doctors may prescribe their use for ill-defined "prevention" rather than for any expected improvement in your condition. If you are feeling well and have no symptoms, you need to ask if these medicines are necessary.

Make sure your doctor is aware of any other existing diseases you may have. Beta blockers, for instance, can change your insulin requirements if you are a diabetic, or can worsen your asthma. Heart medications can also aggravate prostate conditions or peripheral vascular disease. If you have another chronic illness, make certain that all your medicines are coordinated. Otherwise you risk unwanted reactions among the drugs.

Step 2. Look for Shortcomings

I hope that by reading Step 1 you get a good feeling about your treatment and that you understand much of it better. You'll learn even more by calling organizations listed in Step 4. But if you have an uncomfortable feeling that your treatment is not on track, then study this section, which specifies some common and serious shortcomings that experts in the field recognize. If this section confirms your suspicions, you should go on to Step 3. Some of these mistakes you can discover yourself; others only an expert can confirm.

MISTAKES IN DIAGNOSIS

You fail to get early screening tests.

You have had early warning signs of heart disease months to a year or more before seeking medical attention.

You have a more serious stage of the disease than your health care provider diagnosed and are being undertreated as a result.

You have a murmur or other condition that has not been evaluated by a cardiologist and could account for your condition.

You rely on symptoms as an indicator of how severe your disease is.

You ignore a change in symptoms.

Your health care provider doesn't take your symptoms seriously.

You don't see a doctor who is competent to undertake the full range of diagnostic tests and treatments.

Your doctor is unaware of other diseases you have.

You are being treated without a proper diagnosis.

You face long delays in diagnosis and referral to specialists or advanced diagnostic tests so your health plan can save money.

You are a woman over 65 and have not been screened.

You are a man over 50 and have not been screened.

MISTAKES IN TREATMENT

You don't get the medications, surgeries, or procedures required at your stage of the disease.

You take antiarrhythmia drugs that could be harmful to you.

You have a pacemaker, or are scheduled to get one, that you don't need.

You smoke and thereby hasten your disease.

You're a fatalist and assume a passive or pessimistic attitude to your care, assuming that little can be done.

You doctor does not refer you to the specialists you need.

You notice no improvement on your medications, or you feel worse because of side effects that alter your quality of life.

You take a variety of heart medicines without any clear benefit or strategy.

You are put on multiple medications all at the same time.

You are scheduled for bypass surgery at a center that does few of these operations, lacks an experienced operating room team, or has poor outcome.

Step 3. See a Specialist

If, from Step 2, you are concerned that your care is not state-of-the-art, this section will tell you how to choose an expert.

Many physicians have a real reluctance to refer patients to regional medical centers. Sometimes, primary care doctors aren't aware of the leading heart centers in their area or, even if they do know them, they fear that a referral will result in the loss of a patient. But cardiac care is a quickly changing specialty. Unless a doctor is devoting most of her or his time to the treatment of heart disease, it is difficult to keep up.

The Doctor

You will want to begin with a board-certified cardiologist. Almost every community in America has excellent cardiologists. Cardiologists also have different subspecialties. Some supervise coronary intensive care units; others spend much of their time in a catheterization laboratory. If you have a specific problem, you can seek out one of these subspecialties. You will want a doctor who spends most of his or her time with patients who have case histories similar to yours. If you've had a heart attack and have congestive heart failure, you'll want to see a doctor at a major university center that has active research programs in this area. If you are at high risk for coronary artery disease, you'll want a physician who practices preventive medicine and will motivate you to make the necessary lifestyle changes. If you have very high cholesterol, you'll want to see a lipid specialist. If you develop new chest pain, you'll want, at the very least, a referral to a doctor who performs diagnostic testing and can evaluate your need for sophisticated testing. Top academic cardiologists emphasize emphatically that noncardiologists often do not evaluate coronary artery disease accurately.

Centers of Excellence for Coronary Artery Disease

Although community hospitals offer the convenience and expertise to care for many heart disease patients, you want to be certain you are at a center of excellence if complications develop or risky procedures are recommended. That could be your local hospital, but it may not be. See the chapters on Stress Test, Angiogram, Coronary Artery Bypass Surgery, and Angioplasty for the respective lists of centers of excellence. Here is a list of centers of excellence in coronary artery disease.

The following list of hospitals is provided only as a convenient starting place in your search for excellence. These hospitals are recommended on the basis of reputation, not experience and results. The list is not an endorsement. There may be hospitals just as excellent that have been omitted. You should apply the guidelines for experience, results, and other measures of excellence to any hospital you choose, whether or not it is on this list.

Although hospitals from different sources have been combined into one list, the compilation in no way implies that one source has endorsed the hospital list of another source.

ALABAMA
University of Alabama
   Medical Center   BIM
619 So. 19th St/University
   Station
Birmingham, AL 35294

ARIZONA
University of Arizona Health
   Sciences Center   BIM
1501 No. Campbell Ave
Tucson, AZ 85724

CALIFORNIA
Cedars Sinai Medical Center   EX
8700 Beverly Blvd
Los Angeles, CA 90048

Moffitt Hospital   EX
University of California
San Francisco Medical Center
505 Parnassus Ave
San Francisco, CA 94143

San Francisco Cardiovascular
   Institute   EX
UCSF
505 Parnassus Ave
San Francisco, CA 94143

Stanford University School
   of Medicine   BIM/EX
300 Pasteur Dr
Stanford, CA 94305

COLORADO
University of Colorado Health
   Sciences Center   BIM
4200 E Ninth Ave
Denver, CO 80262

CONNECTICUT
Yale–New Haven Hospital   BIM
333 Cedar St
New Haven, CT 06510

DISTRICT OF COLUMBIA
Georgetown University Hospital   EX
3800 Reservoir Rd NW
Washington, DC 20007

FLORIDA
Jackson Memorial Hospital   BIM
1611 NW 12th Ave
Miami, FL 33136

University of Florida College
   of Medicine   EX
Box J-215, J. Hillis Miller
   Health Center
Gainesville, FL 32610

GEORGIA
Emory University Hospital   BIM/EX
1364 Clifton Road NE
Atlanta, GA 30322

ILLINOIS
Northwestern University
   Medical Center   BIM
250 E Superior St
Chicago, IL 60611

University of Chicago Hospitals   EX
5841 So. Maryland Ave
Chicago, IL 60637

MARYLAND
Johns Hopkins Hospital   BIM
600 No. Wolfe St
Baltimore, MD 21205

MASSACHUSETTS
Brigham and Women's Hospital   BIM
75 Francis St
Boston, MA 02115

Children's Hospital   BIM
300 Longwood Ave
Boston, MA 02115

Lown Cardiovascular Center EX
21 Longwood Ave
Brookline, MA 02146

Massachusetts General Hospital BIM/EX
55 Fruit St
Boston, MA 02114

MICHIGAN
University of Michigan Hospitals EX
1500 E Medical Center Dr
Ann Arbor, MI 48109

MINNESOTA
Mayo Clinic BIM/EX
200 First St SW
Rochester, MN 55905

University of Minnesota Medical
School—Minneapolis EX
UMHC Box 293
420 Delaware St SE
Minneapolis, MN 55455

MISSOURI
Mid-America Heart Institute EX
St Luke's Hospital
Wornall Road at 44th St
Kansas City, MO 64111

NEW YORK
Columbia Presbyterian
Medical Center EX
630 W 168th St
New York, NY 10032

Mount Sinai Hospital EX
One Gustave Levy Pl
New York, NY 10029

New York Hospital–Cornell
Medical Center BIM/EX
525 E 68th St
New York, NY 01121

New York University Medical
Center EX
560 First Ave
New York, NY 10016

NORTH CAROLINA
Duke University Medical Center BIM
Box 3005
Durham, NC 27710

Duke University Hospitals EX
Box 3708
Erwin Rd.
Durham, NC 27710

OHIO
Cleveland Clinic Foundation BIM/EX
One Clinic Center
9500 Euclid Ave
Cleveland, OH 44106

Ohio State University College
of Medicine EX
200 Meiling Hall
370 W Ninth Ave
Columbus, OH 43210

University of Cincinnati
College of Medicine EX
231 Bethesda Ave
Cincinnati, OH 45267-0555

PENNSYLVANIA
Children's Hospital of
Philadelphia BIM
34th St at Civic Center Blvd
Philadelphia, PA 19104

Hahnemann University Hospital BIM
Broad and Vine Sts.
Philadelphia, PA 19102

Hospital of the University of
Pennsylvania EX
3400 Spruce St
Philadelphia, PA 19102

University of Pennsylvania
School of Medicine EX
36th and Hamilton Walk
Philadelphia, PA 19104-6015

TENNESSEE
Vanderbilt University Medical
   Center   BIM
1211 22nd Ave S
Nashville, TN 37232

TEXAS
Baylor College of Medicine
   and Hospitals   BIM
One Baylor Plaza
Houston, TX 77030

St Luke's Episcopal Hospital   EX
Texas Heart Institute
1101 Bates St
Houston, TX 77030

VIRGINIA
Virginia Commonwealth
   University   EX
Medical College of Virginia
   School of Medicine
Box 565, MCV Station
Richmond, VA 23298

University of Virginia Hospital   BIM
Jefferson Park Ave
Charlottesville, VA 22908

WASHINGTON
University of Washington
   Hospitals   EX
Harborview Medical Center
325 9th Ave
Seattle, WA 98194

University of Washington
   Medical Center   BIM
1959 NE Pacific St
Seattle, WA 98195

SOURCES

EX   indicates those hospitals recommended by experts interviewed.

BIM   indicates those hospitals recommend by *The Best in Medicine.*

Step 3. Become Your Own Expert

WHO TO CALL

American Heart Association   They can provide educational literature that will help you to understand your disease.

7320 Greenville Ave
Dallas, TX 75231
214/373-6300

Mended Hearts   This is a national group with over 200 chapters and 22,000 members. Volunteers visit people in the hospital before and after cardiac surgery. Individual chapters conduct educational programs and hold support groups once a month. Its publication, *Heartbeat,* covers diet, nutrition, exercise, research updates, new books—anything that might interest the heart patient.

7320 Greenville Ave
Dallas, TX 75231
214/706-1442

Coronary Club   This organization publishes *Heartline* about cardiac care
and a pocket guide to cardiac drugs available for $6.95. The 10 local chapters have
support group and educational meetings once a month.

Cleveland Clinic Foundation
9500 Euclid Ave, Rm. E4-15
Cleveland, OH 44195
216/444-3690

American College of Cardiology   This medical society publishes guidelines
and position papers on cardiac care.

9111 Old Georgetown Rd
Bethesda, MD 20814
800/253-4636

New Heart Society   This is a support group for heart-transplant and heart-
lung-transplant patients. Their newsletter, *Change of Heart*, is published nine
time a year.

10210 No. 32nd St, Ste. C201
Phoenix, AZ 85028
602/867-7172

TRIO   This group provides support before, during, and after organ transplant operations, to patients and families. The 37 chapters meet once a month,
with guest speakers. A national meeting once a year brings together recipients
from all over the world. Patient literature is available.

244 No. Bellefield Ave
Pittsburgh, PA 15213
412/687-2210

United Network for Organ Sharing (UNOS)   This organization holds the
federal contract for allocation and distribution of all organs in the United States.
It maintains a scientific registry of potential patients and tracks recipients to get
quality-of-life studies. It provides information on cost, survival rates, and other
topics. *UNOS UPDATE,* a monthly newsletter, covers all issues relating to transplantation.

1100 Boulders Pkwy, Ste. 500
Richmond, VA 23225
800/243-6667

NIH CRISP System

301/496-7543

University-Affiliated Teaching Hospitals   See Appendix.

Further Resources: NIH Specialized Centers—
National Heart, Lung, and Blood Institute

The following centers have been designated as specialized research centers in specific areas for the treatment of coronary artery disease.

ARTERIOSCLEROSIS

Bowman Gray School of Medicine,
Wake Forest University
Winston-Salem, NC

University of California, San Diego
La Jolla, CA

University of Iowa,
Iowa City, IA

University of California
San Francisco, CA

University of Chicago
Chicago, IL

Columbia University
New York, NY

Baylor College of Medicine
Houston, TX

ARRHYTHMIAS   These centers study the suppression of asymptomatic ventricular arrhythmias in patients who have had a heart attack.

University of Washington
Seattle, WA

Baylor College of Medicine
Houston, TX

University of Alabama
Birmingham, AL

University of Calgary
Calgary, Alberta, Canada

Case Western Reserve
Cleveland, OH

Columbia University
New York, NY

Emory University
Atlanta, GA

University of Gothenburg
Gothenburg, Sweden

Hahnemann University
Philadelphia, PA

Henry Ford Hospital
Detroit, MI

University of Maryland
Baltimore, MD

Medical College of Virginia
Richmond, VA

University of Minnesota
Minneapolis, MN

Montreal Heart Institute
Montreal, Quebec, Canada

Oregon Health Sciences University
Portland, OR

Ottawa Heart Institute
Ottawa, Ontario, Canada

Rhode Island Hospital
Providence, RI

University of Rochester
Rochester, NY

Rush-Presbyterian-St Luke's Medical
    Center
Chicago, IL

Salt Lake Clinic Research Foundation
Salt Lake City, UT

St Louis University Medical Center
St Louis, MO

Vanderbilt University
Nashville, TN

Medlantic Research Foundation of
    Washington Healthcare Corp.
Washington, DC

New York University State Research
    Foundation
Brooklyn, NY

The George Washington University
Washington, DC

University of Kentucky Research
    Foundation
Lexington, KY

CHILDREN AND DIET   These centers study the feasibility, acceptability, efficacy, and safety of dietary intervention in children and adolescents with elevated low-density lipoprotein cholesterol levels.

Northwestern University
Chicago, IL

Maryland Medical Research Institute,
    Inc.
Baltimore, MD

Kaiser Foundation Research Institute
Portland, OR

University of Iowa
Iowa City, IA

University of Medicine and Dentistry of
    New Jersey
Newark, NJ

The Johns Hopkins University
Baltimore, MD

Children's Hospital
New Orleans, LA

CHILD AND ADOLESCENT CARDIOVASCULAR HEALTH   These centers study the effectiveness of school-based risk-reduction interventions involving three components: cardiovascular curriculum, parent participation, and environmental changes in the school.

University of Minnesota
Minneapolis, MN

University of California, San Diego
La Jolla, CA

Boston University
Boston, MA

Louisiana State University Medical
    Center
New Orleans, LA

University of Texas Health Science
    Center
Houston, TX

ISCHEMIC HEART DISEASE   These centers study the underlying basis of ischemic heart disease, from basic to clinical investigations.

Washington University
St Louis, MO (IHD)

The Johns Hopkins University
Baltimore, MD (IHD)

University of Alabama
Birmingham, AL (IHD)

University of Texas
Southwestern Medical School
Dallas, TX (IHD)

Duke University
Durham, NC (IHD)

University of California at San Diego
La Jolla, CA (IHD)

University of Iowa
Iowa City, IA (IHD)

EXPERT SOURCES

Although dozens of experts were interviewed for these chapters, these physicians are acknowledged for their significant contributions to this section.

Dr. Jeffrey S. Borer, Gladys and Roland Harriman Professor of Cardiovascular Medicine, New York Hospital–Cornell Medical Center, New York, NY

Dr. Thomas B. Graboys, Director, Lown Cardiovascular Center, Harvard Medical School, Boston, MA

REFERENCES AND SUGGESTED READING

American Heart Association. *1991 Heart and Stroke Facts.*

Barvik, Stale, and others. Effect of Timolol on Cardiopulmonary Exercise Performance in Men After Myocardial Infarction. *American Journal of Cardiology,* Vol. 69, No. 3 (Jan. 15, 1992), pp. 163–168.

Boehrer, James D., and others. Influence of Collateral Filling of the Occluded Infarct-Related Coronary Artery on Prognosis After Acute Myocardial Infarction. *American Journal of Cardiology,* Vol. 69, No. 1 (Jan. 1, 1992), pp. 10–12.

Bonzheim, Scott C., and others. Physiologic Responses to Recumbent Versus Upright Cycle Ergometry, and Implications for Exercise Prescription in Patients with Coronary Artery Disease. *American Journal of Cardiology,* Vol. 69, No. 1 (Jan. 1, 1992), pp. 40–44.

Boucher, Charles A., and others. Technetium-99ᵐ Sestamibi Myocardial Imaging at Rest for Assessment of Myocardial Infarction and First-Pass Ejection Fraction. *American Journal of Cardiology,* Vol. 69, No. 1 (Jan. 1, 1992), pp. 22–27.

Buxton, Alfred E. Antiarrhythmic Drugs: Good for Premature Ventricular Complexes but Bad for Patients? [editorial] *Annals of Internal Medicine,* Vol. 116, No. 5 (Mar. 1, 1992), pp. 420–422.

Carney, Robert M., and others. Psychosocial Adjustment of Patients Arriving Early at the Emergency Department After Acute Myocardial Infarction. *American Journal of Cardiology,* Vol. 69, No. 3 (Jan. 15, 1992), pp. 160–162.

Chaudhary, Hemant, and others. Tissue Plasminogen Activator Using a Rapid-Infusion Low-Dose Regimen for Unstable Angina. *American Journal of Cardiology,* Vol. 69, No. 3 (Jan. 15, 1992), pp. 173–175.

Chronic Coronary Artery Constriction Leads to Moderate Myocyte Loss and Left Ventricular Dysfunction and Failure in Rats. *Journal of Clinical Investigation,* Vol. 89, No. 2 (Feb. 1992), pp. 618–629.

D'Agostino, Ralph B., and others. A Comparison Between Lovastatin and Gemfibrozil in the Treatment of Primary Hypercholesterolemia. *American Journal of Cardiology,* Vol. 69, No. 1 (Jan. 1, 1992), pp. 28–34.

Effects on Coronary Artery Disease of Lipid-Lowering Diet, or Diet Plus Cholestyramine, in the St. Thomas' Atherosclerosis Regression Study (STARS). *Lancet,* Vol. 339, No. 8793 (Mar. 7, 1992), pp. 563–569.

Graboys, T. B. Antiarrhythmic Drug Selection in the Patient with Malignant Ventricular Arrhythmia—What Is a Realistic Therapeutic Objective? *Proceedings of the 3rd International Symposium on Holter monitoring,* Vienna, 1988, p. 145.

Gressin, Virginie, and others. Holter Recording of Ventricular Arrhythmias During Intravenous Thrombolysis for Acute Myocardial Infarction. *American Journal of Cardiology,* Vol. 69, No. 3 (Jan. 15, 1992), pp. 152–159.

Hilton, Thomas C., and others. Prognostic Significance of Exercise Thallium-201 Testing in Patients Aged >=70 Years with Known or Suspected Coronary Artery Disease. *American Journal of Cardiology,* Vol. 69, No. 1 (Jan. 1, 1992), pp. 45–50.

Hong, Mun K., and others. Effects of Estrogen Replacement Therapy on Serum Lipid Values and Angiographically Defined Coronary Artery Disease in Postmenopausal Women. *American Journal of Cardiology,* Vol. 69, No. 3 (Jan. 15, 1992), pp. 176–178.

How to Choose a Doctor and Hospital If You Have Coronary Artery Disease. Cleveland: Cleveland Clinic Division of Health Affairs, 1992.

Illingworth, D. Roger, and others. Hypocholesterolaemic Effects of Lovastatin in Familial Defective Apolipoprotein B-100. *Lancet,* Vol. 339, No. 8793 (Mar. 7, 1992), pp. 598–600.

King, Kathleen B., and others. Coronary Artery Disease: Patterns of Referral and Recovery in Women and Men Undergoing Coronary Artery Bypass Grafting. *American Journal of Cardiology,* Vol. 69, No. 3 (Jan. 15, 1992), pp. 179–182.

King, Kathleen B., and others. Patterns of Referral and Recovery in Women and Men Undergoing Coronary Artery Bypass Grafting. *American Journal of Cardiology,* Vol. 69, No. 3 (Jan. 15, 1992), pp. 179–182.

Lee, Thomas H., and others. Long-Term Survival of Emergency Department Patients with Acute Chest Pain. *American Journal of Cardiology,* Vol. 69, No. 3 (Jan. 15, 1992), pp. 145–151.

Maublant, Jean C., and others. Comparison Between Thallium-201 and Technetium-99^m Methoxyisobutyl Isonitrile Defect Size in Single-Photon Emission Computed Tomography at Rest, Exercise and Redistribution in Coronary Artery Disease. *American Journal of Cardiology,* Vol. 69, No. 3 (Jan. 15, 1992), pp. 183–187.

National Heart Lung and Blood Institute. *Data Fact Sheet: Morbidity from Coronary Heart Disease in the United States,* June 1990.

Peuhkurinen, Keijo J., and others. Blood Pressure, Plasma Atrial Natriuretic Peptide and Catecholamines During Rapid Ventricular Pacing and Effects of Beta-Adrenergic Blockade in Coronary Artery Disease. *American Journal of Cardiology,* Vol. 69, No. 1 (Jan. 1, 1992), pp. 35–39.

Ramsay, L. E., and others. *Finnish trial of cardiovascular disease prevention* [letters to the editor]. *Lancet,* Vol. 339, No. 8793 (1992), p. 628.

Ranjadayalan, K., and others. Platelet Size and Outcome After Myocardial Infarction [letters to the editor]. *Lancet,* Vol. 339, No. 8793 (Mar. 7, 1992), p. 625.

Results of the Survival and Ventricular Enlargement Study (SAVE), presented at the Symposium of the American College of Cardiology, April 14, 1992, Dallas, TX. Presented by Marc A. Pfeffer and Eugene Braunwald, Brigham and Women's Hospital, Harvard Medical School.

Steinberg, Jonathan S., and others. Predicting Arrhythmic Events After Acute Myocardial Infarction Using the Signal-Averaged Electrocardiogram *American Journal of Cardiology,* Vol. 69, No. 1 (Jan. 1, 1992), pp. 13–21.

Transdermal Nitroglycerin Cooperative Study. Acute and Chronic Antianginal Efficacy of Continuous 24-Hour Application of Transdermal Nitroglycerin. *American Journal of Cardiology,* Vol. 68, No. 13 (Nov. 15, 1991), pp. 1263–1273.

Wong, Wilson, and others. Pharmacology of the Class III Antiarrhythmic Agent Sematilide in Patients with Arrhythmias. *American Journal of Cardiology,* Vol. 69, No. 3 (Jan. 15, 1992), pp. 206–212.

Zaret, Barry L., and others. Assessment of Global and Regional Left Ventricular Performance at Rest and During Exercise After Thrombolytic Therapy for Acute Myocardial Infarction: Results of the Thrombolysis in Myocardial Infarction (TIMI) II Study. *American Journal of Cardiology,* Vol. 69, No. 1 (Jan. 1, 1992), pp. 1–9.

Depression

Risk for Inappropriate Care EXTREMELY HIGH

Up to 90% of persons with depression can be treated successfully, but only one in three ever seeks treatment. Those who seek help may not find it, according to a National Institute of Mental Health Depression Awareness and Recognition Report. The report states, "Current evidence suggests that too often depression is poorly recognized, undertreated, or inappropriately treated by the health care system. The inadequate care, which results from a lack of understanding or a misunderstanding of depression, is expensive and tragic."

Depression can lead to divorce, unemployment, alcohol and drug abuse, and suicide. Among suicide victims, researchers judged that more than half were depressed. One study concluded that among people who have no histories of mental disorder, only 1% attempt suicide. Among those with a lifetime history of depression, up to 24% try to take their own lives.

More than 10 million people in the United States will suffer a depressive illness this year. Women are twice as likely as men to be depressed. Researchers don't fully understand the reason.

What It Is

Depression is a mood disorder. Patients express a loss of interest in life, a lack of pleasure in almost all activities they previously enjoyed, and a feeling of hopelessness and worthlessness. A depressed person seems to look at the world through black glasses that minimize or negate accomplishments and achievements. A depressed person's "gloominess" is vastly different from "the blues" or grief, moods that strike everyone from time to time and that eventually lift. A depressed person suffers from feelings of sadness that, in most severe form, are profoundly incapacitating. One reason sufferers fail to seek help is that, seized by an overwhelming sense of hopelessness, they simply do not believe they can get better. Some depressed people consider depression a sign of personal weakness of character and do not want to admit or seek help.

Three different clinical patterns characterize depression:

MAJOR DEPRESSION This pattern is marked by the symptoms of sadness, dejection, loss of self-esteem, and decreased energy. It interferes with the ability to work, eat, or enjoy otherwise pleasurable activities. People who are depressed have trouble sleeping, often awakening in the early morning. They experience loss of appetite and they lose weight. These are the obvious physiologic signs of depression. Major depression may occur once, twice, or several times in a life-time. This condition is also called *unipolar* illness, since it is characterized by only depression, not mania.

MANIC DEPRESSION   This pattern involves cycles of depression alternating with mania. In the manic phase, symptoms can include hyperactivity, aggressive be-havior, irritability, grandiose notions, and poor judgment leading to excessive drinking, promiscuity, and foolish overspending. Many scientists theorize that the disorder stems from an imbalance of neurochemicals in the brain. Manic depression also has a genetic component. Researchers have found faulty genes in family members who have manic depressive illness but not in relatives without a history of manic depressive illness. Mental health professionals use the term *bipolar* for this combination of manic and depressive components.

DEPRESSIVE NEUROSIS   This is a less severe form of the disease. Chronic symp-toms keep sufferers from functioning at their best or from feeling good. Symp-toms are not disabling. Depressive neurotics may develop major depressive epi-sodes, but the condition is really considered a form of neurosis accompanied by anxiety, tension, and depression.

Step 1. Make Sure You Get the Best Care

Read this section on potential problems with your treatment carefully to deter-mine if there are discrepancies between your care and state-of-the-art care. Use Step 2 to review shortcomings.

Risk Factors

Although psychiatrists don't fully understand the causes of depression, research has uncovered certain risk factors, both social and psychological. People with risk factors are more vulnerable to depression. You may be at higher risk of depression if you have a family history of the disease, low self-esteem, chronic illness, or financial problems. If you are involved in a difficult relationship, are by nature pessimistic, or have gone through unwelcome change in your life, you may be susceptible. In addition, you should be alert to symptoms of depression if you have one of the following illnesses:

- Endocrine disorders, including those of the pituitary, adrenals, and thyroid

- Vitamin and mineral deficiencies and excesses (for example, pellagra, hyper-vitaminosis A, beri-beri, and pernicious anemia)

- Infections (for example, encephalitis, hepatitis, and tuberculosis); even flu and influenza can commonly trigger the onset of depression.

- Neurologic disorders (for example, multiple sclerosis and Wilson's disease)

- Collagen disorders (for example, systemic lupus erythematosis)

- Cardiovascular disease (for example, cardiomyopathy, cerebral ischemia, myocardial infarction)

- Malignancies

Diagnosis

Doctors may fail to diagnose depression because they are not trained in psychiatry or because they concentrate on the physical, rather than the mental, symptoms. Many primary care doctors, such as general or family practitioners, lack the education to detect depression, one of a number of illnesses that are just not taught adequately in most medical schools. There is substantial evidence that primary care doctors diagnose depression properly no more than half the time. They are more likely to look for depression in female patients, which raises the possibility that men are less likely to seek help or to be treated for depression than are women.

Many patients discourage doctors from diagnosing depression by focusing on physical symptoms. Some believe that it's better to have a "real" illness than a mental illness, although a major depression is just as much a "real" illness as any other. In a National Institute of Mental Health poll, respondents said they would not seek treatment for depression because they feared their jobs would be jeopardized if it became known. Their symptoms would markedly improve if they were treated for their true illness.

While primary care doctors underdiagnose depression, psychiatrists may overdiagnose it. Dr. Herbert C. Schulberg of the University of Pittsburgh says that this remains a major concern. "The problem is not as great as the underdiagnoses but it still is an existing issue," he says. Dr. Schulberg is an author of a 1985 report on the subject. According to Dr. Schulberg, psychiatrists diagnose 150% more depression than they would if they strictly followed medical guidelines.

Your diagnosis will be made largely on the basis of the history you give of your illness and the questions your doctor asks and the physical he or she performs. That's different from many illnesses discussed in this book for which laboratory tests, x-rays, and imaging scans are required. Here are the symptoms that characterize depression and those that characterize mania. If you have several of the following symptoms, you will want to discuss them with your doctor.

Symptoms of Depression

- Persistent sad, anxious, or "empty" mood

- Feelings of hopelessness, pessimism

- Feelings of guilt, worthlessness, helplessness

- Loss of interest or pleasure in hobbies and activities once enjoyed, including sex

- Insomnia, early-morning awakening or, conversely, oversleeping (The sleep patterns of both unipolar and bipolar patients are different from those of persons who do not have a mood disorder. For example, the rapid eye movement (REM) phase of sleep associated with dreaming occurs earlier in people with mood disorders. Persons with mood disorders also have more eye movements during REM sleep, less deep (slow-wave) sleep, and more problems staying asleep.)

- Changes in appetite leading to weight loss or gain

- Decreased energy, fatigue, being "slowed down"

- Thoughts of death or suicide, suicide attempts

- Restlessness, irritability

- Difficulty concentrating, remembering, making decisions

- Persistent physical symptoms that do not respond to treatment, such as headaches, digestive disorders, and chronic pain

- Irritability, with anger and deteriorating human relations

Symptoms of Mania

- Inappropriate elation

- Inappropriate irritability

- Grandiose notions

- Increased talking

- Disconnected and racing thoughts

- Increased sexual desire

- Inappropriate social behavior

- Combativeness

- Refusal to listen to family or friends who suggest you have changed from your normal self

TESTS   Depression can be secondary to real physical illness. That's why a complete workup by your family doctor or internist is important. That workup will include tests to rule out thyroid disease, anemia, viral infection, and other disorders. To reach an accurate diagnosis of depression, your doctor should check the following:

- Neurological functioning, including coordination, reflexes, and balance

- Medical and psychiatric history

- Mental status

- General physical appearance

- Orientation to person, place, and time

- Cognitive functioning, such as illogical thinking, racing thoughts or speech, hallucinations or delusions, memory, verbal and abstract reasoning, and overall judgment

- Anxiety levels

- Appetite/sleep disturbances

- Suicidal ideation

- Complete blood and urine laboratory tests

Treatment: Three-Dimensional Psychiatry

My father, Robert E. Arnot, M.D., a graduate of Harvard Medical School and a psychiatrist for 50 years, has long taught that the psychiatrist must treat three separate aspects of each patient's illness: They are the biology, the psychology, and the sociology of the illness. He has named this three-dimensional psychiatry, or "tridomic psychiatry" for these three separate domains. Every diagnosis and treatment plan depends on successfully dealing in these three domains. If your doctor approaches only one of these three, he or she isn't going to properly comprehend or treat your case. Here's what these three different dimensions are.

Biology   These are the real physical factors that can cause your depression. An underactive thyroid, a severe anemia, or side effects of medications can cause depression. Depression itself is a physiologic and biochemical disturbance. Defects in the way that brain chemicals (called neurotransmitters) operate may also cause depression. It is known how medication affects these neurotransmitters; it is not known precisely what the defect is in how these neurotransmitters fail to work properly.

Psychology   These factors are factors purely in the mind. They represent how you look at the world around you and your interpretation of memories of past experiences, such as your relationship with your parents and how you were raised. Standard treatment involves psychotherapy.

Sociology   At a minimum, you need to understand how your marriage, job, and relationships with family, friends, and co-workers affect your depression. Your treatment should help you alter your attitude towards your environment and even encourage you to change it. That could mean finding a new job or apartment if your present job or apartment severely affects your psychology.

The biologic dimension can be treated with medical therapy for illness or with antidepressants for depression in which there is no other physical cause found.

Your treatment should be based on the severity and predominant characteristics of your illness:

TREATMENT FOR MILD DEPRESSION   Numerous individuals experience brief depressive episodes with relatively mild symptoms that may last between a few days and a week. Although these episodes may cause personal distress and discomfort, they ordinarily do not interfere with the ability to function at work or at home. Such episodes often cease without intensive treatment. But you may be helped by counseling or psychotherapy. Although antianxiety and tranquilizer medications are not treatments for depression itself, these can sometimes be helpful. Exercise has been shown to be as effective as an antidepressant in mild depression.

TREATMENT FOR MODERATE DEPRESSION   If your symptoms continue for more than two weeks and include anxiety, sleep difficulty, loss of interest or pleasure in usual activities, difficulty concentrating, headache, backache or other bodily complaints, and some interference with work and family activities, you should seek a comprehensive diagnostic assessment that includes a medical examination. You and your doctor have a choice between medications, particularly tricyclic antidepressants or monoamine oxidase inhibitors, and brief, focused psychotherapy that focuses on current problems and relationships. Often the most effective forms of treatment are a combination of medication and psychotherapy.

TREATMENT FOR SEVERE DEPRESSION   You need more intensive treatment if your depression continues for many weeks and involves thoughts of death, suicidal attempts, impaired judgment, and poor concentration. For this depression antidepressants are generally required, and electroconvulsive therapy may be advisable.

Treatment Medications: Antidepressants

"We really don't know yet how to match the chemistry of the disease to the chemistry of the drug. Selection of drug treatment should be educated trial and error, an informed effort," says Dr. Matthew Rudorfer, Deputy Director for Clinical Psychopharmacology at the National Institute of Mental Health. Despite the gaps in knowledge, antidepressants can be lifesaving. Even after referral to a major medical center, only 75% of patients are given antidepressants. Be sure your doctor is up-to-date on the latest antidepressants.

FINDING THE RIGHT MEDICATION   After you start taking antidepressants, you must be patient and give the drugs adequate time to take effect. With most mood-disorder drugs it will take between one and four weeks before you notice any change. It's important to continue drug treatment until an adequate trial is given. You may be passing up a drug that's appropriate for you. Even when the right drug has been found, it may take some experimentation to determine the dosage that has the most impact on your illness. The National Institute of Mental Health found that only about one in 10 patients was receiving adequate amounts.

You shouldn't terminate a drug unless you've tried the maximum dosage levels considered safe. Correct dosage varies among individuals because of the wide variability in how the body metabolizes antidepressants. Dosage must be tailored to the individual. It's not enough for a doctor simply to go by the reference book. While antidepressants are generally safe, you should be careful about interactions with other medications. Discontinue any medication that is not helping you after more than three or four weeks, and ask for another medication.

You may have to continue your chosen antidepressant for one to three months. If you are subject to recurrent depressions, once you find the right antidepressant for you, you may have to continue it for many years in small doses.

SIDE EFFECTS   All antidepressants control the level of chemicals, called neurotransmitters, in the brain. In doing so they improve mood, sleep, appetite, energy levels, and concentration. They also have similar side effects, which include dry mouth, constipation, bladder problems, blurred vision, sexual problems, dizziness, and drowsiness. Often these side effects will disappear or at least become tolerable as your body adjusts to the drug.

Your doctor should check your blood levels for the correct dosage levels if your depression worsens or if you suffer unpleasant side effects. However, you shouldn't discontinue the drugs abruptly just because of side effects such as dry mouth. Usually an alternative drug can be found. It is important not to stop the drugs abruptly if you are feeling better, either. Your depression may quickly worsen. Research shows that patients who continue their medication for a period after a depression lifts have fewer recurrences.

Other Medications Used to Fight Depression

ANTIANXIETY DRUGS   Frequently in depression there is a moderate to large amount of anxiety and tension. To treat this anxiety, especially until the antidepressant becomes effective, your doctor may need to add an antianxiety drug of the minor tranquilizer group, for example, Librium, or Ativan, or Xanax, although Xanax can be quite habit forming or difficult to terminate. When you are improved or recovered from the depression, the tranquilizer may be discontinued; or it may be continued with an antidepressant, such as Elavil or Marplan, to continue to treat the anxiety. Elavil does have antianxiety and sedative properties in addition to its antidepressant effect.

Sometimes, if depression is mild and anxiety is up, just the minor tranquilizer effect itself will also correct the depression, and the antidepressant may not have to be used.

VITAMINS   Vitamins such as high-potency vitamin B complex with C may be added. The antidepressants require this supplement. Again, in a very mild depression just giving the high-potency B complex may bring improvement. In addition to vitamin B complex, a strong and complete vitamin and mineral combination can also be added.

SEDATIVES   At the beginning of the treatment of depression, some experts add a sedative to correct the symptom of severe sleeplessness, which is a major concern and which may bring the patient to the doctor in the first place. A sleeping pill may be used at bedtime. However, too weak a sedative, one that does not really put the patient to sleep or keep her or him asleep may increase the concern about the illness. The sedative may have to be continued for two to four weeks until the antidepressant becomes effective. It is important not to become dependent on it but to use it wisely.

Inappropriate Drugs

One out of three people is being treated incorrectly for depression because doctors don't know state-of-the-art of psychopharmacology. Even though new medications revolutionizing the treatment of depression are being marketed, some doctors are still relying, totally inappropriately, on Valium to treat a depressive disorder. Valium is sometimes prescribed with antidepressants in patients who are suffering from anxiety as well as depression, but it is not an antidepressant. As many as half of depressed patients are given antianxiety drugs alone, without antidepressants for depression. That's just plain wrong. Sleeping pills and stimulants such as amphetamines are two other drugs often incorrectly prescribed. A person who is sleeping excessively because of depression should not be on a sedating drug; a person who is manic because of bipolar depression should not take a drug that stimulates. These drugs can have unintended effects. For example, bipolar patients on antidepressants can become manic. Therefore, an excessively agitating drug can be risky.

Major Medications for Unipolar Illness

TRICYCLICS   This category of drugs includes Tofranil (imipramine), Elavil (amitriptyline), Desyrel (trazadone), and Pamelor (nortriptyline). Most patients with unipolar disorders are initially treated with tricyclic antidepressants. As with most antidepressants, full-strength doses are impossible to tolerate initially. You need to work up to a high dose gradually.

PROZAC (FLUOXETINE)   This is a new-generation antidepressant that works best for mild depression. Since its introduction it has become the most widely used drug to treat the milder forms of depression because it has been shown to be highly effective and to have relatively few side effects, especially in comparison to the tricyclics. The most frequently reported side effects are nervousness, anxiety, insomnia, headache, and gastrointestinal problems. In February 1990, the *American Journal of Psychiatry* reported that six people on Prozac experienced an intense obsession with suicide, sparking a controversy about its effectiveness that continues unresolved. However, Dr. Rudorfer says, "I believe the concern has been exaggerated. No cause and effect has ever been proven. Correlation is different than cause and effect. You're talking about an enormous number—millions—of prescriptions coupled with the known risk of suicidal ideation as part of the illness. In a sense, it got too popular for it's own good. It is a very safe drug but not innocuous. When the drug works, it really works well."

Still Prozac has become intensely controversial in the national media and has been the subject of magazine cover stories and investigative television reports. The jury is still out. Some prominent psychiatrists are concerned that it is not potent enough for severe depression and may simply lift depression enough for a patient to act on suicidal thoughts. That has not been proven in research literature as of this writing. The key to using Prozac successfully is careful observation of its effect on the patient by a skilled physician and by the patient. If Prozac is not effective fairly quickly, a stronger antidepressant should be used.

MONOAMINE OXIDASE INHIBITORS (MAOIS)   These are in a separate category from other antidepressants. They make you feel better by increasing the amount of neurotransmitters in the brain. They do this by inhibiting the destruction of several neurotransmitters. Neurotransmitters transmit messages from one nerve to the next. (The tricyclics also act at the same sites in the brain, but do so by slowing the absorption of neurotransmitters by the nerve endings.)

MAOIs have fallen out of favor, and may cause apprehension in doctors and pharmacists who do not know them. They are a very powerful and useful kind of antidepressant. In fact, a new study shows they are very effective first-line drugs of choice. The MAOIs are most useful for patients who suffer a marked fatigue. Tricyclics are better used in depression marked by agitation. Your doctor will usually begin by prescribing tricyclics, turning to MAOIs only if the tricyclics fail. Ordinarily doctors will try two or three of the tricyclic-related drugs before they prescribe MAOIs.

Precautions Necessary with MAOIs

■ The systolic blood pressure must be above 106 before starting. MAOIs cannot be used if the systolic blood pressure is under 106 because the drug will drop the blood pressure further and cause the patient to feel weak or faint, particularly upon getting up from a chair or going upstairs.

■ Certain foods and drugs that contain adrenaline or chemicals that can be turned into adrenaline by the body have to be avoided, since they can cause episodes of severely high blood pressure. Such foods are: particularly strong cheeses, red wine, and beer. Cold medicines containing adrenaline-like drugs are to be avoided. Antihistamines, however, may be used. The drugs acquired a bad reputation in the early years, before patients became educated about the foods or drugs that could interact badly with MAOIs. There were some fatalities. A few years ago at a major New York City teaching hospital, a young woman taking a MAOI inhibitor was admitted and given a pain killer that in combination with certain other drugs can cause serious reactions. In this well-publicized case the patient died.

■ Make certain to let your dentist, surgeon, or anesthesiologist know that you take MAOIs, especially if they plan to use Novacaine or a similar local anesthetic.

■ MAOIs cannot be mixed with tricyclics. A 10-day interval off these drugs must be observed before the other type of drug can be taken.

Major Medications for Bipolar Illness

LITHIUM Lithium is an excellent drug for the prevention of recurrent manic attacks, and it may also help to prevent depressions. It is usually the best treatment for manic depressive illness. When manic depression is diagnosed, the patient is typically started on lithium to normalize the mood swings. Lithium may lift the mood of a depressed individual as well.

Although the drug provides effective relief in acute episodes, it does so slowly over a two- to four-week period. About 20–40% of patients on lithium will not be able to tolerate the side effects or will not respond fully. Lithium needs to be taken for years by patients with true recurrent bipolar (manic depressive) illness.

Lithium can be used in treating acute mania, but it may be necessary to add a phenothiazine such as Thorazine. In extreme cases, with a highly disturbed patient, some doctors resort to electric shock treatment. Lithium and the electroconvulsive therapy cannot be given together. In some cases, it may be necessary to continue taking antidepressants and/or a small dose of phenothiazine, in addition to lithium

Before starting lithium, certain laboratory tests need to be done, including a complete blood count, a urine analysis, a determination of thyroid function with T3 and T4 tests, and the creatinine as well as the lithium level. Repeated tests for blood levels of lithium must be taken regularly to be certain the lithium level is in an effective range—between 0.5 mEq/liter and 1.0 mEq/liter—neither so high as to be toxic nor so low as to be ineffective. The initial laboratory tests just mentioned need to be repeated every three to six months. This may sound complicated, but the laboratory tests are taken in the morning before lithium is taken and are easy to obtain.

NEUROLEPTICS   Haloperidol (Haldol) is used in the treatment of acute mania. Because lithium can take weeks to work, Haldol may be prescribed to control the symptoms until lithium can take effect. Then it's withdrawn and lithium is continued alone. It is also used in the short-term treatment of cases of psychotic depression in which the patient withdraws from reality and suffers marked social and intellectual dysfunction, for which the standard antidepressants don't work. Haldol treats the psychotic aspects of the illness. It's given alone or in combination with antidepressants. It acts by blocking dopamine receptors. Although Haldol can produce a pseudo-Parkinsonian state, it cannot cause the disease. However, the long-term side effects include neurologic disorders. About 20% of such patients will develop involuntary movement disorders. Some experts consider Haldol a poor choice because of its side-effect profile.

POTENTIATORS   These are compounds that may be useless on their own but in combination with other medications can increase the effectiveness of the originally prescribed drug. They act by increasing the sensitivity of receptors in the brain to the first drug. Thyroid hormone may be used as a potentiator with any of the antidepressants. Since lithium often slows the thyroid, it may be prescribed for patients on that medication also. Care must be taken, by thyroid blood tests, to avoid chronic high doses of thyroid medication.

Other Treatments for Depression

PSYCHOTHERAPY   Drug therapy often is ineffective on its own. Psychotherapy has long gone hand in hand with drug treatment. Recent studies confirm its effectiveness. Many doctors now recommend a combination of medication for the quick relief of symptoms and psychotherapy to help cope with underlying problems. Depression takes a toll on people's lives and, while mental health experts in the past tended to favor either medication or therapy, these divisions are now less clear-cut. Mental health experts are moving away from that either/or theory, recognizing that patients don't take medications in a vacuum. Recent studies have shown that the following two methods of brief, extremely focused psychotherapy can be very effective in the relief of the symptoms of depression.

Cognitive Therapy This attempts to change self-defeating negative thought patterns.

Intrapersonal Therapy This emphasizes the development of new social skills.

Another method, psychodynamic psychotherapy, delves into the unconscious conflicts that precipitated the depressive symptoms. This treatment has only been proven effective in one case study, although many experienced psychiatrists have established empirically that the traditional interpersonal relationships they develop with their patients in psychodynamic therapy is beneficial. You will probably begin with traditional psychotherapy. Once your medications have begun to take effect, you may want to discuss alternative forms of psychotherapy and different mental health professionals with your doctor. You should learn enough about different kinds of psychotherapy to find what works best for you.

ELECTROCONVULSIVE THERAPY (ECT) In some cases you may want to consider electroconvulsive therapy, an artificially induced seizure that appears to reregulate several disturbed transmitter systems in the brain. While 60% of patients respond to drug therapy, 80% improve after shock therapy. Although ECT has a bad reputation, dating from the early, primitive methods and its portrayal in such movies as "One Flew Over the Cuckoo's Nest," ECT carries little risk in carefully controlled settings. ECT should be considered in cases of severe, life-threatening, or psychotic depression, and severe malnourishment and when medication does not bring relief or cannot be given because of other illnesses.

LIGHT THERAPY This is a new treatment for depression that has sometimes proven helpful, particularly with people who become depressed during the winter, a condition known as seasonal affective disorder, or SAD. Artificial high-intensity lights that simulate daylight help people avoid that kind of depression.

EXERCISE For mild depression, exercise can be as effective as some antidepressants. Exercise works as a mood elevator and helps to increase self-esteem.

WHAT YOU CAN DO FOR YOURSELF Along with your drug or other treatment for depression, you can work on your own to change the negative thoughts that predominate in this disease. You may not see life accurately if you have a depressive disorder. Your pessimism may be a direct consequence of your disease. The National Institute of Mental Health suggests that you will feel better if you:

- Do not set yourself difficult goals or take on a great deal of responsibility during a depression.

- Break large tasks into small ones, set some priorities, and do what you can as you can.

- Do not expect too much from yourself, which will only increase feelings of failure.

- Try to be with other people; it is usually better than being alone.

- Participate in activities that may make you feel better. You might try mild exercise, going to a movie or a ball game, or participating in religious or social activities. Don't overdo it or get upset if your mood is not greatly improved right away. Feeling better takes time.

- Do not make a major life decision, such as changing jobs, getting married, or getting divorced, without consulting others who know you well and who have a more objective view of your situation. In any case it is advisable to postpone important decisions until your depression has lifted.

- Do not blame yourself if you fail to snap out of your depression. People rarely do. Help yourself as much as you can, and do not blame yourself for not being up to par.

- Remember not to accept your negative thinking. It is part of the depression and will disappear as your depression responds to treatment.

Step 2. Look for Shortcomings

I hope that by reading Step 1 you have gotten a good feeling about your treatment and that you understand much of it better. You'll learn even more by calling organizations listed in Step 4. But if you have an uncomfortable feeling that your treatment is not on track, then study this next section, which specifies some common and serious shortcomings that experts in the field recognize. If this section confirms your suspicions, you should go on to Step 3. Some of these mistakes you can discover yourself; others only an expert can confirm.

MISTAKES IN DIAGNOSIS

You have a medical illness and are unaware of its depressive symptoms.

Your symptoms are too disabling to reach out for help.

You are too proud to admit you are depresssed and to seek help.

You are misdiagnosed.

You are not seeking help because you assume it's too expensive.

Your health care provider isn't educated about depression and fails to recognize your symptoms.

MISTAKES IN TREATMENT

You're taking medications that don't mix.

You don't get the state-of-the-art drugs.

You're not being given enough of your medication to be effective.

Your doctor is not checking your medication's dosage and effectiveness regularly.

You don't take your medications regularly or you stop on your own when you feel better.

Your health care provider uses only sleeping pills, amphetamines, or tranquilizers to treat depression.

You are not treated for your depression at all.

You are manic depressive and are not treated for the manic component of your illness.

You take an antidepressant that agitates you and prevents sleep.

You sleep excessively, yet are put on sedating medications.

You have excessive "highs" yet are put on a stimulating medication.

Your medication isn't given an adequate time to take effect (usually 2–4 weeks).

Your insurance coverage influences whether and for how long you are treated.

You no longer want to continue treatment, and stop.

You don't like drug side effects and quit taking your medications.

Your doses are "too frequent" and so you miss taking medication.

Step 3. See a Specialist

If, from Step 2, you are concerned that your care is not state-of-the-art, this section will tell you how to choose an expert.

Choosing a Doctor

There are intense rivalries in the mental health field among psychologists, social workers, psychiatrists, psychopharmacologists, and others for patients. Many mental health specialists are skilled diagnosticians. But remember, primary care physicians properly detect depression only half of the time, whereas in one study patients of mental health specialists were diagnosed with 100% accuracy. If you are severely depressed, the only specialist trained to deal with both the physical and the psychological aspects of depression is a psychiatrist. While a number of people with different types of training can help you, a psychiatrist who has a biological orientation is a good place to start.

Unlike surgery or many internal medicine specialities there is very little concrete, scientific data that can help you to choose an individual doctor. But you can start by asking your family doctor for the name of a board-certified psychiatrist who has a reputation for good results with depressed patients or by seeking a referral from the chief of psychiatry at a major teaching hospital. You will want a psychiatrist who spends the majority of his or her time with depressed patients.

SPECIALISTS IN PSYCHOTHERAPY   Psychotherapy is available from a variety of sources. You may want to consult more than one expert to find the person who appears most likely to help you. Here are the experts who provide psychotherapy and the training that is required for licensure or other certification.

Psychiatrists   Psychiatrists have:

- Four years of college

- Four years of medical school

- One-year internship

Although any licensed physician may practice psychiatry, many psychiatrists undertake an additional three-year residency program in a psychiatric facility. After completing an approved residency program and practicing for two years, a psychiatrist is considered board eligible and may then take a national exam to become board-certified.

Psychoanalysts   A psychoanalyst is generally a psychiatrist or psychologist with a doctorate degree or social worker with a master's degree who has undertaken specialized postgraduate training in psychoanalysis and received extensive supervision as part of the training. The person usually has been psychoanalyzed himself or herself.

Psychologists   These specialists have:

■ Four years of college

■ Four or more years of graduate study in psychology

■ One year of internship to receive a doctorate, usually granted in clinical or counseling psychology which requires the most training and formal supervision

For a psychologist to be licensed or certified to practice independently, most states require the doctoral degree, a national and/or state exam, and an additional one to two years of supervised practice in an approved setting. Psychologists with a master's degree, requiring one to two years of graduate study, may practice independently in some states but usually must be supervised. Psychologists are qualified to administer and interpret psychological tests.

Many people in a National Institute of Mental Health poll said they would not seek treatment for depression because they believed it would be too costly. If you want to find a therapist but cannot afford private counseling, you can contact:

■ A community mental health center (to request an intake interview)

■ A local hospital (to inquire about outpatient mental health services)

■ Area universities (for treatment at their counseling service or psychological clinic, usually located in the Department of Psychology)

■ The director of clinical training at any university that trains therapists (for a referral—try the departments of psychology, psychiatry, and social work)

■ Local psychiatric, psychological, social work, or marriage and family therapy societies for the names of two or three qualified therapists)

Centers of Excellence for Depression

If you need to be hospitalized, you don't have to go to a psychiatric institution specializing in depression. General hospitals with strong psychiatry staffs are an excellent choice. They can also be an ideal setting to diagnose underlying medical illnesses, to monitor blood levels of antidepressants and other drugs, and to undertake a full medical workup. For recommendations, you can call a department of psychiatry at a major teaching hospital. Be certain that hospitalization is needed. In general, many insurance companies discriminate against psychological illnesses. Most companies will reimburse doctor visits and other outpatient care at 80% of charges for most illnesses, but they will pay only 50% of the charges for depression.

However, they will pay a much higher percentage of the charges if you are hospitalized for depression. That creates an incentive to hospitalize depressed patients, when the patient can be treated just as well on the outside.

The following list of hospitals is provided only as a convenient starting place in your search for excellence. These hospitals are recommended on the basis of reputation, not experience and results. The list is not an endorsement. There may be hospitals just as excellent that have been omitted. You should apply the guidelines for experience, results, and other measures of excellence to any hospital you choose, whether or not it is on this list. Although hospitals from different sources have been combined into one list, the compilation in no way implies that one source has endorsed the hospital list of another source.

ALABAMA
University of Alabama   HC
School of Medicine
University Station
Birmingham, AL 35294

University of Southern
  Alabama   HC
College of Medicine
Dept of Psychiatry
307 University Blvd
Mobile, AL 36688

ARIZONA
Southern Arizona Mental
  Health Center   HC
1930 E Sixth St
Tucson, AZ 85719

ARKANSAS
University of Arkansas   HC
4301 W Markham, Ste 506
Little Rock, AR 72205

CALIFORNIA
Langley Porter Neuropsychiatric
  Institute   HC
401 Parnassus Ave
San Francisco, CA 94143

Stanford University   HC
Dept of Psychiatry and
  Behavioral Science
Stanford, CA 94305

University of California at Irvine
  Medical Center   HC
Dept of Psychiatry and Human
  Behavior
101 City Dr S
Orange, CA 92668

University of California at
  Los Angeles   HC
Affective Disorders Clinic
760 Westwood Plaza, Box 18
Los Angeles, CA 90024

University of California, Los
  Angeles, School of Medicine   US
10833 LeConte Ave
Los Angeles, CA 90024

University of California, Los
  Angeles, Medical Center   HC
Building F-5
Torrance, CA 90509

UCSD Gifford Mental
  Health Clinic   HC
3427 Fourth Ave
San Diego, CA 92103

COLORADO
University of Colorado
  Medical Center   HC
4200 E Ninth Ave
Denver, CO 80220

CONNECTICUT
Institute of Living   US
400 Washington St
Hartford, CT 06106

University School of Medicine   HC
Depression Research Unit
350 Congress Ave
New Haven, CT 06519

FLORIDA
Anclote Manor Hospital   HC
P.O. Box 1224
Tarpon Springs, FL 33589

Mount Sinai Medical Center   HC
4300 Alton Rd
Miami Beach, FL 33140

Suncoast Gerontology Center   HC
University of So. Florida
Dept of Psychiatry
12901 No. 30th St, Box 50
Tampa, FL 33612

University of Miami
    Medical Center   HC
Box 016960
Miami, FL 33101

GEORGIA
Emory University School
    of Medicine   HC
Emory Outpatient Clinic
1365 Clifton Rd NE
Atlanta, GA 30322

HAWAII
University of Hawaii   HC
Dept of Psychiatry
1356 Lusitana St
Honolulu, HI 96813

ILLINOIS
Illinois State Psychiatric Institute   HC
1601 W Taylor St
Chicago, IL 60612

Rush Medical College   HC
1720 W Polk St
Chicago, IL 60612

INDIANA
LaRue D. Carter Memorial
    Hospital   HC
1315 W 10th St
Indianapolis, IN 46202

IOWA
University of Iowa   HC
Dept of Psychiatry
500 Newton Rd
Iowa City, IA 52242

KANSAS
Menninger Clinic   US/HC
5800 SW Sixth St
Topeka, KS 66601

University of Kansas   HC
School of Medicine
Dept of Psychiatry
Kansas City, KS 67214

KENTUCKY
University of Kentucky   HC
Dept of Psychiatry
Lexington, KY 40536

LOUISIANA
Louisiana State University   HC
School of Medicine
Dept of Psychiatry
P.O. Box 33932
Shreveport, LA 71130

Tulane Medical Center   HC
Dept of Psychiatry
1415 Tulane Ave
New Orleans, LA 70112

MARYLAND
Johns Hopkins Hospital   US
600 No Wolfe St
Baltimore, MD 21205

National Institute of
Mental Health   HC
Bdg 10, Rm 3N-218
9000 Rockville Pike
Bethesda, MD 20892

Sheppard and Enoch Pratt
Hospital   US
6501 No. Charles St
Baltimore, MD 21204

MASSACHUSETTS
Massachusetts General Hospital   US
55 Fruit St
Boston, MA 02114

Massachusetts Mental
Health Center   HC
74 Fenwood Rd.
Boston, MA 02115

McLean Hospital   HC/US
115 Mill St
Belmont, MA 02178

MICHIGAN
Lafayette Clinic   HC
951 E Lafayette
Detroit, MI 48207

Michigan State University   HC
Psychiatry Clinics
Affective Disorders Clinic
East Lansing, MI 48824

University Hospital   HC
Dept of Psychiatry
7500 E Medical Center Dr
B2964, Box 0704
Ann Arbor, MI 48109

MINNESOTA
Mayo Clinic   US
200 First St SW
Rochester, MN 55905

Paula Clayton, M.D.   HC
University of Minnesota
Medical School
Minneapolis, MN 55455

MISSISSIPPI
University of Mississippi   HC
School of Medicine
Dept of Psychiatry and
Human Behavior
2500 No. State St
Jackson, MS 39216

MISSOURI
Washington University   HC
School of Medicine
4940 Audubon Ave.
St Louis, MO 63110

NEBRASKA
University of Nebraska   HC
Nebraska Psychiatric Institute
602 So. 45th St
Omaha, NE 68106

NEVADA
University of Nevada School
of Medicine   HC
Dept of Psychiatry and
Behavioral Sciences
Reno, NV 89557

NEW HAMPSHIRE
Dartmouth-Hitchcock
Medical Center   HC
Community Mental Health
Center
Hanover, NH 03755

NEW JERSEY
Fair Oaks Hospital   HC
19 Prospect St
Summit, NJ 07901

NEW MEXICO
Robert Kellner, M.D.   HC
University of New Mexico
School of Medicine
Dept of Psychiatry
2400 Tucker NE
Albuquerque, NM 87131

NEW YORK

New York Hospital–Cornell
    University Medical Center   HC
Payne Whitney Clinic,
    Westchester Div
21 Bloomingdale Rd
White Plains, NY 10605

Mount Sinai Services   HC
City Hospital at Elmhurst
Dept of Psychiatry
7901 Broadway
Elmhurst, NY 11373

New York Hospital–Cornell
    Medical Center   US
525 E 68th St
New York, NY 10021

New York University
    Medical Center   HC
560 First Ave
New York, NY 10016

Psychiatric Institute   HC
Frederic Quitkin, M.D.
722 W 168th St
New York, NY 10032

University of Rochester   HC
Dept of Psychiatry
Affective Disorders Clinic
300 Crittenden Blvd
Rochester, NY 14642

NORTH CAROLINA

University of No. Carolina   HC
School of Medicine
Division of Health Affairs
Chapel Hill, NC 27514

NORTH DAKOTA

University of North Dakota   HC
Medical Education Center
1919 No. Elm
Fargo, ND 58102

OHIO

Case Western Reserve University   HC
Dept of Psychiatry
2040 Abington Rd
Cleveland, OH 44106

Central Psychiatric Clinic   HC
Associate Director,
    Adult Division
3259 Elland Ave.
Mail Location 539
Cincinnati, OH 45267

OKLAHOMA

University of Oklahoma   HC
Health Sciences Center and
    Behavioral Sciences
Dept of Psychiatry
P.O. Box 26901
Oklahoma City, OK 73190

OREGON

Portland Division V.A.   HC
3710 So. West U.S.
Veterans Hospital Rd
P.O. Box 1034
Portland, OR 97207

PENNSYLVANIA

Center for Cognitive Therapy   HC
133 So. 36th St
Philadelphia, PA 19104

Hospital of the University
    of Pennsylvania   HC
Depression Research Unit
I-Gibson
36th and Spruce Sts
Philadelphia, PA 19104

Medical College of Pennsylvania
    at Eastern Pennsylvania   HC
Psychiatric Institute
3200 Henry Ave
Philadelphia, PA 19129

V.A. Ambulatory Care Center   HC
Mental Hygiene Clinic 116A
1421 Cherry St
Philadelphia, PA 19102

Western Psychiatric Institute
   and Clinic   HC
University of Pittsburgh
School of Medicine
3811 O'Hara St
Pittsburgh, PA 15213

RHODE ISLAND
V.A. Hospital of Providence   HC
Providence, RI 02908

SOUTH CAROLINA
Medical University of
   South Carolina   HC
Psychiatric Outpatient Dept
171 Ashley Ave
Charleston, SC 29425

TENNESSEE
Vanderbilt University   HC
Dept of Psychiatry
Nashville, TN 37232

TEXAS
Baylor College of Medicine   HC
Texas Medical Center
Dept of Psychiatry
1 Baylor Plaza
Houston, TX 77030

University of Texas   HC
Health Science Center
Dept of Psychiatry
5232 Harry Hines
Dallas, TX 75235

University of Texas   HC
Health Science Center at
   San Antonio Medical School
Dept of Psychiatry
7703 Floyd Curl Dr
San Antonio, TX 78284

University of Texas,
   Medical Branch   HC
Dept of Psychiatry and
   Behavioral Science
1200 Graves Bldg
Galveston, TX 77550

UTAH
University of Utah   HC
College of Medicine
Dept of Psychiatry
50 No. Medical Dr
Salt Lake City, UT 84132

VIRGINIA
Eastern Virginia Medical School   HC
Chairperson
Dept of Psychiatry and
   Behavioral Sciences
P.O. Box 1980
Norfolk, VA 23501

WASHINGTON
Harbor View Medical Center   HC
Psychiatry Dept
2H Harbor View Hall
325 Ninth Ave
Seattle, WA 98104

WISCONSIN
Clinical Sciences Center   HC
Dept of Psychiatry
600 Highland Ave
Madison, WI 53792

SOURCES

HC   indicates those hospitals recommended by *Health Care USA.*
US   indicates those hospitals recommend in *U.S. News & World Report.*

Step 4. Become Your Own Expert

WHO TO CALL

National Institute of Mental Health Through the DART (Depression, Awareness, Recognition and Treatment) program, offers information and education programs.

9000 Rockville Pike
Bethesda, MD 20892
301/443-4513
301/443-4140
800/421-4211

National Depressive and Manic-Depressive Association (NDMDA) Over 200 chapters nationwide offer doctor referral, literature, and support groups.

Merchandise Mart
Box 3395
Chicago, IL 60654
312/642-0049

National Mental Health Association More than 550 chapters nationwide provide patient information, including guidelines on insurance reimbursement, educational programs, and support groups. You can receive referrals to mental health specialists through the local chapters.

1021 Prince St
Alexandria, VA 22314-2971
703/684-7722
800/969-6642

National Alliance for the Mentally Ill This group offers patient information plus brief telephone counseling. More than 1,000 affiliates nationwide provide support groups.

2101 Wilson Blvd, Ste 302
Arlington, VA 22201
703/524-7600
800/950-NAMI

American Association of Retired Persons The AARP provides grief support and information on depression in the elderly.

Widowed Persons Services
Social Outreach and Support
601 E St NW
Washington, DC 20049
202/434-2260

National Foundation for Depressive Illness   This organization will provide brochures, articles, and referrals to doctors specializing in affective disorders, hospitals, and support groups in your state. They request a self-addressed envelope with a 75¢ stamp.

P.O. Box 2257
New York, NY 10116
800/248-4344

NIH CRISP System
301/496-7543

University-Affiliated Teaching Hospitals   See Appendix

EXPERT SOURCES

Although dozens of experts were interviewed for these chapters, these physicians are acknowledged for their significant contributions to this chapter.

Dr. Robert E. Arnot, Wellesley Hills, MA

Dr. Richard Grinker, Chicago, IL

REFERENCES AND SUGGESTED READING

American Psychiatric Association. *DSM-III: Diagnostic and Statistical Manual of Mental Disorders*, 1980.

Frank, E., and others. Three-Year Outcomes for Maintenance Therapies in Recurrent Depression. *Archives of General Psychiatry,* Vol. 47 (1990), pp. 1093–1099.

Hilakivi-Clarke, Leena A. Effects of Tryptophan on Depression and Aggression in STZ-D Mice. *Diabetes,* Vol. 40, No. 12 (Dec. 1991), pp. 1598–1602.

Kehoe, R. F., and Mander, A. J. Lithium Treatment: Prescribing and Monitoring Habits in Hospital and General Practice. *British Medical Journal,* Vol. 304, No. 6826 (Feb. 29, 1992), pp. 552–554.

Klemen, G. L., and Weissman, M. M. Increasing Rates of Depression. *Journal of the American Medical Association,* Vol. 261, No. 15 (April 21, 1989), pp. 2229–2235.

National Institute of Mental Health. *Depressive Illnesses: Treatments Bring New Hope.* NIMH Publication no. ADM, 89-1491 (1989).

Neugebauer, Richard, and others. Depressive Symptoms in Women in the Six Months After Miscarriage. *American Journal of Obstetrics and Gynecology,* Vol. 166, No. 1 (Jan. 1992), pp. 104–109.

Patten, Scott B., and others. Pharmacologic Management of Refractory Depression. *Canadian Medical Association Journal,* Vol. 146, No. 4 (Feb. 15, 1992), pp. 483–487.

Regier, D. A., and others. Comorbidity of Mental Disorders With Alcohol and Other Drug Abuse: Results from the Epidemiologic Catchment Area (ECA) Study. *Journal of the American Medical Association,* Vol. 264, No. 19 (Nov. 21, 1990), pp. 2511–2518.

Regier, D. A., and others. The NIMH Depression Awareness, Recognition, and Treatment Program: Structure, Aims, and Scientific Basis. *Psychiatry,* Vol. 145, No. 11 (Nov. 1988), pp. 1351–1357.

Rudorfer, M. V., and others. The New-Generation Antidepressants. *Hospital Therapy,* June 1990.

Schulberg, H. C., and others. Assessing Depression in Primary Medical and Psychiatric Practices. *Archives of General Psychiatry,* Vol. 42 (1985), pp. 1164–1170.

Stoudemire, A., and others. The Economic Burden of Depression. *General Hospital Psychiatry,* Vol. 8 (1986), pp. 387–394.

Talbott, John, and others (eds). *American Psychiatric Press Textbook of Psychiatry.* Washington, DC: American Psychiatric Press, 1988, pp. 403–441.

Trimble, Michael R. Behaviour Changes Following Temporal Lobectomy, with Special Reference to Psychosis [editorial]. *Journal of Neurology, Neurosurgery and Psychiatry,* Vol. 55, No. 2 (Feb. 1992), pp. 89–91.

U.S. Department of Health and Human Services. *Depressive Illness: Treatments Bring New Hope.* DHHS Publication No. (ADM) 89-1491, 1989.

Wells, K. B., and others. The Functioning and Well-being of Depressed Patients: Results from the Medical Outcomes Study. *Journal of the American Medical Association,* Vol. 262, No. 7 (Aug. 18, 1989), pp. 914–919.

Wells, Kenneth B., and others. Detection of Depressive Disorder for Patients Receiving Prepaid or Fee-for-Service Care: Results from the Medical Outcome of Studies. *Journal of the American Medical Association,* Vol. 262, No. 23 (Dec. 15, 1989), pp. 3298–3302.

Diabetes

Risk for Inappropriate Care VERY HIGH

Many Americans receive medical treatment little better than care given in some Third World countries, say several leading experts on diabetes. Simply put, too few health care providers and patients are adequately trained to care for diabetes the right way. Lack of access to state-of-the-art care decreases your quality of life on a daily basis. It increases your vulnerability to heart attack, kidney failure, blindness, circulatory problems leading to possible loss of one or more limbs, and even premature death. Diabetes is the third leading cause of death in the United States.

What It Is

There are two different kinds of diabetes mellitus: type I and type II. The fear with both kinds is that you will develop complications such as blindness, heart disease, kidney failure, loss of limb due to poor circulation, among others.

TYPE I (INSULIN DEPENDENT) DIABETES   Your pancreas produces a hormone called insulin. Insulin is largely responsible for controlling blood sugar levels. In type I diabetes, researchers believe, your body attacks and destroys the cells of the pancreas that produce insulin. This results in extraordinarily high levels of blood sugar, sometimes ranging from a normal near 100 to over 800! Untreated, this condition is usually fatal. Type I diabetes is therefore managed with insulin injections to control the blood sugar. Doctors believe that the more closely you can control blood sugar with insulin, the fewer complications you will suffer. Type I patients are usually children, adolescents, or young adults at the time of diagnosis.

TYPE II (INSULIN INDEPENDENT) DIABETES   In type II diabetes (formerly called adult-onset diabetes), the pancreas still produces insulin. However, either there is not enough insulin or the insulin works so poorly that your blood sugar rises well above normal. Type II diabetes is a disease of older patients, usually over 40. There is a strong genetic component. For instance, native Hawaiians and the Cherokee nation have a very high incidence of type II diabetes. Overeating and a high amount of body fat overwhelm whatever amount of insulin the body has available.

TYPE I VS. TYPE II   For decades a clear distinction has been made between type I and type II. In medical school we were taught that type II is the "good" diabetes

348

and type I the "bad" diabetes. That's no longer considered true. Type II kills many more Americans than type I. There are more type II patients on insulin than type I. In fact, 60% of type II patients are on insulin! The same principles of multiple daily blood sugar readings and insulin injections hold for these type II patients as for type I patients. Doctors aggressively treat the kidney failure, heart disease, and high blood pressure that type II patients develop.

The wide use of insulin among type II patients has blurred many of the distinctions between type I and type II diabetes. The term *insulin-treated diabetes* has been coined by Dr. Robert E. Ratner of the George Washington University Medical Center. This chapter is written for the patient who is dependent on insulin.

Step 1. Make Sure You Get the Best Care

Read this section on potential problems with your treatment carefully to determine if there are discrepancies between your care and state-of-the-art care. Use Step 2 to review shortcomings.

Diagnosis

Diabetes is diagnosed in three different ways. In one way, patients come to their doctor or an emergency room with a specific set of symptoms, including an increased thirst made worse by sweetened beverages; increased urination, sometimes hourly; losing weight but eating more; fatigue; and weakness. If the blood glucose level is 200 or above, the patient is considered to have diabetes.

In the second manner of diagnosis, you are screened for diabetes with what is called a fasting plasma-glucose test: After an overnight fast, blood is drawn and examined for the level of blood sugar. If it is over 140 on two occasions, you will be diagnosed as having diabetes.

If your doctor suspects you have diabetes but neither of the above methods proves it, a standard oral glucose tolerance test is ordered. In this test, after fasting, you will be asked to swallow a liquid very high in sugar. Your body's ability to handle that high sugar load will be followed over the next several hours. If you do poorly, that is, your blood sugar remains high, you will be diagnosed as a person with diabetes.

Treatment

If you have diabetes, you will want medical care to control your blood sugar levels as tightly as your body allows. The theory is that tight control will keep you freer of symptoms, enable you to enjoy a more normal life, and slow the disease's damage to your body. Studies have found that diabetes patients whose blood sugar was kept consistently normal had none of the eye and kidney disorders commonly associated with the disease. However, individuals with blood sugar 1.5 times normal suffered from typical complications: Almost 30% had kidney problems; nearly 40% had eye problems. Although diabetes is a chronic disease, management can make an enormous difference in the quality and length of your life. Many experts call diabetes the original "do-it-yourself" disease.

I want to add a word of caution, however: Not everyone can succeed in keeping their blood sugar under tight control, despite their best efforts. Tight control is not an absolute guarantee. There are still those under tight control who develop complications with their blood sugar. Studies are still in progress to prove, with absolute certainty, that tight control is as good a preventive treatment measure as many diabetes experts believe it to be.

RISK OF LOW BLOOD SUGAR   As doctors and patients shoot for lower and lower glucose levels, there is the risk of dangerously low blood sugar. In one research trial, patients were kept under exceptionally tight control. Researchers were alarmed to find a three-fold increase in the incidence of low blood sugar, low enough that seizures and loss of consciousness occurred or help from another party was required. You and your doctor need to be very conscious about the frequency with which you suffer low blood sugar.

The key is knowing at what threshold you get symptoms. If you feel weak and shaky at a blood sugar of 80, you have an excellent early warning system for low blood sugar. If, however, your first symptom is much more serious and occurs at a much lower level, tight control of your diabetes will be too dangerous. An example would be mental confusion occurring at a blood sugar count of 30. Very low levels of blood sugar can kill nerve cells in the brain. Repeated such episodes in children can lower their IQ.

Your family and co-workers should know how to treat your low blood sugar should you be unable to help yourself. They can give you an intramuscular injection of a drug called glucagon. There is no longer an excuse for the well-educated family of a person with diabetes to call an ambulance, states Dr. Robert Ratner.

If you feel your blood sugar is too low, you can drink a glass of milk. The lactose in the milk will get your blood sugar up quickly. And the fat and protein in the milk will keep your blood sugar from falling rapidly. Orange juice used to be a treatment of choice until doctors found that the blood sugar went up too rapidly and then fell too rapidly.

DAY-TO-DAY MANAGEMENT   Since you will be responsible for the day-to-day management of your diabetes, you should plan to spend time with a certified diabetes educator. Discuss with him or her the basic concepts of the disease, and request information about the following topics essential to your proper care:

- Administering insulin

- Monitoring blood glucose

- Measuring urine ketones

- Selecting foods and estimating quantities

- Preventing and treating abnormally low blood sugar

- Adjusting insulin, food intake, or both to any changes in usual exercise and eating patterns

Your health care provider should follow the American Diabetes Association recommendations on medications, which call for multiple daily injections of mixed insulins of varying time durations. A recent study of physicians showed that 70% ordered only single-injection or nonmixed insulin prescriptions. Those often result in unsatisfactory control of blood sugar.

Tests to Help Manage Your Diabetes

HOME GLUCOSE TESTING   The last few decades have seen many advances in the day-to-day management of diabetes. But the biggest advance by far has been home glucose testing. In fact, the American Diabetes Association has called the portable blood glucose meter the most important development in the last 60 years. Unfortunately, many physicians do not recommend or teach the correct use of this vital tool.

A certified diabetes educator (CDE) can teach you how to use your home testing device. CDEs are doctors, nurses, pharmacists, exercise physiologists, and other health professionals who have had 2,000 hours of direct patient education followed by a national exam. They are your best source of diabetes education.

It's essential that you understand how to operate the meter properly. While a wide variety of models is sold, you should try to purchase one that your doctor or nurse recommends so they can check your technique. The meter adds to the control of blood sugar a level of precision available previously only in hospitals. You can play an active role in your care by using the portable meter to determine your daily blood sugar patterns. If you set your own blood sugar standards, you're more likely to adhere to them. Here's what to do:

Measure your blood sugar level at least four times a day—six times a day for tight control—once before and once after each meal for best results. At the very minimum, take your blood sugar level three to four times a week. If you are sick with a cold or flu, increase the number of readings to one every two to three hours during the day. Drs. Diana and Richard Guthrie, professors at the University of Kansas School of Medicine, have provided the following chart. Your blood sugar readings should fall within these ranges:

	ACCEPTABLE BLOOD SUGAR	IDEAL BLOOD SUGAR
Fasting	120	80–110
1 hour after meal	180	100–150
2 hours after meal	150	80–130
3 hours after meal	130	80–110

These guidelines were not developed to drive you crazy by setting impossible standards. They are reasonable guidelines, though not within everyone's reach. Many patients feel they are failures if they can't meet these goals. Failure to achieve them can be the result of something that's not your fault. You can't control every variable on every occasion. Where on your body you give yourself an insulin injection or how deep the needle penetrates can alter your blood sugar level. For instance, insulin is absorbed more quickly from the abdomen than from an arm.

Eventually you should be able to monitor your glucose levels without the need to draw blood. Scientists are trying to adapt infrared scanners, now used to measure the amount of sugar in fruit, for use in diabetes. Until that comes on the market, you should continue to take blood samples on a regular basis.

GLUCOSE TESTING AT THE DOCTOR'S OFFICE   Even though you will be checking your blood sugar levels daily, your doctor should also order regular glucose tests to monitor your efforts to control the disease. By measuring the glycosylated hemoglobin (also called glycohemoglobin or hemoglobin A_{1C}), your doctor can assess your diabetes control over the prior six to eight weeks. It's an excellent measure of overall control that should be done far more often. One study surprisingly showed that only four out of ten primary care doctors regularly ordered the test.

OTHER SIGNS THAT DIABETES IS OUT OF CONTROL   While these guidelines are reliable measures of your blood sugar levels, you should be alert to other indications that your diabetes is getting out of control. Watch for: increased thirst; blurred vision; constant fatigue; infections of the urinary tract, skin, or feet; dental problems; or an increase in appetite that is accompanied by weight loss. You should be alert to episodes of hypoglycemia (low blood sugar) and ketoacidosis (a dangerous process in which the body tries to manufacture fuel by burning its own fat and muscle; as fat and muscle are burned, poisonous by-products, ketones, are released into the body, where they can be fatal).

Screening Tests for Complications of Diabetes

Your doctor should screen regularly for a range of potentially life-threatening complications. In a study of seven health care clinics, it was found that doctors measured only blood pressure, omitting entirely the assessment of all the other possible complications.

Screening should include the following

BLOOD TESTS

■ *Fasting plasma glucose,* a measure of blood glucose, usually taken before breakfast

■ *Glycosylated hemoglobin,* a measure of glycemic control for the previous one to two months

■ *Fasting lipid profile,* a measure of blood fats, usually taken before breakfast. Since diabetes increases your risk of heart disease, these tests help rate your risk.

High-density lipoprotein (HDL) cholesterol

Low-density lipoprotein (LDL) cholesterol

Tryglycerides

URINE TESTS

■ *Creatinine test.* Diabetes can damage the kidneys, causing microscopic leaks. Doctors can detect such damage by finding protein that has leaked into the urine. Elevated creatinine is another early warning sign of kidney damage. These patients should have a regular test to look for further decrease in kidney function. Creatinine is the usual serial screening test.

■ *Urinalysis,* an analysis of urine to check kidney function as well as glycemic control, with these specific measures:

Protein

Urinary protein excretion in patients who have had diabetes for five or more years

Glucose

Ketones

Protein

These further evaluate kidney function. High glucose and ketone levels in urine are warning flags that your diabetes is badly out of control.

HEART TESTS

■ *Heart scan and echocardiogram,* to evalute evidence that diabetes is beginning to cause heart disease. If it does, read the chapter on Coronary Artery Disease for aggressive, early steps you can take to slow or stop the progress of your heart disease. Remember, once your diabetes is under moderate control, your chief objective is to prevent the complications of diabetes.

THYROID TESTS

■ *Thyroid function.* People with diabetes have a higher incidence of thyroid disease and should have periodic testing.

GENETIC TESTS   If you have diabetes, the Joslin Diabetes Center in Boston and several other centers offer testing that can determine if members of your family are prone to type I diabetes. If they are, regular testing for specific antibodies can predict when full-blown diabetes is likely to develop. Since there are experimental therapies to prevent diabetes *before* it develops, you should consider testing. Limited studies with limited results for the prevention of diabetes are under way. They are offered at the University of California at Davis, the Joslin Clinic, and the University of Florida at Gainesville.

Managing Your Lifestyle

You can help manage your disease by eating carefully to keep your blood sugar under control. You should be meticulous about your diet. It should be well balanced and with limited amounts of sugar and fat and plenty of fiber. Many patients with diabetes mistakenly eat high-fat diets to avoid eating carbohydrates. That's unnecessary, since there are lots of carbohydrates that will not drive up your blood sugar. And because diabetes already puts you at risk for heart disease, a high-fat diet is counterrecommended.

Avoid fluctuations in your weight. Aerobic exercise will help your weight, contol your diabetes, lower your insulin requirement, and lower your risk of heart disease.

The key to a healthful lifestyle is help. You will need a nutritionist who understands diabetes and can help you plan your meals. You will need a physician who knows and believes in exercise with diabetes and will help adjust your insulin dosages to your workout program.

Step 2. Look for Shortcomings

From your reading of Step 1, I hope you got a good feeling about your treatment and that you understand much of it better. You'll learn even more by calling organizations listed in Step 4. But if you have an uncomfortable feeling that your treatment is not on track, then study this section for some common and serious shortcomings that experts in the field recognize. If this section confirms your suspicions, you should go on to Step 3. Some of these mistakes you can discover yourself; others only an expert can confirm.

MISTAKES IN DIAGNOSIS

You suffer complications associated with diabetes for which no prevention is undertaken.

You eat poorly.

You fail to monitor your own blood glucose.

Your health care provider isn't monitoring your blood glucose control.

Your health care provider isn't referring you to the specialists you need.

Your health care provider is not screening for risk factors.

MISTAKES IN TREATMENT

You are not knowledgeable about diabetes and have not learned to control your blood sugar level adequately.

Your health care provider isn't trained to care for you.

Your health care provider doesn't share and explain lab tests, especially blood glucose, cholesterol, and glycosylated hemoglobin readings.

Your health care provider is not prescribing multiple injections of mixed insulins.

Your pregnancy is not managed by diabetes experts.

Step 3. See a Specialist

If, from Step 2, you are concerned that your care is not state-of-the-art, this section will tell you how to choose an expert.

Choosing a Doctor

DIABETOLOGIST   According to research studies by the American Diabetes Association, more than half of community physicians are unable to provide adequate treatment of diabetes. Even if you have no complications, you should be under the care of a diabetes specialist, that is, a physician board-certified in internal medicine and endocrinology whose practice focuses on diabetes— a diabetologist. That physician should be a certified diabetes educator. You should make an appointment at least four times a year, more often if your diabetes isn't being brought under control.

Even with a superb diabetologist you will need specialized care from time to time. Regrettably, American Diabetes Association studies show that not all doctors treating diabetes patients are refering them to specialists. In one study, only 39% of physicians sent patients to dietitians, for example. You should be referred routinely to the following specialists.

OPHTHALMOLOGIST   Each year 5,000 people lose their sight because of diabetes. You must have an annual eye exam by an ophthalmologist who frequently manages people with diabetes. Some experts believe that no patient with diabetes need lose their vision. Regular exams can find retinal problems in time for a retinal specialist to repair the damage.

NUTRITIONIST   Your diet is a way of controlling your blood sugar. You need to see a nutritionist as soon as your diabetes is diagnosed. Follow-up is strongly encouraged at regular, three- to six-month intervals to establish eating guidelines that are realistic and fit your lifestyle. Follow-up visits with a nutritionist depend on the individual. Children with diabetes, however, should visit a nutritionist at least every two years.

PODIATRIST   Diabetes often leads to poor circulation, numbness, or impaired sensation in the feet. Untreated sores, cuts, ingrown toenails, or blisters can cause infection and need to be recognized early. Regular examinations should be part of your overall program to manage your diabetes. In between visits, you should be certain to baby your feet, avoid anything tight around the legs or ankles that could impair circulation, and never walk barefoot—under any circumstances.

CARDIOLOGIST   People with diabetes are two to four times more likely to develop heart disease. You need to go to a board-certified cardiologist who will run a comprehensive set of screening tests for heart disease. Many symptoms of diabetes-related heart disease are similar to those that appear in the general population with coronary artery disease—but with some important differences. Your cardiologist should be familiar with diabetes and your personal medical history. If you smoke and overeat, you will be at even higher risk of developing heart disease than the population at large.

KIDNEY SPECIALIST   When early diagnostic tests reveal signs of kidney failure, you should consult a nephrologist, who specializes in kidney disease.

NEUROLOGIST   This specialist can evaluate the possibility of nerve damage.

OBSTETRICIAN   Consult one with a special interest in diabetes. If you have diabetes and become pregnant, your chances of giving birth to a healthy baby will be improved dramatically if you are managed by a team. A diabetologist and an obstetrician who has an interest in diabetes should form the heart of that team. Many women who could not otherwise undergo a full-term pregnancy can bear normal children under the care of such specialists.

Centers of Excellence for Diabetes

The following list of hospitals is provided only as a convenient starting place in your search for excellence. These hospitals are recommended on the basis of reputation, not experience and results. The list is not an endorsement. There may be hospitals just as excellent that have been omitted.

PROGRAMS RECOGNIZED BY THE AMERICAN DIABETES ASSOCIATION   More and more programs are being recognized by the ADA every day. Just contact the ADA to see if there is a program near you (see Step 4).

ALABAMA
Providence Hospital
The Diabetes Center
6801 Airport Blvd
Mobile, AL 36685

University of Alabama at Birmingham
Diabetes Research & Education Hospital
1808 7th Ave. So., Rm D-112
Birmingham, AL 35233

ARIZONA
Carondolet St. Joseph's Hospital
Diabetes Care Center
350 No. Wilmot Rd
Tucson, AZ 85711

CIGNA Healthplan of Arizona
Outpatient Diabetes Program
755 E. McDowell Rd
Phoenix, AZ 85006

CALIFORNIA
Contra Costa Endocrine Associates
112 La Casa Via, Ste 120
Walnut Creek, CA 94598

Diabetes Education Associates
5300 Orange Ave
#110 Espalier Square
Cypress, CA 90630

Doctors Hospital of Lakewood
Diabetes Treatment Centers of America
5300 No. Clark Ave
Lakewood, CA 90712

Eisenhower Memorial Hospital
The Diabetes Program
Probst Ste 100
39000 Bob Hope Dr
Rancho Mirage, CA 92270

Foothill Presbyterian Hospital
Diabetes Treatment Centers of America
250 So. Grand Ave
Glendora, CA 91740

Hillside Hospital
Diabetes Outpatient Services
1940 El Cajon Blvd
San Diego, CA 92104-9988

Loma Linda University Medical Center
Diabetes Treatment Center
11255 Mt. View Ave, Ste I
Loma Linda, CA 92354

Mercy Hospital and Medical Center
Diabetes Education Program
4077 Fifth Ave
San Diego, CA 92103-2180

Mt. Diablo Medical Center
Center for Diabetes
2700 Grant St, Ste 104
Concord, CA 94520

Parkview Community Hospital
Diabetes Treatment Centers of America
3865 Jackson St
Riverside, CA 92503

St. Jude Hospital
The Diabetes Life Center
101 E Valencia Mesa Dr
Fullerton, CA 92635

Sutter General Hospital
Sutter Diabetes Care Center
2801 L St
Sacramento, CA 95816

Tarzana Regional Medical Center
Diabetes Treatment Centers of America
18321 Clark St
Tarzana, CA 91356

Warrack Hospital
2449 Summerfield Rd
Santa Rosa, CA 95405

COLORADO
Rose Medical Center
Diabetes Treatment Centers of America
4567 E. Ninth Ave
Denver, CO 80220

CONNECTICUT
St. Francis Hospital and Medical Center
Diabetes Care Center
114 Woodland St
Hartford, CT 06105

DISTRICT OF COLUMBIA
Walter Reed Army Medical Center
Diabetes Education Program
Washington, DC 20307-5001

FLORIDA
Baptist Hospital Diabetes
Education Center
1201 W Moreno St
Pensacola, FL 32501

Baptist Hospital of Miami
The Diabetes Care Program
8900 No. Kendall Dr
Miami, FL 33176-2197

Florida Hospital Medical Center
601 E Rollins St
Orlando, FL 32803

Lee Memorial Hospital
Diabetes Treatment Centers of America
2776 Cleveland Ave
Fort Myers, FL 33901

Mease Health Care
833 Milwaukee Ave
P.O. Box 760
Dunedin, FL 34296-0760

Mercy Hospital
Diabetes Treatment Centers of America
3663 So. Miami Ave
Miami, FL 33133

Methodist Hospital
Diabetes Treatment Centers of America
580 W Eighth St
Jacksonville, FL 32209

North Ridge Medical Center
Diabetes Treatment Centers of America
5757 No. Dixie Hwy
Ft. Lauderdale, FL 33334

Orlando Regional Medical Center
Diabetes Treatment Centers of America
1414 So. Kuhe Ave
Orlando, FL 32806-2093

University Community Hospital
Diabetes Treatment Centers of America
3100 E Fletcher Ave
Tampa, FL 33613

GEORGIA
Doctors Hospital
Diabetes Treatment Centers of America
616 19th St
Columbus, GA 31993

The Emory Clinic
Section on Internal Medicine
1365 Clifton Rd, NE
Atlanta, GA 30322

Georgia Center for Diabetes
4470 No. Shallowford Rd, Ste 101
Atlanta, GA 30338

South Georgia Medical Center Hospital
Diabetes Education Program
P.O. Box 1727
Valdosta, GA 31601-1727

West Paces Ferry Hospital
Diabetes Treatment Centers of America
3200 Howell Mill Rd NW
Atlanta, GA 30327

ILLINOIS
Alexian Brothers Medical Center
Diabetes Treatment Centers of America
800 W Biesterfield Rd
Elk Grove Village, IL 60007

Highland Park Hospital
718 Glenview Ave
Highland Park, IL 60035

Holy Family Hospital
Stable Lives Diabetes Program
100 No. River Rd
Des Plaines, IL 60016

Mercy Hospital and Medical Center
Diabetes Treatment Centers of America
Stevenson Expressway and King Dr
Chicago, IL 60616

INDIANA
Parkview Regional Diabetes Care Center
2200 Randallia Dr
Fort Wayne, IN 46805

St. Joseph Hospital
Taking Charge of Your Diabetes
215 W Fourth St
Mishawaka, IN 46544

IOWA
McFarland Diabetes Center
1215 Duff Ave
Ames, IA 50010

University of Iowa Hospitals and Clinics
(UIHC)
Diabetes - Endocrinology Unit
Iowa City, IA 52242

KANSAS
Bethany Medical Center
Diabetes Education Program
51 No. 12 St
Kansas City, KS 66102

St. Joseph Medical
Diabetes Treatment
3600 E Harry
Wichita, KS 67218

Stormont-Vail Regional Medical Center
Diabetes Learning Center
1500 W 10th St
Topeka, KS 66604

KENTUCKY
Mercy Hospital
Diabetes Education Program
1006 Ford Ave
Owensboro, KY 42301

Methodist Evangelical Hospital
Diabetes Care Center
315 E Broadway
Louisville, KY 40202-1703

Northern Kentucky Control Program
401 Park Ave
Newport, KY 41071

LOUISIANA
Baton Rouge General Med. Center
Diabetes Center
3600 Florida Blvd
Baton Rouge, LA 70821-2511

Glenwood Regional Medical Center
Diabetes Treatment Centers of America
P.O. Box 35805
West Monroe, LA 71294-5805

Medical Center of Baton Rouge
Diabetes Management Center
17000 Medical Center Dr
Baton Rouge, LA 70816

North Monroe Hospital
Diabetes Center
3421 Medical Park Dr
Monroe, LA 71203

St. Francis Medical Center
Diabetes Care Center
309 Jackson St
Monroe, LA 71201

Willis-Knighton Medical Center
2600 Greenwood Rd
Shreveport, LA 71103

MAINE
Cary Medical Center
37 Van Buren Rd
Caribou, ME 04736

Eastern Maine Medical Center
"Managing Your Diabetes"
489 State St
Bangor, ME 04401

Yankee Healthcare, Inc.
152 Dresen Ave
P.O. Box 550
Gardner, ME 04345

MARYLAND
Suburban Hospital
8600 Old Georgetown Rd
Bethesda, MD 20816

MASSACHUSETTS
Joslin Diabetes Center
One Joslin Pl
Boston, MA 02215

Waltham Weston Hospital
Diabetes Treatment Centers of America
5 Hope Ave
Waltham, MA 02254

MICHIGAN
Henry Ford Hospital
Ambulatory Diabetes Regulation/
    Education Program
2799 W Grand Blvd
Detroit, MI 48202

MINNESOTA
Fairview Southdale Hospital
Diabetes Education and Self-
    Management Program
6401 France Ave So.
Edina, MN 55435

Group Health, Inc.
Diabetes Education Program
22829 University Ave SE
Minneapolis, MN 55414

International Diabetes Center
Park Nicollet Medical Foundation
5000 W 39th St
Minneapolis, MN 55416

Mayo Clinic
Diabetes Clinic, N15
200 First St SW
Rochester, MN 55905

Metropolitan–Mt. Sinai Medical Center
Diabetes Treatment Centers of America
900 So. Eighth St
Minneapolis, MN 55404

United Hospital
Diabetes Treatment Centers of America
333 No. Smith Ave
St. Paul, MN 55102

MISSOURI
Barnes Hospital
Diabetes Education Program
1st Floor Peter's Bldg
One Barnes Hospital Plaza
St. Louis, MO 63110

Children's Mercy Hospital
824th at Gillham Rd
Kansas City, MO 64108

Cox Diabetes Center
Lester E Cox Medical Centers
1423 No. Jefferson
Springfield, MO 65802

International Diabetes Center
Kansas City Regional Affiliate
2184 E Meyer Blvd
Kansas City, MO 64132

St. John's Mercy Medical Center
So. Ballas Rd
St. Louis, MO 63141-8221

St. John's Regional Health Center
Diabetes Education Series
1235 E Cherokee
Springfield, MO 65804-2263

St. Mary's Health Center
Diabetes Education Program
6420 Clayton Rd
St. Louis, MO 63117

Trinity Lutheran Hospital
Diabetes Treatment Centers of America
3030 Baltimore
Kansas City, MO 64108

MONTANA
Trinity Hospital
Outpatient Education Program
315 Knapp St
Wolf Point, MT 59102

NEBRASKA
Midlands Diabetes Education and Self-
    Help Center
824 Doctors Bldg., South Tower
4239 Farnum Rd
Omaha, NE 68131

NEVADA
Desert Springs Hospital
Diabetes Education Program
2075 E Flamingo Rd
Las Vegas, NV 89119

NEW HAMPSHIRE
St. Joseph Hospital
172 Kinsley St
Nashua, NH 03061

NEW JERSEY
East Orange VA Medical Center
Diabetes Education & Treatment Center
Tremont Ave
East Orange, NJ 07019

Englewood Hospital Association
Diabetes Program
350 Engle St
Englewood, NJ 07631

Monmouth Medical Center
Diabetes Treatment Center of America
300 Second Ave
Long Branch, NJ 07740

Newark Beth Israel Medical Center
Diabetes Treatment Centers of America
201 Lyons Ave
Newark, NJ 07112

Somerset Medical Center
Diabetes Treatment Centers of America
110 Rehill Ave
Somerville, NJ 08876

NEW MEXICO
Indian Health Service
Albuquerque Service Unit
801 Vassar Dr NE
Albuquerque, NM 87106

NEW YORK
Diabetes Education Associates
600 Northern Blvd, Ste 111
Great Neck, NY 11021

North Shore Co Unity Hospital
Diabetes Education & Treatment Center
300 Community Dr
Manhasset, NY 11030

St. Luke's/Roosevelt Hospital Center
Ambulatory Care Dept
Amsterdam Ave at 114th St
New York, NY 10025

Winthrop-University Hospital
259 First St
Mineola, Long Island, NY 11501

NORTH CAROLINA
The Charlotte-Mecklenburg Authority
Carolinas Diabetes Center
1000 Blythe Blvd
Charlotte, NC 28207

East Carolina University School of
    Medicine
Diabetes Self-Care Program
Section on Endocrinology &
    Metabolism
Greenville, NC 27858

Greensboro Diabetes Self-Care Center
1022 Professional Village
Greensboro, NC 27401

Nalle Clinic
Diabetes Center
1350 So. Kings Dr
Charlotte, NC 28207

Raleigh Community Hospital
Diabetes Treatment Centers of America
3400 Wake Forest Rd
Raleigh, NC 27609

Wesley Long Community Hospital
Diabetes Treatment Centers of America
501 No. Elam Ave
P.O. Drawer X-3
Greensboro, NC 27402

NORTH DAKOTA
Diabetes Center MeritCare
Fargo Clinic MeritCare
737 Broadway
Fargo, ND 58123

Grand Forks Regional Diabetes Education Center
1000 So. Columbia Rd
P.O. Box 6003
Grand Forks, ND 58206-6003

OHIO
Children's Hospital Medical Center
Elland and Bethesda Aves
Cincinnati, OH 45229-2899

Flower Memorial Hospital
5200 Harroun Rd
Sylvania, OH 43560

Lakewood Hospital
Diabetes Center
14519 Detroit Ave
Lakewood, OH 44107

Lorain Community Hospital
Diabetes Comprehensive Care Program
3700 Kolbe Rd
Lorain, OH 44053-1697

Mercy Hospital
2238 Jefferson Ave
Toledo, OH 43624

University MEDNET
Center for Diabetes Care
18599 Lake Shore Blvd
Euclid, OH 44119

OKLAHOMA
Claremore Diabetes Program
U.S. Public Health Service
Indian Hospital
101 So. Moore
Claremore, OK 74017

St. Francis Hospital
Diabetes Center
William Medical Building
6585 So. Yale, Ste. 300
Tulsa, OK 74136

OREGON
Good Samaritan Hospital & Medical Center
Diabetes Institute
1130 NW 22nd Ave, Ste 400A
Portland, OR 97210

Salem Hospital
P. O. Box 14001
665 Winter St SE
Salem, OR 97309-5014

PENNSYLVANIA
Chester County Hospital
Diabetes Learning Center
701 E Marshall St
West Chester, PA 19380

Geisinger Medical Center
Geisinger Diabetes Center
No. Academy Ave
Danville, PA 17822

Guthrie Healthcare System
Guthrie Medical Center
Guthrie Square
Sayre, PA 18840

Montgomery Hospital
Diabetes Treatment Centers
Powell and Fornance Sts
Norristown, PA 19401

Moses Taylor Hospital
Diabetes Treatment Centers
700 Quincy Ave
Scranton, PA 18510

SOUTH CAROLINA
Richland Memorial Hospital
Diabetes Education Program
Five Richland Medical Park
Columbia, SC 29203

SOUTH DAKOTA
McKennan Hospital
Diabetes Education Program
800 E 21st St
Box 5045
Sioux Falls, SD 57117-5045

Sioux Valley Hospital
1100 So. Euclid Ave
P.O. Box 5039
Sioux Falls, SD 57117-5039

TENNESSEE
Baptist Memorial Hospital Medical
Center
899 Madison Ave
Memphis, TN 38146

Endocrinology–Diabetes Associates
Diabetes Care Program
2611 W End Ave., Ste 302
Nashville, TN 37203

Erlanger Medical Center
Regional Diabetes Center
975 E Third St
Chattanooga, TN, 37403

Indian Path Medical Center
Diabetes Treatment Centers of America
2000 Brookside Rd
Kingsport, TN 37660

LeBonheur Children's Medical Center
Diabetes Education Program
One Children's Plaza
Memphis, TN 38103

Regional Medical Center at Memphis
877 Jefferson Ave
Memphis, TN 38103

TEXAS
AMI Park Plaza Hospital
Diabetes Treatment Centers of America
1313 Herman Dr
Houston, TX 77004

Baylor University Medical Center
Ruth Collins Diabetes Center
3500 Gaston Ave
Dallas, TX 75246

Endocrine Associates of Dallas P.A.
5480 La Sierra Dr
Dallas, TX 75231

High Plains Baptist
Center for Diabetes
1600 Wallace Blvd
Amarillo, TX 79106

Irving Hospital
Diabetes Lifestyle Center
1901 No. MacArthur
Irving, TX 75061

St. David's Hospital
Diabetes Center
Box 4039
Austin, TX 78765-4039

Scott & White Clinic
Diabetes Education
240 So. 31st St
Temple, TX 76508

Spohn Hospital
600 Elizabeth St
Corpus Christi, TX 78404

Sun Towers Hospital
Diabetes Treatment Centers of America
1801 No. Oregon St
El Paso, TX 79902

VIRGINIA
Loudoun Healthcare, Inc.
Diabetes Management Program
224 Cornwall St, NW
Leesburg, VA 22075

Memorial Hospital
Diabetes Education Program
142 So. Main St
Danville, VA 24541

Richmond Diabetes Management
   Center
7301 Forest Ave
Richmond, VA 23226

Roanoke Memorial Hospitals
Diabetes Care Unit
Belleview at Jefferson St
Roanoke, VA 24033

WASHINGTON
Virginia Mason Medical Center
Diabetes Center
1100 Ninth Ave
Seattle, WA 98111

WISCONSIN
Columbia Hospital
Diabetes Treatment Centers of America
2025 E Newport Ave
Milwaukee, WI 53211

Froedtert Memorial Lutheran Hospital
Diabetes Care Center
Medical College of Wisconsin
9200 W Wisconsin Ave
Milwaukee, WI 53226

Prairie Clinic, S.C.
Diabetes Focus Program
55 Prairie Ave
Prairie du Sac, WI 53578

WYOMING
DePaul Hospital
Diabetes Education Program
2600 E 18th St
Cheyenne, WY 82001

Step 4. Become Your Own Expert

WHO TO CALL

National Institutes of Health   NIH sponsors numerous research projects on diabetes. To participate you must be referred by your doctor. Physicians can call 301/496-4891, or for severely ill patients 301/496-4181 or 301/495-4658.

9000 Rockville Pike
Bethesda, Maryland 20892

International Diabetes Center

5000 West 39th St
Minneapolis, MN 55416
612/927-3393

American Diabetes Association   This organization offers a broad array of patient information about symptoms, treatments, and prevention. If you want doctor referrals and support group information, call your local affiliate (telephone numbers available through the 800 number).

1660 Duke St
Alexandria, VA 22314
800/232-3472

Juvenile Diabetes Foundation International While JDF's primary focus is to raise money for diabetes research, it also offers patient information on diabetes. Local chapters can provide contacts for specific support groups. The national organization can provide lists of endocrinologists in New York City; local chapters keep lists of area doctors.

432 Park Ave S
New York, NY 10016
800/223-1138

National Diabetes Information Clearinghouse This clearinghouse offers patient information but no doctor referrals. A bulletin, *Diabetes Dateline,* published three times a year, provides articles and brochures from the combined health information database.

P.O. Box NDIC
9000 Rockville Pike
Bethesda, MD 20892
301/468-2162

American Dietetic Assocation This group offers information about nutrition specific to diabetes in addition to referrals to consulting nutritionists.

216 W Jackson
Chicago, IL 60606
312/899-0040

American Association of Diabetes Educators This is primarily a professional organization for nurses, pharmacists, educators, and others in the field. However, it can refer patients to educators in their area. The AADE certifies diabetes educators.

500 No. Michigan Ave, Ste 1400
Chicago, IL 60611
312/661-1700

Joslin Diabetes Center

One Joslin Pl
Boston, MA 02215
617/732-2400

NIH CRISP System
301/496-7543

University-Affiliated Teaching Hospitals   See Appendix

EXPERT SOURCES

Although dozens of experts were interviewed for these chapters, the following are acknowledged for their significant contributions to this section.

Dr. Robert Ratner, George Washington School of Medicine, Washington, DC

The staff of the Joslin Clinic, Boston, MA

The staff of the American Diabetes Association, Alexandria, VA

REFERENCES AND SUGGESTED READING

American Diabetes Association. *Diabetes A to Z,* 1988.

Atkinson, M. A., and Maclaren, N. K. What Causes Diabetes? *Scientific American,* July 1990.

Biermann, J., and Toohey B. *The Diabetics' Book: All Your Questions Answered.* Los Angeles: Jeremy Tarcher, 1990.

Centers for Disease Control. Regional Variation in Diabetes Mellitus Prevalence—U.S., 1988–1989. *Morbidity and Mortality Weekly Report,* Vol. 39, No. 45 (Nov. 16, 1990).

Dills, Diana G., and others. Association of Elevated IGF-I Levels with Increased Retinopathy in Late-Onset Diabetes. *Diabetes,* Vol. 40, No. 12 (Dec. 1991), pp. 1725–1730.

MacFarlane, I. A., and others. Diabetes in Prison: Can Good Diabetic Care Be Achieved? *British Medical Journal,* Vol. 304, No. 6820 (Jan. 18, 1992), pp. 152–155.

National Standards for Diabetes Patient Education and American Diabetes Association Review Criteria. Standards and Review Criteria. *Diabetes Care,* Vol. 9 (1986), pp. XXXVI–XL.

Physician's Guide to Insulin-Dependent (Type I) Diabetes. *Diagnosis and Treatment,* 1988.

Robbins, D., Ed. American Diabetes Association. *Diabetes Care: Clinical Practice Recommendations,* Vol. 13, January 1990.

Schade, David S., and Boyle, Patrick J. Insulin Resistance: Its Role in Health and Disease. *Clinical Diabetes,* Vol. 10, No. 1 (Jan.–Feb. 1992), pp. 3–6.

Zimmerman, B. and Radak, J. T. American Diabetes Association. *Standards of Care for Patients with Diabetes Mellitus,* 1989.

Epilepsy

Risk for Inappropriate Care   HIGH

"Most of the two million Americans with epilepsy still experience a poor quality of life," reports the National Seizure Disorders Survey, released in June 1990. That's unfortunate—and unnecessary. With correct medication, half of these people could be seizure free indefinitely, and most of the remainder would suffer far fewer seizures.

Experts we interviewed estimate that as many as two-thirds of patients are not getting state-of-the-art care. They don't get that care because their health care providers frequently misdiagnose them and don't properly match their diagnosis to the appropriate therapy.

What It Is

Epilepsy is a disorder involving recurrent seizures. A seizure is sudden, excessive electrical discharge in the brain that produces changes in the body that range from abdominal discomfort to convulsions. In about half of the cases the cause is unknown. If no brain damage from birth trauma or tumors is present, it may be the result of a chemical abnormality in the brain. Lead poisoning, meningitis, encephalitis, stroke, head injury, and inherited diseases such as phenylketonuria can all cause epilepsy. Although there is a genetic predisposition to some forms of the disease, epilepsy may be present even without a family history.

Step 1. Make Sure You Get the Best Care

Read this section on potential problems with your treatment carefully to determine if there are discrepancies between your care and state-of-the-art care. Use Step 2 to review shortcomings.

Diagnosis

If you have epilepsy, your goals should be to remain seizure and symptom free and to maintain a normal quality of life. Be aware that not all seizures are caused by epilepsy. In an astounding 20–30% of the cases in which seizures are poorly controlled, the patients do not have epilepsy at all, according to experts I polled.

It requires a real specialist to distinguish between seizures caused by epilepsy and those by other causes, especially if your medical history and diagnostic tests are inconclusive. Not every doctor can make that distinction. A New York City woman who was fainting and suffering seizures consulted a half-dozen doctors. It wasn't until specialists examined her at a center of excellence for epilepsy that doctors correctly diagnosed her. A heart condition, not epilepsy, was her real problem. In a similar case researchers videotaped a woman as she stiffened and fell to the floor. Every doctor who saw the tape believed she had epilepsy. Not one correctly diagnosed her condition—a heart problem that reduced the amount of oxygen reaching her brain. Her previous health care providers had prescribed three different seizure medications, all of which failed to correct the problem. You should remember that if a drug doesn't work, it may be because the diagnosis is wrong.

TESTS   To reach the proper diagnosis your doctor should take an accurate medical history of your seizures. Often patients can't accurately recall their seizures, so it's important to question witnesses as well. Here are tests that doctors rely on.

Magnetic Resonance Imaging (MRI) Scan   An MRI scan looks for signs of cancer, multiple sclerosis, vascular abnormalities, and other problems that can cause seizures. This is a diagnostic procedure of choice.

Electroencephalogram (EEG)   An EEG records abnormal electrical brain wave activity. The EEG complements the MRI. A single EEG tracing may miss any evidence of seizure activity. Many specialists recommend a 24-hour continuous recording if this is so. The continuous EEG is available in the hospital, or at home when a portable recorder is used. When the source of seizures is unknown, a variation of this, called video-EEG monitoring, is performed. With a video camera, specialists can record seizures and EEG recordings simultaneously. This allows them to tie the exact physical motions of the seizure to the abnormal brain wave activity.

You need to be wary if your health care provider won't order an EEG when you are first diagnosed. According to the National Seizure Disorder Survey, 68% of doctors always order an EEG, 26% do so occasionally, and 6% seldom or never order the test.

Positron Emission Tomography (PET) Scan   A PET scan produces color-coded pictures of the brain showing blood flow, glucose use, and oxygen presence. Surgeons plan their operation strategy using the PET scan.

Computed Axial Tomography (CAT) Scan   A CAT scan is used in emergencies. Following a first seizure, doctors need to exclude quickly the possibility of blood clots and other serious abnormalities. In a nonemergency situation, however, it is better to wait until an MRI can be done.

Other Tests   Blood tests rule out as the cause of the seizures medical illnesses, including low blood sugar, meningitis, and liver disease, among others. Tests exist that can rule out an infection.

Overuse of Tests   While tests can be extremely important to your diagnosis, be wary of their excessive use. In the United States, roughly one of every two tests contributes neither to the diagnosis nor to the treatment of the disease.

Doctors should order tests when there is potential to change the treatment. Some doctors will ask you to have an EEG every month. In most instances you will need an EEG during your first workup and again if there is some change in your epilepsy status. If you are doing well, there's no need to spend the $350 that EEGs typically cost.

Treatment

During a Seizure   You should be sure that people close to you know the proper actions to take when you're having a seizure. Most Good Samaritans will try to jam an object, often a tongue depressor, into your mouth when you are having a seizure. They believe this will prevent you from swallowing your tongue. In fact, it is not possible to swallow your tongue. (Even some university teaching hospitals keep tongue depressors next to the beds of seizure patients!) You could break a tooth or even asphyxiate yourself on a depressor. Family, co-workers, and friends should be informed never to put anything into the mouth of a seizure patient. Instead, they should roll the head to one side so the patient doesn't swallow vomit or saliva.

Treatment Medications

Make sure your doctor is prescribing the latest medications. In the National Seizure Disorder Survey 85% of patients continued to receive older medications, including barbiturates such as phenobarbital. Experts now consider them second-line medications. These physicians simply have not caught up with the latest research findings. Studies have shown that when doctors take patients off sedating antiepilepsy drugs, the patients think more clearly and their memory improves. Jerome Engel Jr., Chief of Epilepsy and Clinical Neurophysiology at the University of California's Hospital and Clinics in Los Angeles, says: "Too many patients and doctors are satisfied with termination of seizures. They need to be concerned with quality-of-life issues, as well—some people are walking around like zombies. It's an important issue with kids as well because parents often think that laziness or tiredness is a consequence of the disease when it's really a result of the drug."

Your doctor should counsel you about the interactions of antiseizure and other drugs. Some anticonvulsants cause other drugs to work less well. Phenytoin, carbamazepine, and phenobarbital may decrease the effectiveness of birth control pills, as one example. One woman taking birth control pills became pregnant within a few months of beginning treatment with phenytoin. For another example, erythromycin may cause an abrupt increase in carbamazepine levels, which can create severe side effects.

All epilepsy drugs become toxic at a certain dosage. For that reason doctors frequently test the amount in your blood to make sure levels are high enough to work but not so high as to be dangerous. That doesn't mean doctors should treat the blood level and ignore the patient. Too often doctors, seeing that the blood level is too high, lower the dosage even if the patient is well controlled and isn't experiencing any side effects. Then, again, if the drug level in your blood isn't high enough for the recommended dosage, your doctor may increase the amount of medication even though your seizures are already well-controlled.

If you have tried two or more drugs and are still experiencing seizures, you should confirm your diagnosis. Remember, it may be wrong.

Today, doctors know that antiseizure medications are specific for a particular seizure type and that specific drugs need a trial period to determine whether or not they can control the disorder. Since treatment should be based on your seizure type, you should be sure that the type is identified accurately. Table 4 presents the proper medications for each seizure type (according to Dr. Orrin Devinsky, Chief of the Department of Neurology and the Comprehensive Epilepsy Center at New York University's Hospital for Joint Diseases).

TABLE 4. Epileptic Seizure Medications

Seizure Type	Drugs of Choice	Alternative Drugs
Partial Seizures: simple, complex or secondary generalized	• carbamazepine • phenytoin	• phenobarbital • primidone • valproic acid
Absence Seizures without primary generalized tonic-clonic movements	• ethosuximide	• valproic acid • clonazepam
Absence Seizures with primary generalized tonic-clonic movements	• valproic acid	• ethosuximide • clonazepam
Myoclonic Seizures, atypical absence seizures, atonic seizures	• valproic acid	• clonazepam • acetazolamide
Primary Generalized Tonic-Clonic Seizures	• carbamazepine • phenytoin • valproic acid	• phenobarbital • primidone

MEDICATION SIDE EFFECTS   Since quality of life is such an important issue with epilepsy, you should know if you are suffering excessively from drug side effects.

Read through Table 5, provided by Dr. Devinsky. It lists side effects for medications you may be presently taking. If you have any, consider changing drugs and reducing the number of drugs you take.

TABLE 5. Side Effects of Seizure Medications

Drug	Side Effects	Drug	Side Effects
Phenytoin (*trade name:* Dilantin)	• Rash • Unsteadiness • Hirsutism or excessive hair growth • Sedation • Gum overgrowth • Loss of bone substance • Folate deficiency anemia • Acne	**Primidone** (*trade name:* Mysoline)	• Sedation • Cognitive slowing • Irritability, rash • Loss of bone substance • Anemia • Behavioral changes
Carbamazepine (*trade name:* Tegretol)	• Sedation • Rash • Gastrointestinal discomfort • Liver and bone marrow toxicity • Dizziness • Blurred or double vision	**Valproic acid** (*trade name:* Depakane)	• Nausea • Vomiting • Liver toxicity • Hemorrhage • Pancreatitis • Hair loss • Weight gain • Tremors
Phenobarbital (*trade name:* Luminal)	• Rash • Unsteadiness • Sedation • Gastrointestinal discomfort • Bone marrow damage • Loss of bone substance • Folate deficiency anemia • Cognitive slowing	**Ethosuximide** (*trade name:* Zarontin)	• Gastrointestinal discomfort • Sedation • Unsteadiness • Seizures • Liver and bone marrow toxicity • Rash • Dizziness
		Clonazepam (*trade name:* Clonopin)	• Sedation • Dizziness • Unsteadiness • Behavioral changes

WISE MEDICATION USE   Be careful about multidrug therapy. Here's a common example of how patients end up taking several drugs instead of one: The doctor prescribes a drug for a first seizure. For each additional seizure, the doctor increases the dosage. When the maximum dose for that drug has been prescribed, additional drugs are added for successive seizures. You could be taking three, four, even five drugs. Too many drugs markedly increase the potential side effects. To alleviate those side effects, doctors may subtract drugs without a well-thought-out plan. In that case, there's little chance you will be taking the best drugs for your case. You also won't know which drugs are controlling your seizures and which are causing side effects.

Today the best doctors know that medications are specific for a particular seizure type (see Table 4) and that individual drugs need a trial period to determine whether or not they can control the disorder. Drug treatment should be simplified. Many patients on several medications really need only one. Dr. Devinsky says: "The vast majority of patients with epilepsy can be controlled on a single drug with little or no side effects. Many patients are treated with archaic regimens of two or three drugs which are all in the subtherapeutic dose range. It is wiser to use a single drug and slowly increase the dosage and blood levels. However, there are clearly some patients who do best with two or, rarely, three antiepileptic drugs." Make certain to discuss medication use with your doctor.

Even the best drug regimen will not work if you don't follow it. Compliance is a problem with nearly every chronic disease. Patients frequently don't take medications around the clock, a necessity for many chronic illnesses.

Some patients don't comply because they:

■ Believe drug treatment to be more dangerous than seizures, especially if they've experienced unpleasant side effects.

■ Have no recollection of seizures, so they underestimate their danger.

■ Enjoy the attention they gain from seizures.

■ Assume they no longer need medication if they have been seizure free for a period of time.

■ Find that taking medications is a hassle.

GENERIC DRUGS   You should beware of generic antiseizure drugs. Although some manufacturers of generic drugs produce a consistent product, many pharmacies and distributors buy from the generic company that charges the least. When the formulations vary, blood levels can vacillate. As a result, if you take the same dose of such a generic drug as of a brand-name medication, you may experience side effects from toxic levels or have seizures from subtherapeutic levels.

OLDER DRUGS   Eighty-five percent of all patients continue to receive older, out-of-date medications. Those may include barbiturates such as phenobarbital. Specialists attribute this to low awareness among other physicians.

Alternative Treatments

In addition to your medications, you may want to experiment with alternative forms of therapy. The guideline is simple: They must keep you seizure free and cause no ill effect. A high-fat diet can produce a chemical condition called ketosis that sometimes will control epilepsy in infants or young children. Biofeedback or relaxation therapy can help some patients to create brain-wave patterns that prevent seizures. So far this has been successful in only a small number of patients.

SURGERY   If your seizures are poorly controlled after a number of drug trials, you should contact a center of excellence for epilepsy to consider if surgery could help you. This is one disease where too few operations are performed. While up to 10% of the people who have epilepsy—that's 300,000 patients—could benefit from surgery, only a tiny fraction ever have an operation. That's the result of a number of factors. First, few doctors train to perform the surgery. Then, there are only a limited number of centers that offer surgery for the control of epilepsy. (Many major medical centers in New York City did not begin performing these operations until 1991.) And the cost of the operation is exceedingly high, ranging from $40,000 to $100,000, depending on the operation.

This next section is highly technical. You will need your precise diagnosis to make use of it.

There are three types of seizures that respond favorably to surgery: partial seizures of temporal or extratemporal lobe origin, secondary generalized seizures that begin locally and spread to both sides of the brain, and one-sided, multifocal seizures associated with infantile paralysis.

Before you consent to surgery, you should have a complete neurological evaluation confirming the following:

■ Diagnosis of epilepsy

■ Seizure type and syndrome

■ Well-defined cause of the seizure that has been traced to a small area of the brain and that can be removed without impairing mental or physical function (Patients who have generalized seizures traced simultaneously to both sides of the brain are *not* likely candidates for surgery.)

■ Reasonable trial of medications that are taken properly without success

There are four operations that may help to relieve you of your symptoms. Dr. Devinsky reviews them as follows.

Temporal Lobectomy   This is the most widely used surgical procedure for epilepsy, and offers the greatest rate of success. The anterior temporal lobe is the most common site of the disease in patients with partial seizures. Surgeons remove this part of the brain. Approximately 60% of patients become seizure free, and another 30% enjoy a marked reduction in seizure frequency. Behavioral disorders such as aggressiveness and hyperactivity may improve. In some patients IQ increases of 10 points have been observed in those who emerge from the surgery seizure free.

Extratemporal Resections Surgical therapy can be effective in patients whose seizures are located in the frontal, parietal, or occipital lobes. The surgery is often limited in scope because of risk to nearby areas of the brain that govern such functions as speech and motor control. As a result, the success rate with extratemporal resections is lower than with temporal resections.

Corpus Callostomy In general, corpus callostomy relieves symptoms but is not curative. It reduces the number of severe seizures and prevents secondary seizure activity and in turn cuts the number of injuries from falls. Complications occur in 20% of patients. Likely candidates for callostomy have an extensive area or multifocal areas of epilepogenic tissue.

Hemispherectomy A tabloid once ran a story of a girl with half a brain. In truth, she did have most of one-half her brain removed to control seizures that occurred multiple times each day and could not be treated with medication. The operation, called a subtotal hemispherectomy, is used to treat seizures for which medications don't work in patients with preexisting diffuse injury to one side of the brain. Infantile spasms are one example. Most of these patients have frequent, severe seizures arising from a hemisphere with little or no function already, so the operation does not result in any functional loss. This operation accounts for only about 2% of all patients who are treated surgically.

EPILEPSY AND DEPRESSION At least 20% of seizure patients are depressed. Doctors have an obligation to diagnose and treat these patients.

Step 2. Look for Shortcomings

From reading Step 1, you have, I hope, gotten a good feeling about your treatment and you understand much of it better. You'll learn even more by calling organizations listed in Step 4. But if you have an uncomfortable feeling that your treatment is not on track, then study this section, which specifies some common and serious shortcomings that experts in the field recognize. If this section confirms your suspicions, you should go to Step 3. Some of these mistakes you can discover yourself; others only an expert can confirm.

MISTAKES IN DIAGNOSIS

You haven't had a full diagnostic workup, including a 24-hour EEG.

Your seizures are not caused by epilepsy.

You are depressed and not receiving treatment for depression.

MISTAKES IN TREATMENT

Your health care provider isn't trained to treat epilepsy.

You're treated for the wrong type of epilepsy.

Your treatment is not keeping you completely free of seizures.

You don't take your medicine.

You're not counseled appropriately on interactions between different drugs you are taking.

You continue to have seizures or severe drug side effects and haven't been referred to an epilepsy center.

You are using generic drugs that aren't as effective as brand-name drugs.

You take more than one drug when a single drug will work as well.

You are overtreated with sedating medications.

You get older drugs that are not state-of-the-art.

You are depressed and not receiving treatment for depression.

Your health care provider treats you based on your blood drug levels, not your condition.

You don't consider state-of-the-art surgery if your seizures are still poorly controlled.

Your family, friends, and co-workers don't know what to do when you're having a seizure.

Your obstetrician doesn't know how to manage pregnant seizure patients.

Step 3. See a Specialist

If, from Step 2, you are concerned that your care is not state-of-the-art, this section will tell you how to choose an expert.

As basically an outpatient disease, epilepsy has advantages and disadvantages. You will rarely need care in the hospital, for most of your care will be in a doctor's office or a clinic. Unfortunately, most medical students and residents spend most of their time learning to treat hospitalized patients and may never have worked in an epilepsy outpatient clinic. They tend never to see epilepsy patients and so may be unfamiliar with many aspects of their care. Most doctors don't learn how to prescribe or monitor antiseizure drugs. In addition, most doctors never learned how to observe and recognize the different types of seizures. This was true even at

Harvard Medical School. Yet many family doctors feel threatened by specialists, fearing they will steal their patients and never refer them back.

Some doctors are satisfied if you only suffer a few seizures. Experts say the complete termination of seizures should be your goal. You need to exhaust all possibilities. Your family doctor or general practitioner should refer you to a neurologist if your seizures are not controlled, with minimal side effects, within three months. If doctors cannot control your epilepsy within six months to a year, see an epileptologist. It is particularly important for children to see specialists early on. With children a delay in effective treatment can impair intellectual development.

Doctors practicing at a center of excellence treat a high volume of epilepsy patients. New York University Medical Center's Comprehensive Epilepsy Program, for instance, sees 1,000 patients a year. The National Association of Epilepsy Centers suggests you should seek specialized care if:

- You have a progressive brain tumor.

- You have a tumor near the area of your brain responsible for language, sensory, or motor control.

- You are not seizure free even after changes in medications and dosages.

- You are depressed.

- You are considering becoming pregnant.

DURING PREGNANCY   You will want to consult a center of excellence if you are pregnant or planning on becoming pregnant. Few obstetricians know how to manage women who have epilepsy. Your obstetrician should work with a seizure expert. One New York obstetrician told his patient to have an abortion, simply because she had a history of seizures and was on an antiepileptic drug. Patients should see an epilepsy specialist *before* getting pregnant. While there is no perfect drug for epilepsy, the goal should be to get down to a single drug. Each drug roughly doubles the risk of fetal malformation, so the fewest drugs at the lowest dosages possible is the best solution. Taking folate during pregnancy lowers the risk of birth defects. You should also consider surgery, since that would, if successful, eliminate the need for medications.

Women with epilepsy don't make bad mothers. If they have seizures with impairment or loss of consciousness, they do need to take certain precautions, such as making sure they are sitting down while breastfeeding, and not being alone when bathing the baby.

PSYCHOLOGICAL SUPPORT   Epilepsy can be as much a psychological problem as it is a physical one. Both the disease and the drugs that treat it can cause psychological problems. It's not enough for a physician to diagnose and treat. If you are among the 20–25% of epilepsy patients who are depressed, that is another reason to contact a center of excellence. Although doctors should know their patients and families and be willing to counsel both, most doctors simply don't have the time. That's why an epilepsy center is so helpful. They offer an integrated team approach that can include psychiatrists, social workers, and psychologists who provide psychological testing.

Experience

Right now, there is no specialty board for epileptologists. In fact, nowhere in neurology are there specialty boards for the care of specific categories of patients. You want a doctor who has trained in a residency in neurology and gone through a one-year or ideally two-year fellowship in clinical epilepsy and/or neurophysiology. Some epileptologists become heavily involved in academia (running a research laboratory, for example). You really want to find a clinician, not someone who's only seeing patients on Wednesday afternoons.

Surgeon's Experience

You want a surgeon who has done between 50 and 100 epilepsy surgeries thus far. Unfortunately, there have been no studies on learning curves for surgery for epilepsy.

RISKS WITH SURGERY   There is always the risk that either the dominant or nondominant portion of your brain will be affected. The dominant part of the brain controls language and verbal memory function, while the nondominant portion controls visual memory and spatial abilities. There is also a very small risk of impaired use of limbs or paralysis.

Surgical Centers of Excellence

If you decide on surgery, you should go to a hospital with a proven track record, one where morbidity and mortality rates are low but not zero for the preoperative invasive recording tests. Therefore look for a center with the latest presurgical evaluations. Success depends on the surgeon's ability to localize a particular area in the brain. The surgical team should include an epileptologist, a neurophysiologist, a neurosurgeon, and a neuropsychiatrist. "The team is really what's important. You need the coordination," according to Dr. Devinsky.

As you look for surgical centers of excellence, ask about their success, complication, and death rates. The hospital should be performing a minimum of two to four surgeries each month. According to one expert, your center should be performing at least 30–40 epilepsy surgeries a year. Here are the acceptable statistics for the four operations performed on people with epilepsy.

PROCEDURE	SEIZURE FREE	COMPLICATION RATE	DEATH RATE
Temporal lobectomy	60–70%	5%	Below 0.5%
Extratemporal resection	30–50%	6%	0%
Corpus callostomy	5%	11%	2%
Hemispherectomy	80%	16%	4%

The center's overall rate for death and serious complications should be less than 5%, states Dr. Jerome Engle. Dr. Engle also suggests that you ask about the number of patients rejected by the center. Some centers are more concerned with their success rate than they are with helping patients. If a patient's chance of significant seizure reduction is only 50%, some centers won't take the case, simply because they may look bad. That's true even if the family knows the risks and are willing to take them. You should look, too, at the number of patients who had to return a second time for surgery and find out why.

Centers of Excellence for Epilepsy

The following list of hospitals is provided only as a convenient starting place in your search for excellence. These hospitals are recommended on the basis of reputation, not experience and results. The list is not an endorsement. There may be hospitals just as excellent that have been omitted. You should apply the guidelines for experience, results, and other measures of excellence to any hospital you choose, whether or not it is on this list. Although hospitals from different sources have been combined into one list, the compilation in no way implies that one source has endorsed the hospital list of another source.

CALIFORNIA
Reed Neurology Research Center   EX
University of California, Los Angeles,
    School of Medicine
710 Westwood Plaza
Los Angeles, CA 90024

CONNECTICUT
Yale University   EX
Comprehensive Epilepsy Center
Dept of Neurology
New Haven, CT 06510

FLORIDA
Miami Children's Hospital   EX
Comprehensive Epilepsy Center
6125 SW 31st St
Miami, FL 33155

GEORGIA
Medical College of Georgia   EX
Dept of Neurology
1459 Laney Walker Blvd
Augusta, GA 30912

MICHIGAN
University of Michigan   EX
Comprehensive Epilepsy Center
Dept of Neurology
1914/0316 Taubman Center
1500 E Medical Center Dr
Ann Arbor, MI 48109

MINNESOTA
Mayo Clinic   EX
200 First St SW
Rochester, MN 55905

New York University–Hospital
  for Joint Diseases   EX
Comprehensive Epilepsy Center
Dept of Neurology
301 E 17th St
New York, NY 10003

OREGON
Good Samaritan Hospital &
  Medical Center   EX
Comprehensive Epilepsy Program
1040 NW 22nd Ave, Ste 400
Portland, OR 97210

PENNSYLVANIA
Graduate Hospital   EX
Comprehensive Epilepsy Center
1800 Lombard St
Philadelphia, PA 19146

TENNESSEE
Epicare Center   EX
899 Madison, Ste 404-M
Memphis, TN 38146

WASHINGTON
University of Washington   EX
Comprehensive Epilepsy Center
Dept of Neurosurgery, RI-20
Seattle, WA 98195

SOURCES

EX   indicates the hospitals recommended by experts interviewed.

Step 4. Become Your Own Expert

WHO TO CALL

Epilepsy Foundation of America   The national foundation will direct you to one of its 85 affiliates. You can call about diagnosis, treatment, medications, first aid, community services, parent support groups, self-help support groups, and employment. The National Epilepsy Library operates from 9 am to 6 pm, Eastern time, Monday through Friday.

> 4351 Garden City Dr, Ste 406
> Landover, MD 20785
> 301/459-3700
> 800/EFA-1000

National Association of Epilepsy Centers   This organization provides a list of member hospitals. However, this list is by no means a list of top or designated centers. Hospitals become members by donating a membership fee; there are no criteria for membership. The association has created a list of guidelines for three different levels of epilepsy care centers. You may want to take a look at the guidelines and compare them to the services offered at the center where you are receiving care.

> 5775 Wayzata Blvd
> Minneapolis, MN 55416
> 612/525-1160

NIH CRISP System

301/496-7543

University-Affiliated Teaching Hospitals   See Appendix.

EPILEPSY RESEARCH CENTERS   The National Institute of Neurological and Communicative Disorders and Stroke, which is part of the National Institutes of Health, sponsors research at the following centers.

Stanford University Medical Center
300 Pasteur Dr
Stanford, CA 94305

Duke University School of Medicine
PO Box 3005
Durham, NC 27710

Yale University School of Medicine
333 Cedar St
New Haven, CT 06516

Baylor College of Medicine
1200 Moursund Ave
Houston, TX 77025

Washington University School of
    Medicine
660 S. Euclid Ave
St. Louis, MO 63110

Dixon Woodbury, M.D.
University of Utah College of Medicine
50 No. Medical Dr
Salt Lake City, UT 84132

EPILEPSY CLINICAL RESEARCH CENTERS   The National Institute of Neurological Disorders and Stroke, which is part of the National Institutes of Health, supports epilepsy clinical research centers that focus on genetics, epidemiology, imaging, drug and surgical treatments, and other areas of basic and clinical research. In addition to providing medical and surgical treatment, these centers look after the entire needs of the patient and provide access to all services the patient may need, including rehabilitation, counseling, and training.

University of California, Los Angeles
710 Westwood Plaza
Los Angeles, CA 90024

University of California, Los Angeles
West Los Angeles VA Medical Center
Wilshire and Sawtelle Blvds
Los Angeles, CA 90078

Medical College of Virginia
Virginia Commonwealth University
Box 599, MCV Station
Richmond, VA 23298-0599

Stanford University School of Medicine
Department of Psychiatry and Behav-
    ioral Sciences
Bldg. TD, Rm 114
300 Pasteur Dr
Stanford, CA 94305

Washington University School of
    Medicine
660 So. Euclid Ave
St. Louis, MO 63110

University of Minnesota
Minneapolis Medical School
2701 University Ave SE, Ste 106
Minneapolis, MN 55455

Baylor College of Medicine
1200 Moursund Ave
Houston, TX 77025

Duke University School of Medicine
P.O. Box 3005
Durham, NC 27710

Yale University School of Medicine
333 Cedar St
New Haven, CT 06516

University of Washington School of
    Medicine
Seattle, WA 98195

EXPERT SOURCES

Although dozens of experts were interviewed for these chapters, these physicians are acknowledged for their significant contributions to this section.

Dr. Orrin Devinsky, Chief, Department of Neurology, Hospital for Joint Diseases, New York University, New York, NY

Dr. Jerome Engle, Chief of Epilepsy and Clinical Neurophysiology, Hospital and Clinics, University of California, Los Angeles, CA

REFERENCES AND SUGGESTED READING

Brett, Edward M. (ed). *Paediatric Neurology,* 2nd ed. New York: Churchill Livingstone, 1991.

Ciccone, Patrick E. Control Groups in the Study of Effects of Medication. [letters to the editor] *American Journal of Psychiatry,* Vol. 149, No. 7 (Jan. 1992), pp. 141–142.

Compston, Alistair. Principles of Diagnosis and Management: Clinical Neurology. *Lancet,* Vol. 339, No. 8790 (Feb. 15, 1992), p. 415.

Dam, M., and Gram, L. *Comprehensive Epileptology.* New York: Raven Press, 1990.

Epilepsy Foundation of America. *Current Trends in Epilepsy: A Self-Study Course for Physicians,* 1990.

Fauth, C., and others. Seizure Induction and Magnetic Brain Stimulation After Stroke. [letter to the editor] *Lancet,* Vol. 339, No. 8789 (Feb. 8, 1992), p. 362.

Haas, L. F. Neurological Stamp: William Harvey, 1578–1657. *Journal of Neurology, Neurosurgery and Psychiatry,* Vol. 55, No. 2 (Feb. 1992), p. 111.

Haller, Jerome S. Seizures and Epilepsy in Childhood: A Guide for Parents. [book review] *Journal of Pediatrics,* Vol. 120, No. 1 (Jan. 1992), p. 78.

Hauser, W. A., and Hesdorffer, D. C. *Facts About Epilepsy.* New York: Demos Publications, 1990.

Illis, L. S. Women and Epilepsy. [book review] *Journal of Neurology, Neurosurgery and Psychiatry,* Vol. 55, No. 1 (Jan. 1992), p. 88

Malyk, Bohdan, and Spence, Michael R. Development of New-Onset Seizures in the Peripartum Period: Should Human Immunodeficiency Virus Infection Be Considered a Cause? *Sexually Transmitted Diseases,* Vol. 19, No. 1. (Jan.–Feb. 1992), pp. 25–27.

Mendez, M. F., and others. Depression in Epilepsy. *Archives of Neurology,* Vol. 43 (1986), pp. 766–770.

National Association of Epilepsy Centers. Recommended Guidelines for Diagnosis and Treatment in Specialized Epilepsy Centers. *Journal of the International League Against Epilepsy,* Vol. 31, Supplement 1, 1990.

National Institutes of Health. *Consensus Development Conference on Surgery for Epilepsy.* Vol. 8, No. 2 (March 19–21, 1990).

Pascual, Julio, and others. Role of Lidocaine (Lignocaine) in Managing Status Epilepticus. *Journal of Neurology, Neurosurgery and Psychiatry,* Vol. 55, No. 1 (Jan. 1992), pp. 49–51.

Penry, J. K. *Epilepsy: Diagnosis, Management, Quality of Life.* New York: Raven Press, 1986.

Pisani, F., and others. Elevation of Plasma Phenytoin by Viloxazine in Epileptic Patients: A Clinically Significant Drug Interaction. *Journal of Neurology, Neurosurgery and Psychiatry,* Vol. 55, No. 2 (Feb. 1992), pp. 126–127.

Rao, S. M., and others. Viscosity and Social Cohesion in Temporal Lobe Epilepsy. *Journal of Neurology, Neurosurgery and Psychiatry,* Vol. 55, No. 2 (Feb. 1992), pp. 149–152.

Reutens, David C., and Berkovic, Samuel F. Increased Cortical Excitability in Generalised Epilepsy Demonstrated with Transcranial Magnetic Stimulation. [letters to the editor] *Lancet,* Vol. 339, No. 8789 (Feb. 8, 1992), pp. 362–363.

Robertson, M. M. The Organic Contribution to Depressive Illness in Patients with Epilepsy. *Journal of Epilepsy,* Vol. 2 (1989), pp. 189–230.

Sandstrom, Robert. The Evaluation and Treatment of Seizures. *Physical Therapy,* Vol. 71, No. 12 (Dec. 1991), pp. 1020–1021.

Stormy Onset with Prolonged Loss of Consciousness in Benign Childhood Epilepsy with Occipital Paroxysms. *Journal of Neurology, Neurosurgery and Psychiatry,* Vol. 55, No. 1 (Jan. 1992), pp. 45–48.

Toone, B. K. The Psychoses of Epilepsy. [book review] *Journal of Neurology, Neurosurgery and Psychiatry,* Vol. 55, No. 2 (Feb. 1992), p. 169.

Trimble, Michael R. Behaviour Changes Following Temporal Lobectomy, with Special Reference to Psychosis. [editorial] *Journal of Neurology, Neurosurgery and Psychiatry,* Vol. 55, No. 2 (Feb. 1992), pp. 89–91.

Van Buren, J. M. Complications of Surgical Procedures in the Diagnosis and Treatment of Epilepsy. In *Surgical Treatment of the Epilepsies,* Ed. J. Engle, Jr. New York: Raven Press, 1987, pp. 465–475.

Williamson, P. D., and others. Occipital Lobe Epilepsy: Clinical Characteristics, Seizure Spread Patterns, and Results of Surgery. *Annals of Neurology,* Vol. 31, No. 1 (Jan. 1992), pp. 3–13.

Woody, Robert C. Life-Threatening Epilepsy. [letters to the editor] *Archives of Disease in Childhood,* Vol. 67, No. 1 (Jan. 1992), p. 151.

High Blood Pressure

Risk for Inappropriate Care **VERY HIGH**

Even though nearly one of every three Americans has high blood pressure, 65% are not properly treated. They are either undertreated, mistreated, or simply never diagnosed. The American Heart Association reports the following:

- 46% of the people with high blood pressure don't know they have it

- 66.9% are not on any kind of therapy: drugs, diet, or exercise

- 21% are aware of their condition but aren't on medication

- 22% are on medication, though their condition is inadequately controlled

Millions suffer the ill effects of medications that are poorly suited to them. High blood pressure is often called the silent killer because victims rarely have symptoms. But while hypertension may kill silently, it kills very effectively. It is a contributing factor in 900,000 deaths a year.

According to the National Heart, Lung, and Blood Institute, a 35-year-old man with normal blood pressure can expect to live to age 76. If his blood pressure is mildly elevated, his life expectancy drops to 72 years. If it is severely elevated, his life expectancy falls to 60 years. Without proper treatment, high blood pressure can damage the eyes, heart, brain, blood vessels, and kidneys. A person with even a slightly elevated blood pressure has a significantly increased risk of stroke.

What It Is

When your heart pumps blood into your arteries with a force greater than necessary to maintain the smooth flow of blood, you have hypertension. That added force, maintained over years, can damage many body organs, including your heart, brain, and kidneys

There are two basic kinds of high blood pressure. The first is called essential hypertension. It's the culprit in 90% of patients with high blood pressure.

The other form of hypertension is called secondary hypertension, that is, secondary to some other cause. By testing, your doctor may find that cause and cure your hypertension. Unfortunately, such a good-luck scenario is true 10% or less of the time, according to the American Heart Association. One example would be a crimped or blocked artery supplying blood to one kidney. By correcting that, nowadays with a simple balloon catheter, your hypertension could be cured.

Step 1. Make Sure You Get the Best Care

Read this section on potential treatment problems carefully to determine if there are any discrepancies between your care and state-of-the-art care. Use Step 2 to review shortcomings.

Diagnosis

A detailed medical history and physical examination are essential for diagnosis, because hypertension may have virtually no physical symptoms. Your doctor may uncover easily remediable causes of your high blood pressure. Use of the birth control pill, drinking in excess, another illness, or medication could cause your hypertension.

Some doctors don't order any diagnostic tests for hypertensive patients. When that happens you lose in several ways. You may be the one in 10 hypertensive patients whose high blood pressure can be cured but whose cause will never be discovered. You won't have a well-planned treatment strategy because your doctor won't know what type of high blood pressure you have. You could take medications needlessly for life.

It's not fair to lay the blame on doctors for this failure. The use of expensive tests is discouraged by some private and government health financing plans. They discount the value of diagnostic workups. While some government agencies are willing to concede that certain hypertensive patients who could be cured will be missed, most insist that in the long run it won't matter. Many insurance companies and managed health care firms will restrict your access to diagnostic tests and expensive medications that might be indicated. You may receive a very inexpensive drug with a side-effect profile that is ill suited to the type of high blood pressure you have. This can undermine your quality of life and increase your risk for serious disease. One state's hypertension program delivered the lowest cost per patient in the nation but at the same time had the country's highest death rate. Cut-rate diagnosis is made with a few blood pressure readings and little in the way of diagnostic tests.

Does everybody need a complete set of diagnostic tests? Dr. Michael Horan of the National Heart, Lung, and Blood Institute points out that a first-rate history/ physical exam can distinguish those who really need further tests. For example, the doctor may hear a special sound called a bruit that comes from a narrowed artery.

Diagnostic Tests

BLOOD PRESSURE READINGS   Health care professionals diagnose and define the severity of your disease with simple blood pressure readings. The Joint National Committee on Detection, Evaluation, and Treatment of High Blood Pressure of the National, Heart, Lung, and Blood Institute provided the following classification for those age 18 years or older.

Systolic Pressure   This is the higher number in the reading is presented first. For example, if your blood pressure is 120/80, 120 represents the systolic number. This is the peak pressure in your arterial system. The systolic blood pressure level occurs when your heart contracts and exerts its greatest force.

If you have a diastolic blood pressure of less than 90 but an elevated systolic blood pressure, you have what is called isolated systolic hypertension. This is how it's classified:

SYSTOLIC PRESSURE	CLASSIFICATION
Less than 140	Normal blood pressure
140–159	Borderline isolated systolic hypertension
Greater than 159	Isolated systolic hypertension

Diastolic Pressure   This is the lower number in the reading and is presented second, after the systolic number. For example, if your blood pressure is 120/80, 80 represents the diastolic number. The diastolic level occurs when your heart relaxes and is refilling.

DIASTOLIC PRESSURE	CLASSIFICATION
Less than 85	Normal blood pressure
85–89	High normal blood pressure
90–104	Mild hypertension
105–114	Moderate hypertension
Greater than 114	Severe hypertension

You will want to have your blood pressure rechecked at periodic intervals based on the following:

DIASTOLIC PRESSURE	RECOMMENDED FOLLOW-UP
Less than 85	Recheck within two years
85–89	Recheck within one year
90–104	Confirm within two months
105–114	Evaluate or refer within two weeks
Greater than 114	Evaluate or refer immediately

SYSTOLIC PRESSURE	RECOMMENDED FOLLOW-UP
Less than 140	Recheck within two years
140–199	Confirm within two months
Greater than 200	Evaluate or refer within two weeks

If your doctor suspects you have high blood pressure, he or she will want to find out as much as possible about its severity and type. This makes an enormous difference in treatment. Treatment based only on blood pressure readings is not enough. Your doctor cannot discover curable causes of high blood pressure nor customize treatment for the fewest side effects and greatest benefit without more information. Here are the key additional tests.

AMBULATORY CUFF   This test, measuring blood pressure over a 24-hour period, is the best method to determine if you have hypertension. A cuff is placed around your arm. It will inflate automatically at specified intervals and measure your blood pressure. The unit records each reading and stores it for a 24-hour period. Your doctor can then observe how your blood pressure changes from day to night, from work to home, from play to rest.

This 24-hour monitor is commonly used in borderline cases where the blood pressure is only marginally elevated. In the past many patients were routinely put on medication as a precaution when their doctor was uncertain if their hypertension was real. Some of these patients no doubt suffered instead from "white coat hypertension," in which the blood pressure rises *only* in the doctor's office. While critics sometimes charge that the use of the ambulatory cuff is not cost-effective, these and other borderline patients are saved the expense of a lifetime of medication and medical treatment. By taking around-the-clock readings in a variety of settings, doctors can discard the diagnosis of hypertension in one-third of patients. That's even when several blood pressure readings taken in the doctors office were in the high blood pressure range. Thus, it is important that treatment be based on readings taken in the home, not in the doctor's office.

ECHOCARDIOGRAM   This test bounces sound waves through the chest wall into the heart (the cardiac equivalent of a ship's sonar). It enables doctors to detect any increases in the thickness of the cardiac wall, which indicate damage from hypertension has already occurred. That makes treatment even more imperative. This test is used primarily in borderline hypertensives who might not otherwise be treated with drugs.

RENIN TESTS   Renin levels are too high in many people with hypertension. They are low in only 30%. In hypertensive people, higher renin levels predict a high risk of heart attack. Dr. John H. Laragh, of the New York Hospital–Cornell Medical Center, calls a high renin level a new risk factor for heart disease. Both converting enzyme inhibitors and beta blockers lower blood pressure sharply by cutting renin. Preliminary new research indicates that renin tests may also be used as a way of determining who will benefit most from lifestyle change as a treatment for borderline and mild hypertension.

CARDIAC PROFILE   This reveals the likelihood that you will develop heart disease. The higher your risk, the more aggressively you'll want your blood pressure to be treated. You'll want to pursue a strategy that lowers your blood pressure and reduces the risk for heart disease. The cardiac profile includes tests to screen for high cholesterol and fat levels. These can help your doctor weigh the relative risks and benefits of certain types of high blood pressure drugs, such as diuretics, which may increase fat and blood sugar levels. If your profile shows an elevated fasting blood sugar or cholesterol level, you will probably want to avoid diuretics.

Treatment

You should be wary if your doctor prescribes medications on your first or second visit. If you are one of the 30 million Americans who has mild hypertension, your initial risk of death or disability is comparatively small. You should be observed over the course of several months. Patience is important. The milder your hypertension, the longer you can afford to wait before beginning treatment. The standard drug therapies for hypertension carry risks of their own. You should ask your doctor if your risk of complications from hypertension is sufficient to justify a commitment to a lifetime of drug therapy. While you should try to bring your cholesterol down to the lowest possible levels, the same strategy is not advisable for high blood pressure. If your blood pressure drops too low, there may not be enough blood flow to fill your coronary arteries adequately. At that point overtreatment becomes dangerous and increases your risk of a heart attack. Reducing blood pressure to about 90 diastolic is acceptable, especially when coronary artery disease is present. But if it falls below 85, your risk of cardiovascular disease increases.

LIFESTYLE CHANGES   You may benefit far more by changing your lifestyle. While this therapy may not sound high-tech or state-of-the-art, it can free you from long-term use of antihypertensive drugs. Recent studies show the following steps can be as good as or even better than currently available drugs.

Lose Excess Poundage If You're Overweight   This is easier said than done. Only 5 percent of the people who lose weight keep the pounds off for a five-year period.

Limit Your Alcohol Consumption   If you're hypertensive, you should have no more than two drinks a day. Alcohol boosts blood pressure.

Reduce Your Salt Intake   About half of all people with high blood pressure are extremely sensitive to salt. Unfortunately, medical researchers have yet to discover an accurate method to identify these individuals. For this reason, a trial of salt restriction is undertaken. Even if you have mild hypertension, your doctor will probably recommend a maximum of two grams of sodium a day for a six-week trial period.

Stop Smoking   Although you may not associate smoking with heart disease, there is a connection. The nation's longest-running study of heart disease, known as the Framingham study, has documented a definite correlation between smoking and heart attacks in men. Among 45- to 54-year-old males, the study found the following incidence of heart attacks per 1,000 men:

	HEART ATTACKS
SMOKING STATUS	PER 1,000 MEN
Never smoked	3.9
Quit smoking	3.6
Smoked up to one pack a day	7.5
Smoke one pack a day	11.9

Exercise   Regular exercise alone can lower your blood pressure. It is the single best thing you can do for your health, with the potential of improving your life expectancy and quality of life. Exercise can help you lose weight and stop smoking because it counteracts the stimulant effect of nicotine. You should try exercise for a few months if your diastolic blood pressure is in the 90–95 range. Your trial should be limited to six weeks if the diastolic blood pressure is in the 95–99 range, so that medications can be started if this trial fails to lower your blood pressure. Since high blood pressure puts you at risk of a heart attack, you will need to discuss your exercise program with your doctor before beginning.

Treatment Medications

If lifestyle changes aren't successful in lowering your blood pressure, you may decide to try medication. Your doctor should customize the choice of drugs based on your medical history, a physical examination, and laboratory tests. Unless you have very severe high blood pressure, your doctor should try one drug at a time to gauge your response and any side effects to the medication. The trial of an individual drug may last up to two weeks. Unless you have very severe and uncontrollable high blood pressure, one drug should not be taken along with another.

If your health care insurer is unwilling to pay for diagnostic tests, your doctor can get a sense of how to customize your drug therapy by your response to different drugs. For example, if diuretics lower your blood pressure, you may be retaining fluid as a result of excessive salt in your diet. If they don't work, then your doctor should try other drugs. This is called "single-file testing." It is the state-of-the-art treatment. Doctors can most accurately undertake single-file testing based on complete diagnostic tests. Dr. Michael Horan says that if a complete history and a physical show no obvious reason for more tests, single-file testing may be an elegant and acceptable alternative.

A final note: Beta blockers and diuretics are the only high blood pressure medications proven to save lives in long-term research studies. The same is probably true of the newer medications, calcium channel blockers and ACE inhibitors, but the data is just not there yet.

The most commonly used drugs are the following.

DIURETICS   These are ideal for patients, particularly women who are overweight and the elderly, who retain excess water and salt. They also seem to be particularly effective for African-Americans. In fact, other drugs often work better in African-Americans who are already taking a diuretic. Although they can prevent strokes, diuretics won't avert heart attacks, which are the primary risk for people with high blood pressure. If you have hypertension, you have an 80% chance of a heart attack but only a 20% chance of a stroke. Some experts even believe that diuretics may accelerate the risk of heart attack by increasing your blood fats and thus raising your chance of developing diabetes. (In a trial in Great Britain 14% of patients developed high blood sugars while they were taking diuretics.) Diuretics also carry other risks, such as impotence, changes in magnesium and potassium levels (affecting muscle and heart function), and high uric acid, which can cause gout.

The chief advantage of diuretics is that they are cheap. When they work, they work very well by removing excess salt and water from the body. The National Institutes of Health recommends reducing your dose of hydrochlorothiazide to 12.5 mg/day to minimize problems. If you do take diuretics, make certain your potassium, cholesterol, and blood sugar are checked regularly. Diuretics have also stood the test of time. Long-term research shows they do save lives.

BETA BLOCKERS   Studies show that when beta blockers are given after a heart attack, they can prevent a second heart attack, especially in the first six months. Follow-up suggests the effect extends at least two years, perhaps longer. Some experts would argue that beta blockers can protect patients who have not yet had a heart attack, but the proof is not yet there. Animal studies show that beta blockers can prevent the build-up of blockages in the arteries. But you will not find beta blockers very highly promoted. Since most beta blockers are no longer under patent, they are not marketed aggressively by pharmaceutical companies.

For this reason, you may not be aware of their potential as a good treatment. Many doctors still consider them very good drugs, however.

But beta blockers do have drawbacks. A large number of patients report feeling less energetic and believe that their quality of life has deteriorated. On the other hand, if you have an uncomfortably high metabolism with a rapid pulse and a high level of renin, beta blockers may improve your physical well-being.

ANGIOTENSIN CONVERTING ENZYME INHIBITORS (ACE)   This class of drugs work by blocking the formation of angiotensins, which raise blood pressure. They are promoted as the most palatable drugs because they are highly effective without lowering quality of life. There is nothing wrong with ACE inhibitors as a drug of first choice. In fact, many experts see them as ideal for the initial treatment. Their only real down side is cost. They can also help in diagnosis, since ACE inhibitors work very well against high renin levels in the blood. If you have a dramatic response, you can ask your doctor to check for causes of high renin, such as a narrowing of the renal artery. People with diabetes respond well to these drugs. As this book goes to press, there is fresh evidence that ACE inhibitors can extend life expectancy of patients who have suffered a heart attack.

CALCIUM CHANNEL BLOCKERS   These very powerful drugs cause the blood vessels to relax. While the other drugs mentioned work for specific patients, calcium channel blockers are less well defined. That means they have little value in diagnosis. They have been found, however, to be very effective drugs of first choice for African-Americans, and patients with diabetes are considered very safe. The only side effects are relatively mild— headache, rapid heartbeat, swelling of the ankles, constipation. If this is a good drug for you, make certain cost isn't the reason you're not getting it.

There is also a large variety of animal data that shows calcium channel blockers have a positive effect on the underlying process that causes coronary artery disease. That has not yet been proven in humans, however.

ALPHA BLOCKERS   These drugs also relax blood vessels, but in general this class of drugs is too weak to work well alone. For a small number of patients—those with a high level of sympathetic nervous system activity and African-Americans—they can produce dramatic effects.

WISE DRUG USE   Whatever drug is prescribed, make sure it is the best one for you, not just the one that has been promoted by cost cutters.

If you have been on the same medications for more than 5–10 years and suffer any drug side effects, you should be reevaluated. That's especially true if you have been on two or more drugs for the same length of time. Here's why: Some of the older drugs still in wide use have truly dreadful side effects. You may be able to switch to newer drugs, often far more powerful, and end up on fewer drugs, with minimal side effects.

Be certain to ask your doctor why a particular drug is being prescribed. Much of what doctors know about drug usage comes from clinical trials of drugs. These are experiments matching hundreds of patients who take no drug against those taking an experimental drug. Researchers hope to be able to pinpoint a clear benefit to the experimental drug by comparing the results of the group treated to the group that is not. Good clinical trials show which medicines do and don't work. However, researchers often don't look carefully at specific subgroups, such as African-Americans or women. This can be a danger. If the results are misinterpreted, they can represent a standardized recipe for every patient. As a result doctors aren't encouraged to customize their treatment. Drug selection should be a match between what clinical trials have found out about a drug and what the doctor has learned about you, the patient.

Step 2. Look for Shortcomings

I hope that from reading Step 1, you have gotten a good feeling about your treatment and that you understand much of it better. You'll learn even more by calling organizations listed in Step 4. But if you have an uncomfortable feeling that your treatment is not on track, then study this section, which specifies some common and serious shortcomings that experts in the field recognize. If this section confirms your suspicions, you should go to Step 3. Some of these mistakes you can discover yourself; others only an expert can confirm.

MISTAKES IN DIAGNOSIS

You have undiagnosed hypertension.

Your health care provider has not ordered diagnostic tests to profile your type of hypertension, to pinpoint the kind of treatment you need, and to check for any damage to body organs.

You are unaware of another undiagnosed illness, such as heart or kidney disease, that causes your high blood pressure.

Your health care provider relies only on blood pressure readings taken in his or her office to make a diagnosis.

MISTAKES IN TREATMENT

You have high blood pressure that has been ignored.

Your blood pressure is reduced to below a diastolic pressure of 85.

Your doctor isn't targeting a specific blood pressure level with your treatment.

Your health care provider gives you medication on your first or second visit even though your blood pressure is only mildly elevated, and he or she fails to recommend lifestyle changes.

You are given diuretics only because they are cheap.

Your health care provider hasn't motivated you to make lifestyle changes.

Your condition requires drug treatment but only lifestyle changes have been suggested.

You take out-of-date medications that cause severe side effects.

Your health care provider hasn't prescribed medications that have the lowest side effects and the greatest disease-preventing potential.

You have side effects such as depression, fatigue, impotence, and inability to exercise for a sustained period.

You are given more than one medicine at a time.

You don't adhere to medical therapy because of bad side effects from drugs.

You don't take your medications because you have no apparent symptoms.

You have not been given a fair trial of nondrug therapy.

You have had hypertension for more than five years and haven't had your drug therapy reviewed for more effective and more side-effect-free medicines.

Step 3. See a Specialist

If from Step 2 you are concerned that your care is not state-of-the-art, this section will tell you how to choose an expert.

There is no certification for specialists in high blood pressure. You will want to see a doctor whose practice is devoted primarily to patients who have high blood pressure. Cardiologists, nephrologists (kidney specialists), and endocrinologists all treat high blood pressure.

The doctor who is willing to spend the time to order a complete diagnostic workup is probably the doctor best trained to care for you. Although patients with high blood pressure make up 50% of all office visits, a doctor doesn't need to know anything about high blood pressure to pass state licensure examinations. When specialists take the board exams to be certified in cardiology, endocrinology, or kidney diseases, questions about the causes and treatment of hypertension are limited. In addition, internists and general practitioners may also have little if any formal clinical training in the treatment of high blood pressure. Many doctors learn about treating hypertension from pharmaceutical companies. And they don't always learn what best meets the needs of their patients. For instance, African-Americans respond just as well to relatively inexpensive diuretics as to calcium channel blockers, which are far more expensive. Some drug company representatives only tell doctors that African-American patients should be on calcium blockers. But if a patient can't afford the medication, there will be no benefit. In some communities, 20–25% of patients are unable to fill their prescriptions because they are too costly.

Centers of Excellence for High Blood Pressure

The following list of hospitals is provided only as a convenient starting place in your search for excellence. These hospitals are recommended on the basis of reputation, not experience and results. The list is not an endorsement. There may be hospitals just as excellent that have been omitted. You should apply the guidelines for experience, results, and other measures of excellence to any hospital you choose, whether or not it is on this list. Although hospitals from different sources have been combined into one list, the compilation in no way implies that one source has endorsed the hospital list of another source.

CALIFORNIA
University of Southern
  California   NIH
2025 Zonal Ave
Los Angeles, CA 90033

IOWA
University of Iowa College
  of Medicine   EX/NIH
200 Eckstein Medical
  Research Bldg
Iowa City, IA 52242

MASSACHUSETTS
Brigham and Women's
  Hospital   EX
75 Francis St
Boston, MA 02115

Boston University School
  of Medicine   EX/NIH
80 E Concord St
Boston, MA 02118

NEW YORK
New York Hospital–Cornell
  Medical Center   EX
525 E 68th St
New York, NY 10021

Cornell University   NIH
1300 York Ave
New York, NY 10021

OHIO
Cleveland Clinic Foundation   EX/NIH
One Clinic Center
9500 Euclid Ave
Cleveland, OH 44195

TENNESSEE
Vanderbilt University School
  of Medicine   EX/NIH
21st Ave So. at Garland Ave
Nashville, TN 37232

SOURCES

NIH   indicates those hospitals recommended by the NIH.

EX   indicates those hospitals recommended by experts interviewed.

Step 4. Become Your Own Expert

WHO TO CALL

Citizens for the Treatment of High Blood Pressure

7200 Wisconsin Ave, Suite 1002
Bethesda, MD 20814
301/907-7790

High Blood Pressure Information Center

120/80 National Institutes of Health
9000 Rockville Pike
Bethesda, MD 20892
301/558-4880

Hypertension Center

New York Hospital–Cornell Medical Center
525 E 68th St, K-400
New York, NY 10021
212/472-8300

National Institute of Hypertension Studies

School of Research
7032 Farnsworth
Detroit, MI 48211
313/491-4211

NIH CRISP System

301/496-7543

University-Affiliated Teaching Hospitals   See Appendix.

EXPERT SOURCES

Although dozens of experts were interviewed for these chapters, these physicians are acknowledged for their significant contributions to this section.

Dr. John H. Laragh, Director, Cardiovascular Center and Hypertension Center, and Chief, Division of Cardiology, Department of Medicine, New York Hospital–Cornell Medical Center, New York, NY

Dr. Michael Horan, Associate Director for Cardiology, National Heart, Lung and Blood Institute, National Institutes of Health, Bethesda, MD

REFERENCES AND SUGGESTED READING

American Heart Association. *1991 Heart and Stroke Facts.*

Aronow, Wilbert S., and others. Prognostic Significance of Silent Ischemia in Elderly Patients With Peripheral Arterial Disease With and Without Previous Myocardial Infarction. *American Journal of Cardiology,* Vol. 69, No. 1 (Jan. 1, 1992), pp. 137–139.

Beard, Keith, and others. Management of Elderly Patients with Sustained Hypertension. *British Medical Journal,* Vol. 304, No. 6824 (Feb. 15, 1992), pp. 412–416.

Deleterious Effects of Diuretic Therapy in Diabetes Mellitus. *Clinical Diabetes,* Vol. 10, No. 1 (Jan.–Feb. 1992), pp. 10–11.

Graves, J. W. New Antihypertensive Agents: Part IV. Isradipine in the Treatment of Hypertension and Atherosclerosis. *Practical Cardiology,* Vol. 16, No. 4 (April 1990).

Houghton, Jan Laws, and others. Systemic Hypertension: Morphologic Hemodynamic and Coronary Perfusion Characteristics in Severe Left Ventricular Hypertrophy Secondary to Systemic Hypertension and Evidence for Nonatherosclerotic Myocardial Ischemia. *American Journal of Cardiology,* Vol. 69, No. 3 (Jan. 15, 1992), pp. 219–224.

Johenning, Agnes, and others. Diagnosis and Management of Chronic Hypertension in Pregnancy [letter]. *Obstetrics and Gynecology,* Vol. 79, No. 3 (Mar. 1992), pp. 475–476.

Kowalenko, Terry, and others. Prehospital Diagnosis and Treatment of Acute Myocardial Infarction: A Critical Review. *American Heart Journal,* Vol. 123, No. 1 (Jan. 1992), pp. 181–190.

Medical Research Council Trial of Treatment of Hypertension in Older Adults: Principal Results. *British Medical Journal,* Vol. 304, No. 6824 (Feb. 15, 1992), pp. 405–411.

Moser, Marvin. *High Blood Pressure and What You Can Do About It.* Elmsford, NY: Benjamin Company, 1989.

National Institutes of Health. *National Heart, Lung, and Blood Institute Fifteenth Report of the Director.* NIH Publication No. 89-2206, Feb. 1989.

National Institutes of Health. *National High Blood Pressure Education Program (NHBPEP) Working Group Report on Blood Pressure Monitoring.* NIH Publication No. 90-3028, Aug. 1990.

National Institutes of Health. Statement on Hypertension in the Elderly. The Working Group on Hypertension in the Elderly. National High Blood Pressure Education Program. *Journal of the American Medical Association,* Vol. 256, No. 1 (July 4, 1986), pp. 70–74.

National Institutes of Health. *The 1988 Report of the Joint National Committee on Detection, Evaluation and Treatment of High Blood Pressure.* NIH Publication No. 89-1088, Nov. 1989.

National Institutes of Health. *The Fifteenth Report of the National Heart, Lung, and Blood Advisory Council. Progress and Challenge.* NIH Publication No. 988-2734, Sept. 1988.

Peoples Medical Society. *Blood Pressure: Questions You Have . . . Answers You Need.* 1984.

Potkin, Benjamin N., and others. Late, Out-of-Laboratory, Abrupt Closure After Angiographically Successful Directional Coronary Atherectomy. *American Journal of Cardiology,* Vol. 69, No. 3 (Jan. 15, 1992), pp. 263–265.

Schnall, P.L., and others. The Relationship Between "Job Strain," Workplace Diastolic Blood Pressure and Left Ventricular Mass Index. Results of a Case-Control Study. *Journal of the American Medical Association,* Vol. 263, No. 14 (April 11, 1990), pp. 1929–1935.

Silagy, Christopher A., and McNeil, John J. Systemic Hypertension: Epidemiologic Aspects of Isolated Systolic Hypertension and Implications for Future Research. *American Journal of Cardiology,* Vol. 69, No. 3 (Jan. 15, 1992), pp. 213–218.

Smith, David H. G., and others. Systemic Hypertension: Impact of Left Ventricular Hypertrophy on Blood Pressure Responses to Exercise. *American Journal of Cardiology,* Vol. 69, No. 3 (Jan. 15, 1992), pp. 225–228.

Subcommittee on Nonpharmacological Therapy of the 1984 Joint National Committee on Detection, Evaluation, and Treatment of High Blood Pressure. Nonpharmacological Approaches to the Control of High Blood Pressure. *Hypertension,* Vol. 8, No. 5 (May 1986), pp. 444–467.

U.S. Preventive Services Task Force. Physical Activity Counseling. *Journal of the American Medical Association,* Vol. 261, No. 24 (June 23–30, 1989), pp. 3588–3589.

Osteoporosis

Risk for Inappropriate Care   HIGH

The treatment of osteoporosis is still an emerging field in medicine. If you're one of the 25 million Americans with osteoporosis, the risk is substantial that you will not be treated at all. A large number of women are under the care of an internist or a gynecologist who may not be educated in the prevention or treatment of osteoporosis. Top academic researchers estimate that 95% of doctors were never taught about osteoporosis in medical school. Doctors generally have become aware of the disease only in the last 10 years, and many still fail to appreciate its seriousness.

Unfortunately, patients pay a high price for this lack of knowledge. Osteoporosis frequently leads to wrist, spine and hip fractures. Forty percent of all women will have at least one spinal fracture by the time they reach 80, and about 15% of white women will fracture a hip at some time during their lives, reports the National Osteoporosis Foundation. The Foundation also estimates that up to 20% of the people who suffer hip fractures will die, within a year, from complications such as pneumonia or blood clots in the lungs. While osteoporosis is considered a disease that affects women, one out of five patients with hip fractures are men and they are twice as likely to die as a result. Even if you have been hospitalized for a hip fracture, you are likely to leave the hospital without medication or treatment for the underlying problem. Five percent of all patients are in hospitals for hip fractures.

What It Is

In osteoporosis, bone density and strength decrease as more and more calcium is lost from the bone. Normal bone is continually remodeled—old bone is destroyed and new bone manufactured. In osteoporosis, this normal balance between bone destruction and bone formation is upset, and bone is destroyed at a faster rate than the body can make new bone. The resulting loss of strength makes bones more susceptible to fracture. The advanced form of the disease is characterized by back pain, shrinking height, spinal deformity, and multiple fractures, most frequently of the vertebrae, hip, and wrist. There are a total of 1.3 million fractures a year due to osteoporosis.

Step 1. Make Sure You Get the Best Care

Read this section on potential problems with your treatment carefully to determine if there are discrepancies between your care and state-of-the-art care. Use Step 2 to review shortcomings.

Here's what state-of-the-art medicine hopes to accomplish by treating osteoporosis: prevent debilitating and painful fractures, especially those to the hip and spine; stop further bone loss, thus reducing the risk of fracture; stimulate the development of bones that are strong enough to resist fracture. If your family doctor or gynecologist is knowledgeable about osteoporosis, you may be happy with that care. You should schedule regular office visits, every one to three months, to monitor your case. If there are complications, you will want to go more often. If your condition is stable, you may reduce the frequency of office visits to once a year.

Risk Factors

Until you have an actual fracture, it can be difficult to know that you have osteoporosis. While risk factors remain rather muddy, some people are more likely to develop the disease than others. Women who enter menopause before age 45 or who take steroids run the highest risk. The other risk factors are not particularly good predictors, but the more of them apply to you, the more likely you should be screened for the disease. The National Osteoporosis Foundation suggest you should be aware of the following risk factors for osteoporosis, since many health care providers are insufficiently alert to symptoms of the disease:

- Advanced age

- Being female (women develop osteoporosis a decade or more before men)

- Being a white or Asian woman with a family history of the disease

- Small bone structure or low body weight (for women, wearing a size 6 or smaller dress)

- Being postmenopausal (estrogen deficiency is the main cause of rapid postmenopausal bone loss)

- Presence of the following diseases: hyperthyroidism, primary hyperparathyroidism, or multiple myelomas (At a minimum, you should undergo basic thyroid testing to determine if you have too much thyroid hormone, for too much robs bones of calcium. This testing is recommended if your bone density is low.)

- Scoliosis

- Taking any of the following medications:

  Thyroid hormone   If you take the thyroid preparation Synthroid, you may be robbing your bones of calcium. That's exactly what happens with patients who have hyperthyroid disease. Thyroid testing will determine if this is true. The precise dose that becomes dangerous is not known. Some doctors become quite concerned with a dose of 0.125 mg and above. Excessive doses should be corrected downwards. A sensitive thyroid-stimulating hormone assay is necessary to ascertain if your dose is excessive.

  Steroids   Prednisone can rapidly accelerate bone loss. There is not a known "safe" dose or schedule. Some doctors believe prednisone should be taken every other day instead of once a day, to minimize its effect on bone. Since long-term, regular use places you at high risk, you will want to have bone-density testing to see if you need special or even experimental treatment. You should take the lowest dose possible. If you take steroids for asthma, consider high doses of inhaled steroids.

- The following lifestyle characteristics:

  Inadequate calcium intake   Patients who develop osteoporosis have almost always eaten insufficient amounts of calcium during their lifetime. Few adolescents eat three dairy servings a day; pregnant women seldom get enough.

  General malnourishment   One-third of the patients admitted to the Hospital for Special Surgery with hip fractures are malnourished, even though they may have adequate-to-substantial incomes.

  Smoking   Tobacco smoke leads to a rapid decrease in estrogen levels. Women who smoke can deplete one-half of their available estrogen.

  Alcohol abuse   This is the number-one cause of osteoporosis in men. Since alcohol slows down the production of new bone, you could be in trouble if your consumption exceeds more than two ounces a day.

  Lack of exercise   Exercise helps the body actively incorporate calcium into bone in younger people. In older women, exercise combined with calcium and estrogen replacement appears to add new bone, according to preliminary reports. Regular, weight-bearing aerobic exercise combined with adequate calcium intake is your best bet to maintain your present level of bone calcium, according to the Osteoporosis Center at the Hospital for Special Surgery. New studies are looking at weight training as an additional benefit, since researchers believe that stressing bone may be beneficial.

Diagnosis

BONE-DENSITY TESTS   If you have a number of risk factors, your doctor may order bone-density tests, which are the only way to confirm the presence of the disease. If you have lost significant amounts of calcium from your bones, they will be thinner. Bone-density tests are used not only for diagnosis but also for assessing the effectiveness of the treatment. These represent the best objective measure. If they are performed regularly, the tests can determine whether you have inherently thin bones or are losing mass rapidly. That information can help your doctor to customize therapy. Unfortunately, most people aren't screened until at least age 65, too late for that distinction to be made.

You should compare costs at different screening centers, because the charges, which shouldn't be more than a few hundred dollars, can be outlandish. (If the test were cheaper, screening could be more widespread.) You should have your test done at a reputable center, asking beforehand about its patient education programs and the number of research studies being undertaken.

Dual-Energy X-Ray (Photon) Absorptiometry   This is the state-of-the-art bone-density test. It is most accurate when used to assess bone loss in the spine, for which its precision rate is 1%. It is less precise in the measurement of hip bone density. This test is precise enough to see gains or losses in bone density with drug treatment, and is the gold standard for scientific research. It is also the test you should demand if you are taking experimental medications.

Single-Photon Absorptiometry   Though this is a less accurate measure, the government and many managed care companies will pay for this test and not for the more reliable dual-photon variation. Ironically, the government relies on the accuracy of the dual-photon test to determine if new osteoporosis drugs work, but won't pay for its use in patients. The disadvantage is that single-photon is a much less precise way of following the course of your illness and the results of treatment.

X-Ray Tests   X-rays are often misread and frequently misused because they are not exposed properly. About one-quarter of bone mass must be lost before it can be detected by an x-ray. The only legitimate use is for the examination of broken bones. This is not a good screening test.

Computed Axial Tomography (CAT) Scan   A more expensive test, the CAT scan uses 20 times the radiation of the dual-photon test and is less precise. You should insist on having a dual-photon or single-photon test instead.

OTHER TESTS   After a bone scan suggests osteoporosis and your doctor reviews your risk factors and medical history, he or she may want to order some of the following tests, which can help your doctor better understand your illness and how to customize treatment for you. For instance, if the calcium in your bones metabolizes quickly, you will consider different medications than if it turns over slowly. Other tests, such as thyroid function tests, may uncover an illness which, if treated, will also treat your osteoporosis.

- Chemistry profile

- Thyroid function

- 24-hour urine calcium and hydroxyproline

- Vitamin D metabolites

- Parathyroid hormone

- Follicle stimulating hormone and estradiol

- Serum and urine immunoelectrophoresis (in select cases)

Treatment Through Prevention

HEALTHFUL LIVING   You can change the course of your disease with a healthful lifestyle. Five thousand years ago osteoporosis didn't exist. Our ancestors did a tremendous amount of lifting, pushing, running, and hiking. In addition, they had enormous calcium intakes, more than 3,000 mg a day, from the water supply in the limestone caves where they lived. Healthful habits from childhood on would eliminate most cases of osteoporosis. Once you have osteoporosis, a healthful lifestyle can still slow bone loss. Modest exercise, meaning 30 minutes of exercise three to four times a week, strengthens the skeleton. Weight-bearing exercise can improve muscular function and agility. Smoking, consuming more than two alcoholic beverages a day, and drinking more than three or four cups of coffee or tea daily can contribute to the disease.

AVOIDING FALLS   As you age, your risk of falling and breaking a hip increases. Many of these falls are caused by poor coordination. Sleep medications and tranquilizers only add to the problem. Sleeping pills alone are responsible for one-third of falls. In a study of nursing home patients, sedatives and hypnotics, such as Seconal, Dalmane, and Halcion, were found to be associated with strikingly higher risk of falls: 36.6 times greater than in patients not taking these kinds of drugs. Vasodilators were associated with a five-fold greater risk of falls. The best way to prevent hip and wrist fractures is to eliminate falls. Here are other steps that the National Osteoporosis Foundation recommends.

Medications

- Reduce the total number of medications taken.

- Assess the risks and benefits of each medication.

- Select medication that is the least centrally acting, is least associated with a sudden drop in blood pressure , and has the shortest action.

- Avoid medications that cause dizziness or light-headedness.

- Take the lowest effective dose.

- Then reassess risks and benefits.

Other Recommendations

- Have your vision and hearing tested regularly.

- Limit alcohol intake.

- Use a cane or walking stick when needed, particularly if walking outdoors on wet or icy pavement.

- Wear supportive, rubber-soled, low-heeled shoes.

- Reduce home hazards that might cause falls; for example, install thick carpeting, bathroom safety bars, and bright stairway lighting.

To sum up, here are the preventive measures that you can take: Avoid the medications that increase your bone loss, including thyroid hormone and corticosteroids; avoid smoking and excessive alcohol intake. Undertake a program of regular exercise. Make certain your daily diet has at least 1,000 mg of calcium, unless you are postmenopausal, in which case you require 1,500 mg per day. Consider a daily multivitamin that contains up to 400 IU of vitamin D to help you better absorb calcium.

CALCIUM INTAKE   At The Hospital for Special Surgery, patients generally receive one-third their daily calcium intake through their diets and the other two-thirds through supplements, the two most popular being calcium carbonate and calcium citrate. If you take calcium carbonate, you need to take fewer tablets. You can even take Tums. Calcium citrate will be more effective if you are not taking estrogen, since it is better absorbed. Patients with a history of kidney stones should seek further guidance. Such individuals should be monitored closely for the development of kidney stones. A common side effect of calcium carbonate supplements is constipation. An increasing number of studies show that calcium is an important part of most therapies. Remember that calcium is the most basic building block of bone. Exercise and estrogen treatment are both proven to be more effective with calcium. Women who have regular bone-density tests seem to take calcium supplements more conscientiously. They want to see results on the bone-density test. It's like members of Weight Watchers who are motivated by changes in weight they see on a scale.

Beyond these general measures, if you have osteoporosis, you may wish to consider drug therapy with your doctor.

Treatment Medications

Although there is no fixed therapy for osteoporosis, there are medications that can help. The most commonly prescribed of these drugs inhibit the resorption (destruction) of existing bone or stimulate the production of new bone.

INHIBITORS OF BONE RESORPTION While these drugs don't build new bone, they will slow the loss of existing bone. The earlier you can take them, the more bone you can preserve, which is another reason to undertake early screening.

Estrogen This is the drug of choice for women who have gone through menopause or have impaired ovarian function, such as that which follows a hysterectomy. The medication should be prescribed for at least a five-year period. Prescribed early enough, estrogen can reduce vertebral, hip, and Colles' fractures by about 50%. (A Colles' fracture is a fracture of the wrist usually caused by falling forward with an outstretched hand.) Some evidence suggests that estrogen decreases the risk of cardiovascular disease by about 50% and deaths from heart attack by 30%. That's the up side. But there's a down side, too. There's little question that estrogen may increase the risk of breast cancer in certain high-risk individuals. What's not clear is whether it causes a correspondingly higher death rate from the disease. In addition, many women develop side effects, and others dislike the accompanying weight gain and the continuation of menstrual bleeding. (Researchers are looking for ways to eliminate this.)

Estrogen used alone also increases the risk of uterine cancer. Women who take only estrogen have nine times the risk of cancer of the uterine lining or endometrium. However, when it is prescribed in low-to-moderate doses and combined with adequate doses of progesterone, the risk is minimized. The osteoporosis center at the Hospital for Special Surgery recommends that patients always take estrogen *with* Provera (progesterone) if they have an intact uterus. (There are rare exceptions.) If you aren't taking estrogen therapy with progesterone, be certain to have regular cancer detection tests.

Estrogen remains a controversial therapy because there are no long-term study results comparing the cardiovascular benefits to the potential cancer risks in women who take estrogen. Those studies are under way. Estrogen therapy remains a hot political issue. Some women complain that estrogen therapy is a panacea put forth by a male-dominated research establishment. These critics can pick legitimate holes in the research. Here's an example: One famous study concluded that the incidence of heart disease in those women who took hormone replacement therapy decreased dramatically. However those women taking estrogen were more physically active and more health conscious. Those good health habits—not necessarily the hormone replacement therapy—could explain the reduced incidence of osteoporosis and the lowered risk of heart disease. This is not meant to confuse you. You should simply be aware that study design for estrogen treatment is far from perfect and that the results are not absolutely conclusive. The bottom line is this: Taking into account your individual risks of breast cancer, heart disease and osteoporosis, you should make a decision with your physician based on the best possible evidence.

While many women begin taking estrogen at the time of menopause, new research suggests that estrogen can help women over the age of 65 also.

Women Who Should Take Estrogen   The women who are the best candidates for estrogen therapy have one or more of the following characteristics:

■ Cardiovascular disease

■ Unpleasant and significant changes that may accompany menopause, such as vasomotor symptoms (once called hot flashes)

■ Menopause before the age of 45

■ History of osteoporosis in all female family members

■ Very low bone mass

■ Rapid loss of bone mass (in which case bone density should be measured every two years)

■ Light, thin frame

■ Medical illness or treatment that may lead to osteoporosis (for example, steroids)

Women Who Shouldn't Take Estrogen   There are some women who shouldn't use estrogens. According to the National Osteoporosis Foundation, they include patients with any of the following:

- Known or suspected cancer of the breast, unless prescribed by your doctor (Very preliminary studies suggest tamoxifen might be an effective alternative to estrogen in breast cancer patients.)

- Known or suspected cancer that needs estrogen to grow

- Known or suspected pregnancy

- Undiagnosed vaginal bleeding

- Active liver disease

- Severe, uncontrolled high blood pressure

- Active thrombophlebitis (inflammation of the veins that can lead to blood clots, a portion of which could break off and make its way to the lungs or somewhere else in the circulatory system)

Be wary if your doctor dismisses estrogen replacement treatment. While not all patients belong on estrogens, your doctor should have a rationale for your particular case. If the doctor says, "Everybody gets osteoporosis and nothing can be done about it," watch out!

Calcitonin   Calcitonin prevents further bone loss in the back and hip. It is used to relieve acute bone pain due to spinal column fractures and can be given by injection or nasal spray; in either form it is expensive. The nasal spray form is not available in the United States as of this writing. Calcitonin provides an alternative to women who are unable or unwilling to use estrogen therapy. Only calcitonin and estrogen are approved by the FDA for use in osteoporosis.

Etidronate   Initial studies found that etidronate can reduce bone loss and back deformities in the immediate postmenopausal years. Critics believe it may cause bone to remodel poorly, making bad bone, which is more susceptible to fractures. These critics say that after a third year of use, fractures may occur. Proponents say that this data is misleading and ask doctors to stay tuned for further results in the fourth and fifth years of the study. The Food and Drug Administration has not approved its use for osteoporosis, although it is available (because approval was granted for treatment of another illness). Critics are concerned that large numbers of women take etidronate for osteoporosis without regular testing's having proven its effectiveness and without FDA approval.

Calcitriol   This is the active form of vitamin D. It helps your intestine absorb calcium better, thereby slowing bone destruction. A new study has found that postmenopausal patients taking calcitriol had a threefold reduction in the number of vertebral compression fractures. This is still an experimental medicine.

STIMULATORS OF BONE FORMATION   The ideal treatment for osteoporosis would be a drug that produces new bone both strong and fracture resistant. While that drug does not yet exist, the following drugs appear to have bone-building properties.

Fluorides   Fluorides stimulate bone-building cells, although intestinal disorders and joint pains remain a problem. The quality of bone may, unfortunately, be of a lower quality than researchers would like.

Anabolic Steroids   Anabolic steroids, the same drug used by body builders, increase bone mass by encouraging the formation of new bone. The FDA has not approved their use for osteoporosis. Some experts theorize that they may turn out to be an excellent choice for male patients. One-third of men with osteoporosis have low testosterone, and testosterone is an anabolic steroid. Side effects such as liver disease and masculinization limit long-term use of anabolic steroids.

Parathyroid Hormone   Parathyroid hormone is still in the experimental stages.

WISE DRUG USE   Be sure to take your medications in a way that will maximize their benefits. Here are examples of common mistakes.

COMMON MISTAKES

■ All calcium is taken at bedtime. (Instead it should be divided up during the day.)

■ Calcium is taken with a fatty meal. (Calcium is poorly absorbed with a fatty meal.)

■ Etidronate is taken at the same time as a calcium supplement. (This inhibits its absorption into your bone. Etidronate must be taken on an empty stomach.)

■ Calcium is taken with iron. (Taking calcium with iron hampers absorption from the intestine. Many patients take one in the morning, the other at night.)

■ Too much vitamin D is taken. (In large dosages, vitamin D works against good bone quality.)

You may unknowingly take drugs that worsen your disease. One expert told me that every osteoporosis patient who comes into his office is on at least five different drugs, for varying illnesses. So many interactions are possible among such an array of drugs, and many interactions can affect the amount of calcium lost by your bones or absorbed by your body. If several doctors prescribe medicines for you, beware! You run the risk of each doctor's adding more medications without a clearly thought-out, well-coordinated strategy. The best solution is to have each specialist recommend specific drugs to your family doctor, who then writes the actual prescriptions.

Even if a drug is working well for you, don't stay on it for years without periodic reevaluation. At least once a year all your medications should be discontinued, to be prescribed again as they are needed. Your doctor should establish a baseline before prescribing each drug. The bone-density test serves as an excellent baseline. Your doctor can order additional tests to check for progress. The best marker is a bone-density test of the spine.

Step 2. Look for Shortcomings

I hope that from reading Step 1, you have gotten a good feeling about your treatment and that you understand much of it better. You'll learn even more by calling organizations listed in Step 4. But if you have an uncomfortable feeling that your treatment is not on track, then study this section, which specifies some common and serious shortcomings that experts in the field recognize. If this section confirms your suspicions, you should go to Step 3. Some of these mistakes you can discover yourself; others only an expert can confirm.

MISTAKES IN DIAGNOSIS

You are at high risk and have not been tested.

You have your testing done at a storefront bone-density center.

MISTAKES IN TREATMENT

You drink too much alcohol.

You smoke.

You are malnourished.

Your diet includes too little calcium.

You take steroids.

You take too much thyroid hormone for another illness.

You take drugs for other illnesses that make your osteoporosis worse.

You stay on drugs for years at a time.

Your health care provider is unfamiliar with screening, diagnosis, and treatment of osteoporosis.

Your doctor doesn't believe in estrogen replacement treatment.

Your health care provider does not customize treatment.

Your doctor doesn't recommend calcium.

Your doctor fails to educate you about diet, exercise, and reducing risk factors.

Your doctor uses unapproved drugs and doesn't do baseline and follow-up testing.

You do not undertake the appropriate exercises to slow the loss of bone.

Your nutrition is not properly managed by your health care provider.

You've had a fracture due to osteoporosis and leave the hospital with no treatment.

Step 3. See a Specialist

If, from Step 2, you are concerned your care is not state-of-the-art, this section will tell you how to choose an expert.

Choosing a Doctor

Your family doctor can certainly oversee the treatment of your osteoporosis if he or she is knowledgeable about the disease, and its treatment is a regular part of your doctor's practice. If your case is more complex, there are several doctors that may treat you. If you have significant bone loss, you will want to see a metabolic bone specialist, which is a specialty or subspecialty of a number of different fields: rheumatology, endocrinology, orthopedics, nephrology, and gerontology. This type of specialist can perform a diagnostic workup to rule out any primary cause of bone loss. For example, bone loss may be the result of a malfunctioning thyroid gland. If hormone replacement therapy is your treatment of choice, your gynecologist can manage your disease. You will want to consult an orthopedist if you've had a spinal, wrist, or hip fracture. Office visits should be scheduled every one to three months initially. After a stable protocol is established, once or twice a year should be sufficient.

Centers of Excellence for Osteoporosis

The following list of hospitals is provided only as a convenient starting place in your search for excellence. These hospitals are recommended on the basis of reputation, not experience and results.

OSTEOPOROSIS RESEARCH CENTERS   The following centers have been designated by the NIH as Specialized Centers of Research in Osteoporosis. They were established to make contributions to the national research effort to combat the disease.

Specialized Centers of Research in Osteoporosis

PENNSYLVANIA
Department of Orthopaedic Surgery
University of Pennsylvania School of
   Medicine
425 Medical Education Bldg
36th and Hamilton Walk
Philadelphia, PA 19104-6081

NEBRASKA
Department of Medicine
Creighton University
Center for Hard Tissue Research
601 North 30th Street
Omaha, NE 68131

NEW YORK
Helen Hayes Hospital
Regional Bone Center
Route 9W
Wester Haverstraw, NY 10993

NIH-DESIGNATED CENTERS STUDYING THE EFFECT OF ESTROGEN REPLACE-
MENT THERAPY (ON BOTH OSTEOPOROSIS AND HEART DISEASE)

CALIFORNIA
Stanford University School of Medicine
300 Pasteur Dr
Stanford, CA 94305

University of California, Los Angeles,
   (UCLA) Medical Center
10833 LeConte Ave
Los Angeles, CA 90024

University of California, San Diego,
   School of Medicine
La Jolla, CA 92093

DISTRICT OF COLUMBIA
George Washington University School of
   Medicine
2300 I St NW
Washington, DC 20037

IOWA
University of Iowa
College of Medicine
200 Eckstein Medical Research Bldg
Iowa City, IA 52242

MARYLAND
Johns Hopkins University
School of Medicine
720 Rutland Ave
Baltimore, MD 21205

NORTH CAROLINA
Bowman Gray School of Medicine of
   Wake Forest University
300 South Hawthorne Rd
Winston-Salem, NC 27103

TEXAS
University of Texas School of Medicine
   at San Antonio
7703 Floyd Curl Dr
San Antonio, TX 78284-7790

Step 4. Become Your Own Expert

WHO TO CALL

National Osteoporosis Foundation

2100 M St NW
Washington, DC 20037
202/223-2226

National Institute of Arthritis and Musculoskeletal and Skin Diseases

9000 Rockville Pike
Bethesda, MD 20892
301/496-4000

National Arthritis and Musculoskeletal and Skin Diseases Information Clearinghouse This organization publishes the booklet *Osteoporosis Prevention and Education: A Resource Guide,* which offers a list of services provided by 130 national, state, and local organizations. Single copies of the document are available free from them.

Box AMS
9000 Rockville Pike
Bethesda, MD 20892

NIH CRISP System
301/496-7543

University-Affiliated Teaching Hospitals See Appendix.

EXPERT SOURCES

Although dozens of experts were interviewed for these chapters, these specialists are acknowledged for their significant contributions to this section.

Dr. Joseph M. Lane, Chief, Metabolic Bone Disease, Hospital for Special Surgery, New York, NY

Dr. William A. Peck, Dean, Washington University School of Medicine, St. Louis, MO

Theresa Galsworthy, R.N., Director, Osteoporosis Center, Hospital for Special Surgery, New York, NY

Staff of the National Osteoporosis Foundation

REFERENCES AND SUGGESTED READING

Bhambhani, M. M., and others. Plasma Ascorbic Acid Concentrations in Osteoporotic Outpatients. [letter to the editor] *British Journal of Rheumatology*, Vol. 31, No. 2 (Feb. 1992), pp. 142–143.

Block, J. E., and others. Does Exercise Prevent Osteoporosis? *Journal of the American Medical Association* Vol. 257, No. 22 (June 12, 1987), pp. 3115–3117.

Consensus Development Conference. Prophylaxis and Treatment of Osteoporosis. *American Journal of Medicine*, Vol. 90 (Jan. 1991), pp. 107–110.

Faulkner, Kenneth G., and others. Noninvasive Measurements of Bone Mass, Structure, and Strength: Current Methods and Experimental Techniques. [review] *American Journal of Roentgenology*, Vol. 157, No. 6 (Dec. 1991), pp. 1229–1237.

Fiatarone, M. A., and others. High-Intensity Strength Training in Nonagenarians: Effects on Skeletal Muscle. *Journal of the American Medical Association*, Vol. 263, No. 22 (June 13, 1990). pp. 3029–3034.

Fleming, Barbara J., and others. Postmenopausal Estrogen Therapy and Cardiovascular Disease. [letter] *New England Journal of Medicine*, Vol. 326, No. 10 (Mar. 5, 1992), pp. 705–708.

Greenfield, Marjorie. Reduced Spinal Bone Mass in Patients with Uterine Cervical Cancer. [letter] *Obstetrics and Gynecology*, Vol. 79, No. 3 (Mar. 1992), pp. 479–480.

Ham, Richard J. Nutrition Screening Initiative: Indicators of Poor Nutritional Status in Older Americans. *American Family Physician*, Vol. 45, No. 1 (Jan. 1992), pp. 219–228.

Hughes, Janey, and Norman, Richard W. Diet and Calcium Stones. [review] *Canadian Medical Association Journal*, Vol. 146, No. 2 (Jan. 15, 1992) pp. 137–143.

Laan, R. F. J. M., and others. Vertebral Osteoporosis in Rheumatoid Arthritis Patients: Effect of Low-Dose Prednisone Therapy. *British Journal of Rheumatology*, Vol. 31, No. 2 (Feb. 1992), pp. 91–96.

Lechky, Olga. Toronto-Based Foundation Tries to Combat Underfunding in Women's Health Research. *Canadian Medical Association Journal*, Vol. 146, No. 2 (Jan. 15, 1992), pp. 261–263.

Lipschitz, David A., and others. Nutrition Screening Initiative: An Approach to Nutrition Screening for Older Americans. *American Family Physician*, Vol. 45, No. 2 (Feb. 1992), pp. 601–608.

Magrini, Nicola, and others. The Italian Way of Osteoporosis. [letter to the editor] *Lancet*, Vol. 339, No. 8791 (Feb. 22, 1992), pp. 499–500.

Marslew, U., and others. Two New Combinations of Estrogen and Progestogen for Prevention of Postmenopausal Bone Loss: Long-Term Effects on Bone, Calcium and Lipid Metabolism, Climacteric Symptoms, and Bleeding. *Obstetrics and Gynecology*, Vol. 79, No. 2 (Feb. 1992), pp. 202–210.

Munnings, F. Exercise and Estrogen in Women's Health: Getting a Clearer Picture. *The Physician and SportsMedicine*, Vol. 16, No. 5 (1988).

National Osteoporosis Foundation. Clinical Indications for Bone Mass Measurements. *Journal of Bone and Mineral Research*, Vol. 4, Supplement 2 (Nov. 1989).

National Osteoporosis Foundation. *Physician's Resource Manual on Osteoporosis: A Decision-Making Guide*, 1987.

Pamidronate. *Medical Letter on Drugs and Therapeutics*, Vol. 34, No. 861 (Jan. 10, 1992), pp. 1–2.

Patel, U., and others. Clinical Profile of Acute Vertebral Compression Fractures in Osteoporosis. *British Journal of Rheumatology*, Vol. 30, No. 6 (Dec. 1991), pp. 418–421.

Plunkett, Earl R., and Wolfe, Bernard M. Prolonged Effects of a Novel, Low-Dosage Continuous Progestin–Cyclic Estrogen Replacement Program in Postmenopausal Women. *American Journal of Obstetrics and Gynecology*, Vol. 166, No. 1 (Jan. 1992), pp. 117–121.

Prince, R. L., and others. Prevention of Postmenopausal Osteoporosis: A Comparative Study of Exercise, Calcium Supplementation, and Hormone-Replacement Therapy. *New England Journal of Medicine*, Vol. 325, No. 17 (Oct. 24, 1991), pp. 1189–1195.

Reid, David M., and Purdie, David W. Bone-Density Measurement. [letter to the editor] *Lancet*, Vol. 339, No. 8789 Feb. 8, 1992), p. 370

Reiter, Robert C., and others. Ovarian Cancer in Women with Prior Hysterectomy: A 14-Year Experience at the University of Miami. *Obstetrics and Gynecology*, Vol. 79, No. 2 (Feb. 1992), pp. 317–319.

Rodigues-Canteras, Rafael, and others. Menopausal Hormone Replacement Therapy and Breast Cancer: A Meta-Analysis. [review] *Obstetrics and Gynecology*, Vol. 79, No. 2 (Feb. 1992), pp. 286–294.

Sato, Masahiko, and others. Bisphosphonate Action: Alendronate Localization in Rat Bone and Effects on Osteoclast Ultrastructure. *Journal of Clinical Investigation*, Vol. 88, No. 6 (Dec. 1991), pp. 2095–2105.

Sheldon, Trevor, and others. Bone-Density Measurement. [letter to the editor] *Lancet*, Vol. 339, No. 8790 (Feb. 15, 1992), p. 425.

Sherman, Frederick T. "Transfer" and "Turning" Fractures in Nursing Home Patients. [letter] *American Journal of Medicine*, Vol. 91, No. 6 (Dec. 1991), pp. 668–669.

Smith, E. L. Exercise for the Prevention of Osteoporosis: A Review. *The Physician and Sports Medicine*, Vol. 10, No. 3 (March 1982).

Stampfer, Meir J., and others. Postmenopausal Estrogen Therapy and Cardiovascular Disease: Ten-Year Follow-Up from the Nurses' Health Study. *Obstetrical and Gynecological Survey*, Vol. 47, No. 2 (Feb. 1992), pp. 135–137.

Tazuke, Salli, and others. Exogenous Estrogen and Endogenous Sex Hormones. *Medicine*, Vol. 71, No. 1 (Jan. 1992), pp. 44–51.

Treatment of Postmenopausal Osteoporosis with Calcitrol or Calcium. *New England Journal of Medicine*, Vol. 326, pp. 357–62.

Peptic Ulcer Disease

Risk for Inappropriate Care HIGH

As an ulcer patient you may be your own worst enemy. Too many Americans do what Madison Avenue tells them to do: They self-medicate their own ulcers. If you treat your own ulcerlike symptoms for longer than a week or two, you could seriously endanger your health. But there is good news—new medications can treat most ulcers without the need for surgery, once a mainstay of ulcer treatment. To get those medications you must see a doctor who will prescribe them for you. If surgery is recommended to you, be quite certain that it is appropriate. Often it is not.

What It Is

Twenty years ago most of us thought of an ulcer as just a hole in the lining of the stomach. Because doctors now investigate most serious stomach pain by looking at the stomach itself with a device called an endoscope, we now realize that peptic ulcer disease covers a spectrum of conditions. At one end of that spectrum is a benign, slight discoloration of the stomach's lining. At the other extreme is a life-threatening condition in which a hole passes through the lining of the stomach into the blood vessels or the abdomen itself. Any area of the gastrointestinal system exposed to harsh stomach acid may be affected. The areas most often affected are: the esophagus (the long, narrow passageway from the mouth into the stomach); the stomach itself; the duodenum (the area of the intestine into which the stomach first empties). You probably have some form of the disease if you suffer recurrent or episodic abdominal pain, particularly if it's sharp and burning, worsens at night, and improves upon eating. The disease includes:

- *Esophagitis:* irritation of the esophagus

- *Gastroesophageal reflux disease (GERD):* condition in which acid from the stomach backs up into the esophagus

- *Gastritis:* irritation of the stomach lining

- *Duodenitis:* irritation of the duodenum

- *Ulcer:* actual break in the lining of the gastric tract (In the stomach, it's called a *gastric ulcer*; in the beginning of the intestine, it's called a *duodenal ulcer*.)

The disease ranges in severity from mild irritation to erosion to an ulcer. Ulcers occur most frequently in the duodenum, followed by the stomach, and then the esophagus.

Step 1. Make Sure You Get the Best Care

Read this section on potential problems with your treatment carefully to determine if there are discrepancies between your care and state-of-the-art care. Use Step 2 to review shortcomings.

Risk Factors

One of every 10 Americans has ulcers. However, some individuals are more susceptible than others. You should be alert to ulcer symptoms if you have any of the following risk factors, which should prompt you to seek early medical attention.

MOST COMMON RISK FACTORS FOR DUODENAL ULCERS
- Elevated serum pepsinogen (An inherited trait, this is found in 50% of patients with duodenal ulcer. People with this characteristic are eight times as likely to have a duodenal ulcer than those who do not.)
- Smoking (People who smoke cigarettes not only have more duodenal ulcers but also are less responsive to therapy and are more likely to die of the disease.)
- Chronic kidney failure
- Regular consumption of alcohol combined with the use of aspirin (Together the two are a severe stomach irritant.)
- Alcoholic cirrhosis
- Kidney transplantation
- Hyperparathyroidism
- Chronic obstructive pulmonary disease
- Having a close relative with a duodenal ulcer (Duodenal ulcers are three times as common in first-degree relatives of duodenal ulcer patients than in the general population.)

While there is some evidence that duodenal ulcer patients may view stress more negatively, there is no characteristic "ulcer personality" for any kind of ulcer. Chronic anxiety and psychological stress may exacerbate ulcer activity, however.

MOST COMMON RISK FACTORS FOR GASTRIC ULCERS

■ Smoking (Rates of gastric ulcers are higher in smokers than in nonsmokers. Smoking also retards ulcer healing. In one study, gastric ulcer healing rate was 80% in nonsmokers and 50% in smokers.)

■ Alcohol consumption (Whether this is truly a risk for gastric ulceration remains uncertain. Alcohol is known to be a gastric irritant and can cause acute gastritis. By itself, alcohol may not cause ulcers directly.)

■ NSAIDs, or nonsteroidal antiinflammatory drugs (Drugs such as aspirin, Motrin, Nuprin, ibuprofen, and Advil are a major cause of stomach irritation and ulceration. If you take any of these medications on a daily basis, be certain to read the Safe Drug Use section in this chapter and the chapter on Arthritis.)

Diagnosis

You can't be diagnosed properly unless you consult a doctor. Many people are reluctant to see a doctor for simple ulcer symptoms. Advertisers promote the belief that nothing could be easier than self-treatment. For a mild stomach upset that's true, but a delay in seeking medical treatment can cause a number of problems. It carries the risks of recurrent and continuous pain, enlargement of an ulcer, perforation of the stomach wall, and bleeding in the gastrointestinal tract. Even if you seek medical treatment, misdiagnosis is extremely common. There is some danger that your symptoms are being caused by colon or stomach cancer, gallbladder or pancreatic disease that then goes undiagnosed. Your doctor should be willing to consider other diagnoses even if you have the classic ulcer symptoms. Then, too, many ulcers are silent, in that they don't produce classic symptoms and may be missed. This is true even if you've had an ulcer before. About 60% of ulcers that heal reoccur within one year; 50% produce no symptoms.

WHEN TO STOP SELF-MEDICATION AND SEE A DOCTOR   Lots of us suffer mild indigestion or abdominal pain that we treat ourselves. However, if you do have these or other ulcerlike symptoms, here's when you should stop treating yourself and see a doctor:

■ Antacids haven't eliminated mild, ulcerlike symptoms after one week of use.

■ You are losing weight without dieting or without an increase in activity.

■ You are experiencing nausea and vomiting.

■ Your stomach is distended.

- You are experiencing a significant change in bowel movement patterns or the color of your stool has turned black.

- You have back pain.

- You have difficulty swallowing.

- You experience fever or chills.

- You're weak, your complexion is pale, or you have chest pain.

- You experience the sudden onset of new, more severe abdominal pain.

Diagnostic Tests

If you have any of the symptoms just listed, your doctor should order diagnostic tests to find the exact cause. Should you have ulcer disease, tests can help gauge the extent of your treatment and the effectiveness of your therapy. There are two basic tests that can make the definitive diagnosis. The first, the upper gastrointestinal series, is less expensive and less physically draining. In general the sicker you are, the more likely you will need the more expensive test, endoscopy.

UPPER GASTROINTESTINAL (GI) SERIES   The upper GI series, a comparatively inexpensive x-ray test (about $200), is reasonably accurate. About 97% of ulcers will be found via this method. A hard copy of the results can be kept on permanent file. The x-rays involve a modest amount of radiation exposure.

Here's how the test works: You are asked to swallow a chalky liquid called barium. (Some patients complain about the taste.) The barium helps illuminate the stomach on x-rays. As you swallow the barium and it makes its way down the esophagus into the stomach and out into the duodenum, x-rays are taken at regular intervals. The x-ray can "see" the barium. If there is anything that protrudes from or recedes into the lining of the stomach, esophagus, or duodenum, this will show on the x-ray as a defect. Skilled radiologists can diagnose ulcers, cancers, narrowings called strictures, and other conditions. They can't, however, see simple irritation of the stomach lining; endoscopy is required for that.

ENDOSCOPY   This is a more sensitive technique. Patients need to be sedated as a long, narrow tube is threaded through the digestive tract and into the small intestine. There is a small risk that stomach fluid will be sucked into the lungs, causing serious problems, or that the scope will perforate part of the digestive system, necessitating surgery. These complications are very rare in the hands of a skilled operator.

While the upper GI series will locate large ulcers, the endoscope is better at finding more subtle disease, such as minor discolorations, erosion, and inflammation of the stomach. During endoscopy, a doctor can biopsy an ulcer to determine if cancer is present. Endoscopy can be repeated in order to follow an ulcer until it is healed. At a minimum, after eight weeks of drug or other therapy the test should be repeated. But endoscopy is more expensive than the GI series, currently costing as much as $1,200, as well as more uncomfortable.

Treatment Medications

H-2 BLOCKERS   The treatment of peptic ulcer disease was altered radically by the introduction of H-2 blockers. These medicines literally turn off the production of stomach acid, in effect drying up ulcers, gastritis, stomach irritation, or related problems. In general, they have eliminated the need for surgery or the continuous use of antacids. Before H-2 blockers, antacids were widely prescribed for ulcers. Antacids can be effective, but they need to be taken frequently and in high dosages, levels at which they can produce other gastrointestinal side effects. While patients still use them heavily, long-term, regular use is less convenient and less effective than H-2 blockers. If you feel better after taking antacids, you are likely to respond to H-2 blockers. They have eliminated the need for a special diet. You needn't cut down on caffeine and spicy and other irritating foods because they make little difference in most patients. Some doctors prescribe H-2 blockers to prevent ulcers in patients who are on ulcer-producing medications such as non-steroidal antiinflammatory drugs. The usual therapy period with H-2 blockers is three to four weeks for gastritis and six weeks when an ulcer is present.

Don't be surprised if your doctor prescribes an H-2 blocker without ordering any diagnostic tests. Your doctor may prescribe H-2 blockers without such tests for two weeks. That's only if you are young or middle-aged and have no history of peptic ulcer disease or symptoms of ulcer disease, weight loss, stools with blood, anemia, systemic illness, previous stomach surgery, or other complicating factors.

You should consult with your doctor after a week or 10 days to ensure that the therapy is working. The single biggest prescribing error that doctors make is allowing a trial of H-2 blockers to continue beyond two weeks without ordering diagnostic tests, which are needed to make certain you are not suffering from a more serious illness. The biggest patient management problem with H-2 blockers is that patients just don't return to the doctor's office after their first visit and are lost to follow-up. If you are not much better by the end of two weeks, it's time to consider diagnostic tests. You could have cancer, a stricture of the esophagus, or some other condition that cannot be cured by the drug. I know of a psychologist who had trouble swallowing and was losing weight. He continued taking H-2 blockers for several months until he was ultimately diagnosed—correctly—with terminal stomach cancer.

H-2 blockers should not be prescribed without diagnostic tests in patients who are elderly or anemic, especially if the anemia is caused by iron deficiency. They are also ill-advised if you have a previous history of ulcers; they should be used cautiously if you are taking nonsteroidal antiinflammatory drugs or are losing weight. Patients who smoke also need to be evaluated carefully.

PROTON PUMP INHIBITOR   A new class of ulcer drug, called a proton pump inhibitor, was introduced in 1991. This is far more potent than the H-2 blockers and may be warranted in selected patients. Since it has been associated with cancer in laboratory rats, many feel it is a second-line drug of choice, after the H-2 blockers. But its use undoubtedly will change as doctors have a more realistic assessment of the risk in humans.

ANTIBIOTICS   Your doctor may prescribe antibiotics as part of your treatment if a bacteria known as H. pylori has played a role in the development of your ulcer. Your doctor can make the diagnosis by using an endoscope to retrieve a stomach specimen to test for the bacteria or using newer high-tech tests for the bacteria. While many doctors are uncertain about the importance of this bacteria, they are willing to use antibiotics or Peptobismol if conventional treatment is unsuccessful. Both can kill the bacteria. Some trials show antibiotics to be very useful when the bacteria is present in your stomach, and to prevent relapse much better than H-2 blockers alone.

SAFE DRUG USE   Before starting any medications, your doctor should inquire about your current use of drugs. If you have a history of ulcers, you should be cautioned about medications such as nonsteroid antiinflammatory drugs (NSAID) that can cause a recurrence. A good rule is that anything good for a joint is bad for the stomach. While NSAIDs or aspirin may relieve the pain, this could muffle the one symptom that signals that your stomach is in trouble. At the same time they can worsen the condition by irritating the stomach lining. Even one NSAID or aspirin tablet can cause an ulcer in certain circumstances. The simultaneous use of many medications obviously multiplies the risk. (If you've had ulcers in the past, for instance, and have asthma, you may be put on steroids for the asthma. If you also take aspirin for joint aches and pains, you run a real risk that your ulcer will return.)

If you take NSAIDs, aspirin, or the steroid prednisone, stool should be checked for blood at least twice a year and your blood hemoglobin measured regularly. You should be aware that massive internal bleeding, which can be fatal, is the most serious and frequent complication of NSAIDs. Doctors are astounded by the number of patients who develop erosions of the stomach after taking just a small dose of NSAIDs. Your doctor may prescribe Cytotec or misoprostol as a preventive measure if you are elderly, smoke, drink, or have a history of bleeding. H-2 blockers are prescribed as a precaution.

Treatment Surgery

Although 20 years ago surgery was fairly common for a hiatal hernia (reflux of stomach acid into the esophagus) and chronic ulcers, new medical treatments have largely superseded this therapy. It is extremely rare for patients to be operated on for a benign ulcer condition. In fact, if surgery is suggested, gastroenterologists would seriously question that recommendation. Some surgeons disagree. Dr. Paul Jordan, of Baylor College of Medicine in Houston, believes that surgery should be presented more often as a possible therapy: "General practitioners and the public don't look at surgery as an option. Surgery is an option and in some cases a necessity." Dr. Jordan believes that just as medications are getting better, surgery is getting better as well.

But the problem is finding a surgeon to operate. "There is a whole generation of surgeons who have not had to perform benign ulcer surgery due to the success of H-2 blockers," says Dr. Paul Miscovitz of the New York Hospital–Cornell Medical Center. Dr. Miscovitz claims that in a busy practice for a gastroenterologist, not more than one patient a year is referred for surgery. "For intractable pain and failure to heal, sometimes you are forced to operate, but there's no guarantee of a cure," he warns. No patient should undergo surgery without an exhaustive trial of medications, including antibiotics.

Step 2. Look for Shortcomings

I hope that, from reading Step 1, you have gotten a good feeling about your treatment and that you understand much of it better. You'll learn even more by calling organizations listed in Step 4. But if you have an uncomfortable feeling that your treatment is not on track, then study this section, which specifies some common and serious shortcomings that experts in the field recognize. If this section confirms your suspicions, you should go to Step 3. Some of these mistakes you can discover yourself; others only an expert can confirm.

MISTAKES IN DIAGNOSIS

You have pain in your upper abdomen that is food related, or worse at night, or made worse by medications, and you have not seen a doctor.

You experience weight loss, an inability to eat, or a change in your digestion and mistakenly believe the cause is indigestion.

Your health care provider ignores signs and symptoms of colon cancer, gallbladder disease, pancreatic disease, or stomach cancer.

Your health care provider is too comfortable with a diagnosis of ulcer and is unwilling to consider other diagnoses when your situation doesn't fit the picture.

You are not properly screened for a past history of ulcers.

Your health care provider orders a CAT scan or MRI to diagnose an ulcer (neither test has a role in diagnosing benign ulcers).

Your stool is not regularly checked for blood if you take aspirin, prednisone, or NSAIDs on a regular basis.

MISTAKES IN TREATMENT

You are given an NSAID but your doctor does not know you are already taking another NSAID, aspirin, or an anticoagulant that could cause your ulcer to bleed.

Your symptoms are being treated, but not your underlying illness.

You use H-2 blockers for more than two weeks without a proper diagnosis.

You take too many NSAIDs.

You take aspirin or NSAIDs for stomach pain.

You take NSAIDs regularly and aren't supervised by a doctor.

Your health care provider recommends elective surgery before an exhaustive trial of medical therapy.

Your surgeon has not had extensive training and experience in performing the superselective parietal vagotomy.

You drink alcohol and take aspirin regularly, thereby putting yourself at risk for ulcer disease.

You self-medicate, delaying proper treatment and risking enlargement of your ulcer, bleeding, or perforation.

You eat different foods or even change your job due to myths about ulcers.

You stop taking your medication after the pain subsides.

Your doctor treats your ulcers with antacids alone.

You fail to stop smoking (smokers have bigger ulcers and more recurrences than nonsmokers).

Step 3. See a Specialist

If, from Step 2, you are concerned that your care is not state-of-the-art, this section will tell you how to choose an expert.

Choosing a Gastroenterologist

You first need to see a gastroenterologist, a specialist in stomach disorders. If he or she recommends surgery, see the next section, Choosing a Surgeon.

SEE AN EXPERT IF:

- Endoscopy is ordered.

- You suffer complications.

- Surgery is advised.

- The diagnosis is unclear.

- Your symptoms are not typical of ulcer disease.

- You don't improve after several weeks of treatment for mild disease. If your symptoms are severe, you should be referred sooner.

The majority of patients refer themselves to stomach specialists. You should select a doctor who is board-certified in internal medicine and gastroenterology, trained at a university-affiliated teaching hospital or a good community hospital that maintains a university affiliation.

SEEK *EMERGENCY CARE* FROM A SPECIALIST IF:

- The pain stays constant, no longer relieved by food or antacids, or radiates to the back or the upper one-quarter of the body. (This can indicate penetration of the ulcer.)

- The pain is increased rather than decreased by food or antacids and/or there is vomiting. (The gastric outlet may be obstructed, which happens in about 2–4% of patients.)

- You experience abrupt, severe or generalized abdominal pain. (This can mean that the ulcer has perforated into the peritoneal cavity, which happens in about 6% of duodenal ulcers. In 5–10% of patients there are no prior symptoms of ulcer. In about 10% of cases there is accompanying hemorrhage, greatly increasing the mortality risk. There can also be penetration into the pancreas and less commonly into the liver, biliary tract, or colon.)

- There is vomiting of blood, passage of black, tarry stools, or bleeding from the rectum. (This indicates hemorrhage, which occurs in about 15% of duodenal ulcers.)

If you are referred for surgery, make certain to get a second opinion from a gastroenterologist who works closely with a surgeon. This doctor will try his or her hardest to avoid surgery, but is not blind to it.

TESTS MANDATORY PRIOR TO SURGERY

- Serum gastrin level (to look for gastrin-secreting tumors)

- Endoscopy (to confirm that the ulcer has not healed)

Choosing a Surgeon

There is no certification program for gastric surgery, although the American Board of Surgery is in the early stages of developing a training program. Your best choice is a board-certified general surgeon who specializes in gastric or digestive surgery. He or she should have performed a minimum of 20–30 ulcer operations during residency. This is one case where you will want to seek out a senior surgeon, trained before the late 1970s, who has wide experience with ulcer surgery. Many younger surgeons did little ulcer surgery in training.

RESULTS   In addition, the general guidelines on mortality and recurrence rates presented in Table 6 can help locate a qualified surgeon. Listed are the average mortality rates and the recurrence rates for the three most commonly performed operations. You will want a surgeon who has mortality rates and success rates better than average.

TABLE 6. Average Mortality and Recurrence Rates for the Most Common Gastric Surgeries

Operation	Mortality Rate	Recurrence Rate
Proximal gastric vagotomy (a severing of the nerves that control acid production, in the upper part of the stomach)	0.3%	10–15%
Antrectomy (removal of the ulcer and the acid-secreting area of the stomach)	2%	3%
Pyloroplasty (a widening of the stomach outlet)	1%	5%

Centers of Excellence for Gastroenterology

The following list of hospitals is provided only as a convenient starting place in your search for excellence. These hospitals are recommended on the basis of reputation, not experience and results. The list is not an endorsement. There may be hospitals just as excellent that have been omitted. You should apply the guidelines for experience, results, and other measures of excellence to any hospital you choose, whether or not it is on this list. Although hospitals from different sources have been combined into one list, the compilation in no way implies that one source has endorsed the hospital list of another source.

CALIFORNIA

Stanford University School
of Medicine NIH
Digestive Disease Center
300 Pasteur Dr
Stanford, CA 94305

University of California, Los
Angeles, School of Medicine EX/NIH/US
Center for Ulcer Education
10833 LeConte Ave
Los Angeles, CA 90024

University of California,
San Diego, Medical Center EX
225 W Dickinson St
San Diego, CA 92103

University of California, San
Francisco, Medical Center EX/NIH
505 Parnassus Ave
San Francisco, CA 94143

COLORADO

University Hospital NIH
Hepatobiliary Research Center
4200 E Ninth Ave
Denver, CO 80262

CONNECTICUT

Yale Liver Research Center NIH
333 Cedar St
P.O. Box 3333
New Haven, CT 06510

FLORIDA

Shands Hospital EX
University of Florida
1600 SW Archer Rd
Gainesville, FL 32610

University of Miami EX
1600 NW 10th Ave
P.O. Box 016099 (R59)
Miami, FL 33101

ILLINOIS

Northwestern University
School of Medicine EX
303 E Chicago Ave
Chicago, IL 60611-3008

University of Chicago
Hospitals EX/NIH/US
5841 S Maryland Ave
Chicago, IL 60637

MARYLAND

Johns Hopkins Hospital EX/US
600 No. Wolfe St
Baltimore, MD 21205

MASSACHUSETTS

Beth Israel Hospital EX
330 Brookline Ave
Boston, MA 02215

Tufts University NIH
Center for Gastrointestinal
Research on Absorptive
and Secretory Processes
136 Harrison Ave
Boston, MA 02111

Lahey Clinic Foundation EX
41 Mall Rd
Burlington, MA 01805

Massachusetts General
Hospital EX/NIH/US
55 Fruit St
Boston, MA 02114

MICHIGAN
University of Michigan
Gastrointestinal Peptide
   Research Center   NIH
1301 Catherine Rd
Ann Arbor, MI 48109-0624

MINNESOTA
Mayo Clinic   EX/US
200 First St SW
Rochester, MN 55905

University of Minnesota
   Hospital and Clinic   EX
Harvard St at East River Rd
Minneapolis, MN 55455

MISSOURI
Barnes Hospital   EX
One Barnes Hospital Plaza
St. Louis, MO 63110

University Hospital and
   Clinics   EX
One Hospital Dr
Columbia, MO 65212

NEW YORK
Albert Einstein Liver
   Research Center   NIH
1300 Morris Park Ave
Bronx, NY 10461

Columbia Presbyterian
   Medical Center   EX
633 W 168th St
New York, NY 10032

Memorial Sloan-Kettering
   Cancer Center   EX
1275 York Ave
New York, NY 10021

Mount Sinai Medical Center   EX/US
One Gustave Levy Pl
New York, NY 10029

New York Hospital–Cornell
   Medical Center   EX
525 E 68th St
New York, NY 10021-4885

NORTH CAROLINA
University of North Carolina   NIH
Center for Gastrointestinal
   Biology and Disease
Chapel Hill School of Medicine
Chapel Hill, NC 27599

OHIO
Cleveland Clinic Foundation   EX/US
One Clinic Center
9500 Euclid Ave
Cleveland, OH 44106

PENNSYLVANIA
Hospital of the University
   of Pennsylvania   EX
3400 Spruce St
Philadelphia, PA 19104

Presbyterian-University
   Hospital   EX
De Soto and O'Hara Sts
Pittsburgh, PA 15213

TENNESSEE
Vanderbilt University
   Medical Center   EX
1161 21st Ave S
Nashville, TN 37232

TEXAS
M. D. Anderson Hospital
   and Tumor Institute   EX
6723 Bertner Dr
Houston, TX 77030

University of Texas Southwestern Medical Center   EX
5323 Harry Hines Blvd
Dallas, TX 75235

VIRGINIA
Medical College of Virginia
  Hospital   EX
401 No. 12th St
Richmond, VA 23219

WASHINGTON
University of Washington
  Medical Center   EX
1959 NE Pacific St
Seattle, WA 98195

SOURCES

EX   indicates the hospitals recommended by experts interviewed.

US   indicates the hospitals recommended in *U.S. News & World Report.*

NIH indicates those centers funded by the NIH's National Institute of Diabetes and Digestive and Kidney Diseases.

Step 4. Become Your Own Expert

WHO TO CALL

CURE (Center for Ulcer Research and Education)
University of California at Los Angeles
Building 115, Rm 212
Los Angeles, CA 90073
213/825-9366

NIH CRISP System
301/496-7543

University-Affiliated Teaching Hospitals   See Appendix.

EXPERT SOURCES

Although dozens of experts were interviewed for these chapters, these physicians are acknowledged for their significant contributions.

Dr. Paul F. Miskovitz, New York Hospital–Cornell Medical Center, New York, NY

Dr. Seymour M. Sabesin, Director, Digestive Diseases, Rush-Presbyterian-St. Luke's Medical Center, Chicago, IL

Dr. Frank G. Moody, Director, Trauma Research Center, University of Texas Health Science Center, Houston, TX

Dr. Jeffrey L. Ponsky, Director, Department of Surgery, Mount Sinai Medical Center, Cleveland, OH

Dr. Paul H. Jordan, Baylor College of Medicine, Houston, TX

REFERENCES AND SUGGESTED READING

American College of Physicians. Endoscopy in the Evaluation of Dyspepsia. *Annals of Internal Medicine,* Vol. 102 (1985), pp. 226–269.

Baker, P. N., and others. Possible Low-Dose-Aspirin-Induced Gastropathy [letter to the editor]. *Lancet,* Vol. 339, No. 8792 (Feb. 29, 1992), p. 550.

Bell, N. J. V., and Hunt, R. H. Role of Gastric Acid Suppression in the Treatment of Gastro-Oesophageal Reflux Disease. *Gut,* Vol. 33, No. 1 (Jan. 1992), pp. 118–124.

Brown, Colin, and Rees, W. D. W. Drug Treatment for Acute Upper Gastrointestinal Bleeding [editorial]. *British Medical Journal,* Vol. 304, No. 6820 (Jan. 18, 1992), pp. 135–136.

Clearfield, Harris R. Management of NSAID-Induced Ulcer Disease. *American Family Physician,* Vol. 45, No. 1 (Jan. 1992), pp. 255–258.

Collen, Martin J. Ulcer Disease: Investigation and Basis for Therapy [review]. *Annals of Internal Medicine,* Vol. 116, No. 4 (Feb. 15, 1992), p. 352.

Cotton, P. B., and Shorvon, P. J. Analysis of Endoscopy and Radiography in the Diagnosis, Follow-Up, and Treatment of Peptic Ulcer Disease. *Clinical Gastroenterology,* Vol. 13 (1984), pp. 383–403.

Craanen, M. E., and others. Intestinal Metaplasia and Helicobacter pylori: An Endoscopic Bioptic Study of the Gastric Antrum. *Gut,* Vol. 33, No. 1 (Jan. 1992), pp. 16–20.

Feldman, Mark. Helicobacter pylori and the Etiology of Duodenal Ulcer: Necessary but not Sufficient [editorial]. *American Journal of Medicine,* Vol. 91, No. 6 (Dec. 1991), pp. 563–565.

Fries, James F., and others. The Relative Toxicity of Nonsteroidal Antiinflammatory Drugs. *Arthritis and Rheumatism,* Vol. 34, No. 11 (Nov. 1991), pp. 1353–1360.

Greenberger, N. J., and Moody, F. G. *Yearbook of Digestive Diseases 1990.* St. Louis: Mosby Year, 1990.

Gustavsson, S., and others. Trends in Peptic Ulcer Surgery: A Population-Based Study in Rochester, Minnesota, 1856–1985. *Gastroenterology,* Vol. 94 (1988), pp. 688–94.

Koretz, Ronald L., and others. Prevention of NSAID-Induced Gastric Ulcer. [letter] *Annals of Internal Medicine,* Vol. 115, No. 11 (Dec. 1, 1991), pp. 911–913.

Kummer, A. F., and others. Changes in Nocturnal and Peak Acid Outputs After Duodenal Ulcer Healing with Sucralfate or Ranitidine. *Gut,* Vol. 33, No. 2 (Feb. 1992), pp. 175–178.

Kurata, J. H., and Halie, B. M. Epidemiology of Peptic Ulcer Disease. *Clinical Gastroenterology,* Vol. 13 (1984), pp. 289–307.

McGuire, H. H., Jr., and Horsley, J. S., III. Emergency Operations for Gastric and Duodenal Ulcers in High-Risk Patients. *Annals of Surgery,* Vol. 203 (1986), pp. 551–557.

Nonsteroidal Antiinflammatory Drug Usage and Requirement in Elderly Acute Hospital Admissions. *British Journal of Rheumatology,* Vol. 31, No. 1 (Jan. 1992), pp. 45–48.

Paulus, Harold E. FDA Guidelines on Analgesics. *Arthritis and Rheumatism,* Vol. 34, No. 12 (Dec. 1991), p. 1619.

Penn, I. The Declining Role of the Surgeon in the Treatment of Acid-Peptic Diseases. *Archives of Surgery,* Vol. 15 (1980), pp. 134–135.

Rabeneck, Linda, and Ransohoff, David F. Is Helicobacter pylori a Cause of Duodenal Ulcer? A Methodologic Critique of Current Evidence. *American Journal of Medicine,* Vol. 91, No. 6 (Dec. 1991), pp. 566–572.

Reese, Jeffrey, and others. Peptic Ulcer Disease Following Renal Transplantation in the Cyclosporine Era. *American Journal of Surgery,* Vol. 162, No. 6 (Dec. 1991), pp. 558–562.

Richter, Joel E. Surgery for Reflux Disease—Reflections of a Gastroenterologist [editorial]. *New England Journal of Medicine,* Vol. 326, No. 12 (Mar. 19, 1992), pp. 825–827.

Somerville, K., and others. Nonsteroidal Antiinflammatory Drugs and Bleeding Peptic Ulcers. *Lancet,* Vol. i (1986), pp. 462–464.

Spechler, Stuart Jon. Comparison of Medical and Surgical Therapy for Complicated Gastroesophageal Reflux Disease in Veterans. *New England Journal of Medicine,* Vol. 326, No. 12 (Mar. 19, 1992), pp. 786–792.

Stanghellini, V., and others. Fasting and Postprandial Gastrointestinal Motility in Ulcer and Nonulcer Dyspepsia. *Gut,* Vol. 33, No. 2 (Feb. 1992), pp. 184–190.

Taha, A. S., and others. Chemical Gastritis and Helicobacter Pylori–Related Gastritis in Patients Receiving Nonsteroidal Antiinflammatory Drugs: Comparison and Correlation with Peptic Ulceration. *Journal of Clinical Pathology,* Vol. 45, No. 2 (Feb. 1992), pp. 135–139.

Thomas, J. M., and Misiewicz, G. Histamine H-2-Receptor Antagonists in the Short- and Long-Term Treatment of Duodenal Ulcer. *Clinical Gastroenterology,* Vol. 13 (1984), pp. 501–541.

Wagner, S., and others. Bismuth Subsalicylate in the Treatment of H-2-Blocker-Resistant Duodenal Ulcers: Role of Helicobacter pylori. *Gut,* Vol. 33, No. 2 (Feb. 1992), pp. 179–183.

Walt, R., and others. Rising Frequency of Ulcer Perforation in Elderly People in the United Kingdom. *Lancet,* Vol. i (1986), pp. 489–492.

Wilson, G. D., and others. *Harrison's Principles of Internal Medicine,* 12th ed. New York: McGraw-Hill, 1991.

Appendix

University-Affiliated Teaching Hospitals

Alabama

Birmingham

Baptist Medical Centers
2000-B.S. Bridge Pky
P.O. Box 830605
Birmingham, AL 35283

Carraway Methodist Medical Center
1600 No. 26th St
Birmingham, AL 35234

University of Alabama Hospitals
619 So. 19th St
Birmingham, AL 35233

Dept of Veteran Affairs Medical Center
700 So. 19th St
Birmingham, AL 35233

Mobile

University of So. Alabama Medical
    Center
2451 Fillingim St
Mobile, AL 36617

Arizona

Phoenix

Good Samaritan Regional Medical
    Center
P.O. Box 2989
Phoenix, AZ 85062

Maricopa Medical Center
2601 E Roosevelt
Phoenix, AZ 85008

St. Joseph Hospital and Medical Center
350 W Thomas Rd
Phoenix, AZ 85013

Tucson

Tucson Medical Center
5301 E Grant Rd
Tucson, AZ 85712

University Medical Center
1501 No. Campbell
Tucson, AZ 85724

Veterans Administration Medical Center
Tucson, AZ 87523

Arkansas

Little Rock

Arkansas Children's Hospital
800 Marshall
Little Rock, AR 72202

Dept of Veteran Affairs Medical Center
4300 W 7th St
Little Rock, AR 72205

University Hospital of Arkansas
4301 W Markham St
Little Rock, AR 72205

California

Bakersfield

Kern Medical Center
1830 Flower St
Bakersfield, CA 93305

Fresno

Valley Medical Center of Fresno
445 So. Cedar Ave
Fresno, CA 93702

Loma Linda

Loma Linda University Medical Center
11234 Anderson St
P.O. Box 2000
Loma Linda, CA 92354

Veterans Administration Medical Center
Jerry L. Pettis Memorial Hospital
11202 Benton St
Loma Linda, CA 92357

Long Beach

Memorial Medical Center of Long Beach
2801 Atlantic Ave
Long Beach, CA 90801

Veterans Affairs Medical Center
5901 E Seventh St
Long Beach, CA 90822

Los Angeles

Cedars-Sinai Medical Center
8700 Beverly Blvd
Los Angeles, CA 90048

Children's Hospital of Los Angeles
4650 Sunset Blvd
Los Angeles, CA 90027

Hospital of the Good Samaritan
616 So. Witmer St
Los Angeles, CA 90017

Los Angeles County–USC Medical Center
1200 No. State St
Los Angeles, CA 90033

Martin Luther King Jr. General Hospital
12021 So. Wilmington Ave
Los Angeles, CA 90059

UCLA Medical Center
10833 Le Conte Ave
Los Angeles, CA 90024

Veterans Affairs Medical Center, West Los
  Angeles
Wilshire and Sawtelle Blvds
Los Angeles, CA 90073

Martinez

Veterans Administration Medical
  Center
150 Muir Rd
Martinez, CA 94553

Orange

University of California, Irvine,
  Medical Center
101 The City Dr
Orange, CA 92668

Pasadena

Huntington Memorial Hospital
100 Congress St
Pasadena, CA 91105

Sacramento

University of California, Davis,
  Medical Center
2315 Stockton Blvd
Sacramento, CA 95817

San Diego

University of California, San Diego,
  Medical Center
225 Dickinson St
San Diego, CA 92103

Veterans Administration Medical
  Center
3350 La Jolla Village Dr
San Diego, CA 92161

San Francisco

Children's Hospital of San Francisco
3700 California St
San Francisco, CA 94118

Dept of Veteran Affairs Medical Center
4150 Clement St
San Francisco, CA 94121

University of California, San Francisco,
  Medical Center
505 Parnassus Ave
San Francisco, CA 94143

Pacific Presbyterian Medical Center
2333 Buchanan St
San Francisco, CA 94115

San Francisco General Hospital and
　　Medical Center
1001 Potrero Ave
San Francisco, CA 94110

St. Mary's Hospital and Medical Center
450 Stanyan St
San Francisco, CA 94117

Stanford
Stanford University Hospital
300 Pasteur Dr
Stanford, CA 94305

Torrance
Harbor-UCLA Medical Center
1000 W Carson St
Torrance, CA 90509

Colorado

Denver
AMI Presbyterian-St. Luke's Medical
　　Center
1601 E 19th Ave
Denver, CO 80218

University Hospital
4200 E Ninth Ave
Denver, CO 80262

Veterans Administration Medical Center
1055 Clermont St
Denver, CO 80220

Connecticut

Bridgeport
Bridgeport Hospital
267 Grant St
Bridgeport, CT 06610

St. Vincent's Medical Center
2800 Main St
Bridgeport, CT 06606

Danbury
Danbury Hospital
24 Hospital Ave
Danbury, CT 06810

Farmington
John Dempsey Hospital
University of Connecticut Health Center
Farmington Ave
Farmington, CT 06032

Hartford
Hartford Hospital
80 Seymour St
Hartford, CT 06115

Saint Francis Hospital and Medical
　　Center
114 Woodland St
Hartford, CT 06105

New Britain
New Britain General Hospital
100 Grand St
New Britain, CT 06050

New Haven
Hospital of St. Raphael
1450 Chapel St
New Haven, CT 06511

Yale-New Haven Hospital
20 York St
New Haven, CT 06504

Newington
Veterans Administration Medical Center
555 Willard Ave
Newington, CT 06111

Stamford
Stamford Hospital
Shelburne Rd and W Broad St
Stamford, CT 06904

Waterbury

St. Mary's Hospital
56 Franklin St
Waterbury, CT 06706

Waterbury Hospital
64 Robbins St
Waterbury, CT 06721

West Haven

Veterans Affairs Medical Center
950 Campbell Ave
West Haven, CT 06516

Delaware

Wilmington

Medical Center of Delaware
P.O. Box 1668
Wilmington, DE 19899

District of Columbia

Children's Hospital National Medical
    Center
111 Michigan Ave NW
Washington, DC 20010

George Washington University Hospital
901 23rd St NW
Washington, DC 20037

Georgetown University Hospital
3800 Reservoir Rd NW
Washington, DC 20007

Howard University Hospital
2041 Georgia Ave NW
Washington, DC 20060

Veterans Administration Medical
    Center
50 Irving St NW
Washington, DC 20422

Washington Hospital Center
110 Irving St NW
Washington, DC 20010

Florida

Gainsville

Shands Hospital
Box J-326, JHMHC
Gainesville, FL 32610

Veterans Administration Medical Center
Archer Rd
Gainesville, FL 32602

Jacksonville

University Hospital of Jacksonville
655 W 8th St
Jacksonville, FL 32209

Miami

Jackson Memorial Hospital
1611 NW 12th Ave
Miami, FL 33136

Veterans Administration Medical Center
1201 NW 16th St
Miami, FL 33125

Miami Beach

Mount Sinai Medical Center
4300 Alton Rd
Miami Beach, FL 33140

Orlando

Orlando Regional Medical Center
1414 So. Kuhl Ave
Orlando, FL 32806

St. Petersburg

All Children's Hospital
801 Sixth St S
St. Petersburg, FL 33701

Tampa

Tampa General Hospital
P.O. Box 1289
Tampa, FL 33601

Veterans Administration Medical Center
James A. Haley Veterans Hospital
13000 Bruce B. Downs Blvd
Tampa, FL 33612

Georgia

Atlanta

Crawford Long Hospital of Emory
    Hospital
550 Peachtree St NE
Atlanta, GA 30365

Emory University Hospital
1364 Clifton Rd NE
Atlanta, GA 30322

Georgia Baptist Medical Center
300 Boulevard NE
Atlanta, GA 30312

Grady Memorial Hospital
80 Butler St SE
Atlanta, GA 30335

Henrietta Egleston Hospital for Chil-
    dren, Inc.
1405 Clifton Rd NE
Atlanta, GA 30322

Augusta

Dept of Veterans Affairs Medical Center
2460 Wrightsboro Rd
Augusta, GA 30910

Medical College of Georgia Hospital and
    Clinics
1120 15th St
Augusta, GA 30912

Decatur

Veterans Administration Medical Center
1670 Clairmont Rd
Decatur, GA 30033

Macon

Medical Center of Central Georgia
777 Hemlock St
Macon, GA 31201

Hawaii

Honolulu

Queen's Medical Center
1301 Punchbowl St
Honolulu, HI 96813

Illinois

Berwyn

MacNeal Hospital
3249 So. Oak Park Ave
Berwyn, IL 60402

Chicago

Children's Memorial Hospital
2300 Children's Plaza
Chicago, IL 60614

Cook County Hospital
1825 W Harrison St
Chicago, IL 60612

Illinois Masonic Medical Center
836 Wellington Ave
Chicago, IL 60657

Mercy Hospital and Medical Center
Stevenson Expressway at King Dr
Chicago, IL 60616

Michael Reese Hospital and Medical
    Center
31st at Lakeshore Dr
Chicago, IL 60616

Mount Sinai Hospital Medical Center
California and 15th Sts
Chicago, IL 60608

Northwestern Memorial Hospital
250 E Superior St
Chicago, IL 60611

Rush-Presbyterian-St. Luke's Medical
    Center
1653 W Congress Pky
Chicago, IL 60612

Schwab Rehabilitation Center
1401 So. California Blvd
Chicago, IL 60608

University of Chicago Hospitals
5841 So. Maryland Ave
Box 430
Chicago, IL 60637

University of Illinois Hospital
1740 W Taylor St
Chicago, IL 60612

Veterans Administration Medical
    Center—Lakeside
333 E Huron St
Chicago, IL 60611

Veterans Administration Medical
    Center—West Side
820 So. Danen Ave
Chicago, IL 60612

Evanston

Evanston Hospital Corporation
2650 Ridge Ave
Evanston, IL 60201

Hines

Edward Hines Jr. Veterans
    Administration Hospital
Hines, IL 60141

Maywood

Foster G. McGraw Hospital
2160 So. First Ave
Maywood, IL 60153

Oak Lawn

Christ Hospital
4440 W 95th St
Oak Lawn, IL 60453

Park Ridge

Lutheran General Hospital
1775 Dempster St
Park Ridge, IL 60068

Springfield

Memorial Medical Center
800 No. Rutledge
Springfield, IL 62781

St. John's Hospital
800 E Carpenter St
Springfield, IL 62769

Indiana

Indianapolis

Indiana University Hospitals
926 W Michigan St
Indianapolis, IN 46202

Methodist Hospital of Indiana, Inc.
1701 No. Senate Blvd
P.O. Box 1367
Indianapolis, IN 46206

Richard L. Roudebush Dept of Veterans
    Affairs Medical Center
1481 W 10th St
Indianapolis, IN 46202

William N. Wishard Memorial Hospital
1001 W 10th St
Indianapolis, IN 46202

Iowa

Des Moines

Iowa Methodist Medical Center
1200 Pleasant St
Des Moines, IA 50308

Iowa City

University of Iowa Hospitals and Clinics
Newton Rd
Iowa City, IA 52242

Dept of Veterans Affairs Medical Center
Iowa City, IA 52246

Kansas

Kansas City

University of Kansas Hospital
39th and Rainbow Blvd
Kansas City, KS 66103

Kentucky

Lexington

University Hospital
University of Kentucky Medical Center
800 Rose St
Lexington, KY 40536

Veterans Affairs Medical Center
Lexington, KY 40511

Louisville

Humana Hospital–University of
    Louisville
530 So. Jackson St
Louisville, KY 40202

Veterans Administration Medical Center
800 Zorn Ave
Louisville, KY 40206

Louisiana

New Orleans

Alton Ochsner Medical Foundation
1516 Jefferson Hwy
New Orleans, LA 70121

Charity Hospital of Louisiana at New
    Orleans
1532 Tulane Ave
New Orleans, LA 70140

Touro Infirmary
1401 Foucher St
New Orleans, LA 70115

Tulane Medical Center Hospital
1415 Tulane Ave
New Orleans, LA 70112

Veterans Administration Medical Center
1601 Perdido St
New Orleans, LA 70146

Shreveport

Louisiana State University Hospital
1541 Kings Hwy
P.O. Box 33932
Shreveport, LA 71130

Veterans Administration Medical Center
510 E Stoner Ave
Shreveport, LA 71101

Maine

Portland

Maine Medical Center
22 Bramhall St
Portland, ME 04102

Maryland

Baltimore

Baltimore Dept of Veterans Affairs
    Medical Center
3900 Loch Raven Blvd
Baltimore, MD 21218

Francis Scott Key Medical Center
4940 Eastern Ave
Baltimore, MD 21224

Franklin Square Hospital
9000 Franklin Square Dr
Baltimore, MD 21237

Greater Baltimore Medical Center
6701 No. Charles St
Baltimore, MD 21204

Johns Hopkins Hospital
600 No. Wolfe St
Baltimore, MD 21205

Maryland General Hospital
827 Linden Ave
Baltimore, MD 21205

Sinai Hospital of Baltimore, Inc.
Belvedere at Greenspring
Baltimore, MD 21215

University of Maryland Medical System
22 So. Greene St
Baltimore, MD 21201

Bethesda

Warren E Magnuson Clinical Center
National Institutes of Health
9000 Rockville Pike
Bethesda, MD 20892

Silver Spring

Holy Cross Hospital
1500 Forest Glen Rd
Silver Spring, MD 20910

Massachusetts

Belmont

McLean Hospital
115 Mill St
Belmont, MA 02178

Boston

Beth Israel Hospital
330 Brookline Ave
Boston, MA 02215

Brigham and Women's Hospital
75 Francis St
Boston, MA 02115

Children's Hospital
300 Longwood Ave
Boston, MA 02115

Faulkner Hospital
1153 Centre St
Boston, MA 02130

Massachusetts General Hospital
Fruit St
Boston, MA 02114

New England Deaconess Hospital
185 Pilgrim Rd
Boston, MA 02215

New England Medical Center, Inc.
750 Washington St
Boston, MA 02111

St. Elizabeth's Hospital of Boston
736 Cambridge St
Boston, MA 02135

St. Margaret's Hospital for Women
90 Cushing Ave
Boston, MA 02125

University Hospital
88 E Newton St
Boston, MA 02118

Veterans Administration Medical Center
150 So. Huntington Ave
Boston, MA 02130

Brockton

Department of Veterans Affairs Medical
    Center (West Roxbury/Brockton)
940 Belmont St
Brockton, MA 02401

Cambridge

Mount Auburn Hospital
330 Mount Auburn St
Cambridge, MA 02238

Pittsfield

Berkshire Medical Center
725 North St
Pittsfield, MA 01201

Springfield

Baystate Medical Center
759 Chestnut St
Springfield, MA 01199

Worcester

Medical Center of Central Massachu-
    setts–Memorial Hospital
119 Belmont St
Worcester, MA 01605

St. Vincent Hospital, Inc.
25 Winthrop St
Worchester, MA 01604

University of Massachusetts Hospital
55 Lake Ave N
Worchester, MA 01655

Michigan

Allen Park

Veterans Administration Medical Center
Southfield and Outer Dr
Allen Park, MI 48101

Ann Arbor

Catherine McAuley Health Center
P.O. Box 992
Ann Arbor, MI 48106

University of Michigan Hospitals
1500 E Medical Center Dr
Ann Arbor, MI 48109

Veterans Affairs Medical Center
2215 Fuller Rd
Ann Arbor, MI 48105

Dearborn

Oakwood Hospital Corporation
18101 Oakwood Blvd
Dearborn, MI 48124

Detroit

Children's Hospital of Michigan
3901 Beaubien
Detroit, MI 48201

Detroit Receiving Hospital and University Health Center
4201 St. Antoine Blvd
Detroit, MI 48201

Harper-Grace Hospitals
3990 John R St
Detroit, MI 48201

Harper-Grace Hospitals
Grace Hospital Division
18700 Meyers Rd
Detroit, MI 48235

Harper-Grace Hospitals
Harper Hospital Division
3990 John R St
Detroit, MI 48201

Henry Ford Hospital
2799 W Grand Blvd
Detroit, MI 48202

Hutzel Hospital
4707 St. Antoine Blvd
Detroit, MI 48201

Sinai Hospital
6767 W Outer Dr
Detroit, MI 48235

St. John's Hospital and Medical Center
22101 Moross Rd
Detroit, MI 48236

Flint

Hurley Medical Center
One Hurley Plaza
Flint, MI 48502

Grand Rapids

Blodgett Memorial Medical Center
1840 Wealthy St, SE
Grand Rapids, MI 49506

Lansing

Edward W Sparrow Hospital
P.O. Box 30480
1215 E Michigan Ave
Lansing, MI 48909

Ingham Medical Center Corporation
401 W Greenlawn
Lansing, MI 48910

Pontiac

St. Joseph Mercy Hospital
900 Woodward Ave
Pontiac, MI 48053

Southfield

Providence Hospital
16001 Nine Mile Rd
Southfield, MI 48075

Minnesota

Minneapolis

Dept of Veterans Affairs Medical Center
One Veterans Dr
Minneapolis, MN 55417

Hennepin County Medical Center
701 Park Ave S
Minneapolis, MN 55415

University of Minnesota Hospital and
    Clinic
Harvard St at East River Rd
Minneapolis, MN 55455

Rochester

St. Mary's Hospital
1216 Second St SW
Rochester, MN 55902

St. Paul

St. Paul-Ramsey Medical Center
640 Jackson St
St. Paul, MN 55101

Mississippi

Jackson

Dept of Veterans Affairs Medical Center
1500 E Woodrow Wison Dr
Jackson, MS 39216

University Hospitals and Clinics
Hospital of Mississippi
    Medical Center
2500 No. State St
Jackson, MS 39216

Missouri

Columbia

Harry S. Truman Memorial Veterans
    Hospital
800 Hospital Dr
Columbia, MO 65201

University of Missouri Hospital and
    Clinics
One Hospital Dr
Columbia, MO 65212

Kansas City

St. Luke's Hospital of Kansas City
Wornall Rd at Forty-Fourth
Kansas City, MO 64111

Truman Medical Center
2301 Holmes St
Kansas City, MO 64108

Veterans Affairs Medical Center
4801 E Linwood Blvd
Kansas City, MO 64128

St. Louis

Barnes Hospital
Barnes Hospital Plaza
St. Louis, MO 63110

Jewish Hospital of St. Louis
216 So. Kingshighway Blvd
P.O. Box 14109
St. Louis, MO 63178

St. John's Mercy Medical Center
615 So. New Ballas Rd
St. Louis, MO 63141

St. Louis Children's Hospital
400 So. Kingshighway Blvd
St. Louis, MO 63110

St. Louis University Hospital
3635 Vista at Grand Blvd
P.O. Box 15250
St. Louis, MO 63110

St. Mary's Health Center
6420 Clayton Rd
St. Louis, MO 63117

Veterans Affairs Medical Center
St. Louis, MO 63125

Nebraska

Omaha

St. Joseph's Hospital
601 No. 30th St
Omaha, NE 68131

University of Nebraska Hospital
600 So. 42nd St
Omaha, NE 68198

Veterans Administration Medical Center
4101 Woolworth Ave
Omaha, NE 68105

New Hampshire

Hanover

Mary Hitchcock Memorial Hospital
Hanover, NH 03756

New Jersey

Camden

Cooper Hospital–University Medical
    Center
One Cooper Plaza
Camden, New Jersey 08103

East Orange

Veterans Administration Medical Center
Center and Tremont Aves
East Orange, NJ 07019

Hackensack

Hackensack Medical Center
30 Prospect Ave
Hackensack, NJ 07601

Livingston

St. Barnabas Medical Center
Old Short Hills Rd
Livingston, NJ 07039

Long Branch

Monmouth Medical Center
300 Second Ave
Long Branch, NJ 07740

Morristown

Morristown Memorial Hospital
100 Madison Ave
P.O. Box 1956
Morristown, NJ 07960

Neptune

Jersey Shore Medical Center, Inc.
1945 Route 33
Neptune, NJ 07754

New Brunswick

Robert Wood Johnson University
    Hospital
One Robert Wood Johnson Place
New Brunswick, NJ 08901

Newark

Newark Beth Israel Medical Center
201 Lyons Ave
Newark, NJ 07112

St. Michael's Medical Center
268 Dr. Martin Luther King Jr. Blvd
Newark, NJ 07102

University of Medicine and Dentistry of
    New Jersey
University Hospital
150 Bergen St
Newark, NJ 07103

Paterson

St. Joseph's Hospital and Medical Center
703 Main St
Paterson, NJ 07503

Plainfield

Muhlenberg Regional Medical Center,
    Inc.
Park Ave and Randolph Rd
Plainfield, NJ 07061

Summit

Overlook Hospital
99 Beauvoir Ave at Sylvan Rd
Summit, NJ 07901

New Mexico

Albuquerque

University of New Mexico Hospital
2211 Lomas Blvd NE
Albuquerque, NM 87106

Veterans Administration Medical Center
2100 Ridgecrest Dr SE
Albuquerque, NM 87108

New York

Albany

Albany Medical Center Hospital
New Scotland Ave
Albany, NY 12208

Veterans Administration Medical Center
113 Holland Ave
Albany, NY 12208

Binghampton

United Health Services
Mitchell Ave
Binghampton, NY 13903

Buffalo

Buffalo General Hospital
100 High St
Buffalo, NY 14203

Erie County Medical Center
462 Grider St
Buffalo, NY 14215

Millard Fillmore Hospitals
3 Gates Circle
Buffalo, NY 14209

Veterans Administration Medical Center
3495 Bailey Ave
Buffalo, NY 14215

Cooperstown

Mary Imogene Bassett Hospital
One Atwell Rd
Cooperstown, NY 13326

East Meadow

Nassau County Medical Center
2201 Hempstead Turnpike
East Meadow, NY 11554

Elmhurst

Elmhurst Hospital Center
79-01 Broadway
Elmhurst, NY 11373

Manhasset

North Shore University Hospital
300 Community Dr
Manhasset, NY 11030

Mineola

Winthrop-University Hospital
259 First St
Mineola, NY 11501

New Hyde Park

Long Island Jewish Medical Center
New Hyde Park, NY 11042

New York

Bellevue Hospital Center
27th and First Ave
New York, NY 10016

Beth Israel Medical Center
First Ave at 16th St
New York, NY 10003

Booth Memorial Medical Center
56-45 Main St
Flushing, NY 11355

Bronx Lebanon Hospital Center
1276 Fulton Ave
Bronx, NY 10456

Bronx Municipal Hospital Center
Pelham Pky So. and Eastchester Rd
Bronx, NY 10461

Brookdale Hospital Medical Center
Linden Blvd at Brookdale Plaza
Brooklyn, NY 11212

Brooklyn Hospital–Caledonian Hospital
121 Dekalb Ave
Brooklyn, NY 11201

Cabrini Medical Center
227 E 19th St
New York, NY 10003

Catholic Medical Center of Brooklyn
    and Queens, Inc.
88-25 153rd St
Jamaica, New York 11432

Harlem Hospital Center
506 Lenox Ave
New York, NY 10037

Hospital for Joint Diseases–Orthopaedic
    Institute
301 E 17th St
New York, NY 10021

Hospital for Special Surgery
535 E 70th St
New York, NY 10021

Kings County Hospital Center
451 Clarkson Ave
Brooklyn, NY 11203

Lenox Hill Hospital
100 E 77th St
New York, NY 10021

Long Island College Hospital
Brooklyn, NY 11201

Maimonides Medical Center
4802 10th Ave
Brooklyn, NY 11219

Memorial Sloan-Kettering Cancer
    Center
1275 York Ave
New York, NY 10021

Methodist Hospital
506 Sixth St
Brooklyn, NY 11215

Metropolitan Hospital Center
1901 First Ave
New York, NY 10029

Montefiore Medical Center
111 E 210th St
Bronx, NY 10467

Mount Sinai Hospital
One Gustave L. Levy Place
New York, NY 10029

New York Hospital
525 E 68th St
New York, NY 10021

New York University Medical Center
560 First Ave
New York, NY 10016

Our Lady of Mercy Medical Center
600 E 233rd St
Bronx, NY 10466

Presbyterian Hospital in the City of New
    York
Columbia-Presbyterian Medical Center
New York, NY 10032

St. Luke's-Roosevelt Hospital Center
Amsterdam Ave at 114th St
New York, NY 10025

St. Vincent's Hospital and Medical
    Center of New York
153 W 11th St
New York, NY 10011

University Hospital of Brooklyn
SUNY Health Science Center
445 Lenox Rd
Box 23
Brooklyn, NY 11203

Veterans Administration Medical Center
800 Poly Place
Brooklyn, NY 11209

Veterans Administration Medical Center
First Ave at E 24th St
New York, NY 10010

Veterans Administration Medical Center
130 W Kingsbridge Rd
Bronx, NY 10468

Northport

Veterans Administration Medical Center
Middleville Rd
Northport, NY 11768

Rochester

Genesee Hospital
224 Alexander St
Rochester, NY 14607

Rochester General Hospital
1425 Portland Ave
Rochester, NY 14621

St. Mary's Hospital
89 Geneseee St
Rochester, NY 14611

Strong Memorial Hospital
601 Elmwood Ave
Rochester, NY 14642

Stony Brook

University Hospital
SUNY at Stony Brook
Stony Brook, NY 11794

Syracuse

University Hospital
SUNY Health Science Center at
    Syracuse
750 E Adams St
Syracuse, NY 13210

Veterans Administration Medical Center
800 Irving Ave
Syracuse, NY 13210

Valhalla

Westchester County Medical Center
Valhalla, NY 10595

North Carolina

Chapel Hill

University of North Carolina Hospitals
Manning Dr
Chapel Hill, NC 27514

Charlotte

Carolina Medical Center
P.O. Box 32861
Charlotte, NC 28232

Durham

Duke University Hospital
Box 3708
Durham, NC 27710

Veterans Administration Medical Center
508 Fulton St
Durham, NC 27705

Greensboro

Moses H. Cone Memorial Hospital
1200 No. Elm St
Greensboro, NC 27401

Greenville

Pitt County Memorial Hospital
200 Stantonsburg Rd
Greenville, NC 27835

Winston-Salem

No. Carolina Baptist Hospitals, Inc.
300 So. Hawthorne Rd
Winston-Salem, NC 27103

Ohio

Akron

Akron City Hospital
525 E Market St
Akron, OH 44309

Akron General Medical Center
400 Wabash Ave
Akron, OH 44307

Children's Hospital Medical Center of
Akron
281 Locust St
Akron, OH 44308

St. Thomas Medical Center
Summa Health System
444 No. Main St
Akron, OH 44310

Cincinnati

Children's Hospital Medical Center
Elland and Bethesda Aves
Cincinnati, OH 45229

Dept of Veterans Affairs Medical Center
3200 Vine St
Cincinnati, OH 45220

Good Samaritan Hospital
3217 Clifton Ave
Cincinnati, OH 45220

University of Cincinnati
234 Goodman St
Cincinnati, OH 45267

Cleveland

Cleveland Clinic Hospital
9500 Euclid Ave
Cleveland, OH 44106

MetroHealth Medical Center
3395 Scranton Rd
Cleveland, OH 44109

Mount Sinai Medical Center
One Mount Sinai Dr
Cleveland, OH 44106

St. Luke's Hospital
11311 Shaker Blvd
Cleveland, OH 44104

University Hospitals of Cleveland
University Circle
Cleveland, OH 44106

Veterans Affairs Medical Center
10701 E Blvd
Cleveland, OH 44106

Columbus

Children's Hospital
700 Children's Dr
Columbus, OH 43205

Grant Medical Center
111 So. Grant Ave
Columbus, OH 43215

Ohio State University Hospitals
410 W Tenth Ave
Columbus, OH 43210

Riverside Methodist Hospital
3535 Olentangy River Rd
Columbus, OH 43214

Dayton

Children's Medical Center
One Children's Way
Dayton, OH 45404

Dept of Veterans Affairs Medical Center
4100 W Third St
Dayton, OH 45428

Miami Valley Hospital
1 Wyoming St
Dayton, OH 45409

St. Elizabeth Medical Center
Franciscan Health System
601 Edwin C. Moses Blvd
Dayton, OH 45408

Kettering

Kettering Medical Center
3535 Southern Blvd
Kettering, OH 45429

Toledo

Medical College of Ohio Hospitals
C.S. 10008
Toledo, OH 43699

Toledo Hospital
2142 No. Cove Blvd
Toledo, OH 43606

Youngstown

St. Elizabeth Hospital Medical Center
1044 Belmont Ave
Youngstown, OH 44501

Oklahoma

Oklahoma City

Dept of Veterans Affairs Medical Center
921 NE 13th St
Oklahoma City, OK 73104

Oklahoma Medical Center
800 NE 13th St
Oklahoma City, OK 73104

Tulsa

St. Francis Hospital
6161 So. Yale
Tulsa, OK 74136

Oregon

Portland

Oregon Health Sciences University
    Hospital
3181 SW Sam Jackson Park Rd
Portland, OR 97201

Veterans Administration Medical Center
P.O. Box 1034
Portland, OR 97207

Pennsylvania

Allentown

Allentown Hospital–Lehigh Valley
    Hospital Center
1200 So. Cedar Crest Blvd
Allentown, PA 18105

Bryn Mawr

Bryn Mawr Hospital
130 So. Bryn Mawr Ave
Bryn Mawr, PA 19010

Chester

Crozer-Chester Medical Center
15th St and Upland Ave
Chester, PA 19013

Danville

Geisinger Medical Center
Academy Ave
Danville, PA 17822

Darby

Mercy Catholic Medical Center
Lansdowne Ave and Bailey Rd
Darby, PA 19023

Erie

Hamot Medical Center
201 State St
Erie, PA 16550

Hershey

Penn State University Hospital
500 University Dr
P.O. Box 850
Hershey, PA 17033

Philadelphia

Albert Einstein Medical Center (Northern Division)
York and Tabor Rds
Philadelphia, PA 19141

Children's Hospital of Philadelphia
34th and Civic Center Blvd
Philadelphia, PA 19104

Episcopal Hospital
Front St and Lehigh St
Philadelphia, PA 19125

Frankford Hospital of the City of
Philadelphia
Knights and Red Lion Rds
Philadelphia, PA 19114

Germantown Hospital and Medical
Center
One Penn Blvd
Philadelphia, PA 19144

Graduate Hospital
One Graduate Plaza
Philadelphia, PA 19146

Hahnemann University Hospital
Broad and Vine
Philadelphia, PA 19102

Hospital of the Medical College of
Pennsylvania
3300 Henry Ave
Philadelphia, PA 19129

Hospital of the University of
Pennsylvania
3400 Spruce St
Philadelphia, PA 19104

Lankenau Hospital
Lancaster Ave, W of City Line
Philadelphia, PA 19151

St. Christopher's Hospital for Children
Division United Hospitals, Inc.
5th and Lehigh Ave
Philadelphia, PA 19133

Temple University Hospital
Broad and Ontario Sts
Philadelphia, PA 19140

Thomas Jefferson Univerisity Hospital
11th and Walnut Sts
Philadelphia, PA 19107

Veterans Administration Medical Center
University and Woodland Aves
Philadelphia, PA 19104

Pittsburgh

Allegheny General Hospital
320 E North Ave
Pittsburgh, PA 15212

Children's Hospital of Pittsburgh
3705 Fifth Ave
Pittsburgh, PA 15213

Eye and Ear Hospital of Pittsburgh
230 Linthrop St
Pittsburgh, PA 15213

Magee-Womens Hospital
Forbes Ave and Halket St
Pittsburgh, PA 15213

Mercy Hospital of Pittsburgh
1400 Locust St
Pittsburgh, PA 15219

Montefiore Hospital Assoc. of Western
Pennsylvania
3459 Fifth Ave
Pittsburgh, PA 15213

Presbyterian-University Hospital
DeSoto at O'Hara Sts
Pittsburgh, PA 15213

Shadyside Hospital
5230 Centre Ave
Pittsburgh, PA 15232

St. Francis Medical Center
45th St at Penn Ave
Pittsburgh, PA 15201

Veterans Administration Medical Center
University Dr C
Pittsburgh, PA 15240

Western Pennsylvania Hospital
4800 Friendship Ave
Pittsburgh, PA 15224

Western Psychiatric Institute and Clinic
3811 O'Hara St
Pittsburgh, PA 15213

York

York Hospital
1001 So. George St
York, PA 17405

Puerto Rico

Rio Piedras

University Hospital
Rio Piedras, PR 00935

San Juan

Veterans Administration Medical Center
One Veterans Plaza
San Juan, PR 00927

Rhode Island

Pawtucket

Memorial Hospital
Prospect St
Pawtucket, RI 02860

Providence

Miriam Hospital
164 Summit Ave
Providence, RI 02906

Rhode Island Hospital
593 Eddy St
Providence, RI 02903

Roger Williams General Hospital
825 Chalkstone Ave
Providence, RI 02908

Women and Infants Hospital of Rhode
Island
101 Dudley St
Providence, RI 02905

South Carolina

Charleston

Medical University Hospital
171 Ashley Ave
Charleston, SC 29425

Veterans Administration Medical Center
109 Bee St
Charleston, SC 29403

Greenville

Greenville Hospital System
701 Grove Rd
Greenville, SC 29605

Tennessee

Memphis

Baptist Memorial Hospital
899 Madison Ave
Memphis, TN 38146

Methodist Hospital of Memphis
1265 Union Ave
Memphis, TN 38104

Regional Medical Center at Memphis
877 Jefferson
Memphis, TN 38103

Veterans Administration Medical Center
1030 Jefferson Ave
Memphis, TN 38104

Mountain Home

Dept of Veterans Affairs Medical Center
Mountain Home, TN 37684

Nashville

George W Hubbard Hospital of
   Meharry Medical College
1005 D. B. Todd Jr. Blvd
Nashville, TN 37208

Vanderbilt University Hospital
1211 22nd Ave S
Nashville, TN 37232

Veterans Administration Medical Center
1310 24th Ave S
Nashville, TN 37203

Texas

Dallas

Baylor University Medical Center
3500 Gaston Ave
Dallas, TX 75246

Dallas County Hospital District
Parkland Memorial Hospital
5201 Harry Hines Blvd
Dallas, TX 75235

Dept of Veterans Affairs
4500 So. Lancaster Rd
Dallas, TX 75216

Methodist Hospitals of Dallas (MHD)
301 W Colorado
Dallas, TX 75208

Presbyterian Hospital of Dallas
8200 Walnut Hill Lane
Dallas, TX 75231

St. Paul Medical Center
5909 Harry Hines Blvd
Dallas, TX 75235

Galveston

University of Texas Medical Branch–
   Hospitals at Galveston
301 University Blvd
Galveston, TX 77550

Houston

Harris County Hospital District
726 Gillette
Houston, TX 77019

Herman Hospital
6411 Fannin St
Houston, TX 77030

Methodist Hospital
6565 Fannin St
Houston, TX 77030

St. Luke's Episcopal Hospital
6720 Bertner
Houston, TX 77030

Texas Children's Hospital
6621 Fannin
Houston, TX 77030

University of Texas
M.D. Anderson Cancer Center
1515 Holcombe Blvd
Houston, TX 77030

Veteran Affairs Medical Center
2002 Holcombe Blvd
Houston, TX 77030

San Antonio

Audie L. Murphy Memorial Veterans
   Hospital
7400 Merton Minter Blvd
San Antonio, TX 78284

Bexar County Hospital District
4502 Medical Dr
San Antonio, TX 78229

Temple

Scott and White Memorial Hospital
2401 So. 31st St
Temple, TX 76508

Utah

Salt Lake City
University of Utah Hospital
50 No. Medical Dr
Salt Lake City, UT 84132

Vermont

Burlington
Medical Center Hospital of Vermont
Colchester Ave
Burlington, VT 05401

White River Junction
Veterans Administration Medical Center
and Regional Office
White River Junction, VT 05001

Virginia

Charlottesville
University of Virginia Medical Center
Jefferson Park Ave
Charlottesville, VA 22908

Falls Church
Fairfax Hospital
3300 Gallows Rd
Falls Church, VA 22046

Hampton
Veterans Affairs Medical Center
Hampton, VA 23667

Norfolk
Children's Hospital of the King's
Daughters
800 W Olney Rd
Norfolk, VA 23507

Sentara Health System
6015 Poplar Hall Dr
Norfolk, VA 23502

Richmond
Medical College of Virginia Hospitals
401 No. 12th St
Richmond, VA 23298

Salem
Veterans Administration Medical Center
1970 Boulevard
Salem, VA 24153

Washington

Seattle
Children's Hospital and Medical Center
4800 Sand Point Way NE
Seattle, WA 98105

University of Washington Hospitals
Harborview Medical Center
325 9th Ave
Seattle, WA 98194

University of Washington Medical
Center
BB318 NE Pacific R-35
Seattle, WA 98195

Veterans Administration Medical Center
1660 So. Columbian Way
Seattle, WA 98108

West Virginia

Charlestown
Charlestown Area Medical Center
501 Morris St
Charlestown, W Virginia 25326

Morgantown
W Virginia University Hospitals, Inc.
Morgantown, WV 26506

Wheeling
Ohio Valley Medical Center
2000 Eoff St
Wheeling, WV 26003

Wisconsin

Madison

University of Wisconsin Hospital and
Clinics
600 Highland Ave
Madison, WI 53792

William S. Middleton Memorial
Veterans Hospital
2500 Overlook Terrace
Madison, WI 53705

Milwaukee

Children's Hospital of Wisconsin
9000 W Wisconsin Ave
Milwaukee, WI 53226

Clement J. Zablocki Veterans Administration Medical Center
Milwaukee, WI 53295

Froedtert Memorial Lutheran Hospital
9200 W Wisconsin Ave
Milwaukee, WI 53226

Milwaukee County Medical Complex
8700 W Wisconsin Ave
Milwaukee, WI 53226

Sinai Samaritan Medical Center
950 No. 12th St
Milwaukee, WI 53201

St. Joseph's Hospital
5000 W Chambers St
Milwaukee, WI 53210

St. Luke's Medical Center
2900 W Oklahoma Ave
Milwaukee, WI 53215

Index